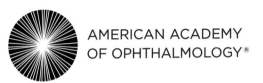

AMERICAN ACADEMY
OF OPHTHALMOLOGY®

MW00845183

Practical Ophthalmology

Eighth Edition | **A Manual for Beginning Residents**

Executive Editor
Preston H. Blomquist, MD

Contributing Authors
Andrew J. Barkmeier, MD
Charline S. Boente, MD, MS
Todd J. Mondzelewski, MD
Misha F. Syed, MD, MEHP
Fasika A. Woreta, MD, MPH

Protecting Sight. Empowering Lives.®

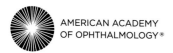

AMERICAN ACADEMY
OF OPHTHALMOLOGY®

American Academy of
  Ophthalmology
Box 7424
San Francisco, CA 94120-7424

Clinical Education Secretaries
Christopher J. Rapuano, MD,
  *Senior Secretary for Clinical
  Education*
J. Timothy Stout, MD, PhD, MBA,
  *Secretary for Lifelong Learning
  and Assessment*

Academy Staff
Dale E. Fajardo, EdD, MBA,
  Vice President, Education
Beth Wilson, *Director, Continuing
  Professional Development*
Susan Malloy, *Manager,
  Acquisitions and Development*
Amanda Fernandez, *Publications
  Editor*
Denise Evenson, *Director,
  Brand & Creative*
James Frew, *Senior Designer*
Daniel Mummert, *Director, Online
  Education*
Jasmine Chen, *Manger, E-learning*
Eric Gerdes, *Interactive Designer*
Donna Scism, *E-Editor and
  Proofreader*

AAO, AAOE, American Academy of Ophthalmology, Basic and Clinical Science Course, BCSC, EyeCare America, EyeNet, EyeSmart, EyeWiki, Femtocenter, Focal Points, IRIS, ISRS, OKAP, ONE, Ophthalmic Technology Assessments, Ophthalmology, Ophthalmology Retina, Preferred Practice Pattern, ProVision, The Ophthalmic News & Education Network, and the AAO logo (shown on cover) and tagline (Protecting Sight, Empowering Lives) are, among other marks, the registered trademarks and trademarks of the American Academy of Ophthalmology.

The Academy provides this material for educational purposes only. It is not intended to represent the only or best method or procedure in every case, nor to replace a physician's own judgment or give specific advice for case management. Including all indications, contraindications, side effects, and alternative agents for each drug or treatment is beyond the scope of this material. All information and recommendations should be verified, prior to use, with current information included in the manufacturers' package inserts or other independent sources, and considered in light of the patient's condition and history. Reference to certain drugs, instruments, and other products in this publication is made for illustrative purposes only and is not intended to constitute an endorsement of such. Some materials may include information on applications that are not considered community standard, that reflect indications not included in approved FDA labeling, or that are approved for use only in restricted research settings. The FDA has stated that it is the responsibility of the physician to determine the FDA status of each drug or device he or she wishes to use, and to use them with appropriate patient consent in compliance with applicable law. The Academy specifically disclaims any and all liability for injury or other damages of any kind, from negligence or otherwise, for any and all claims that may arise from the use of any recommendations or other information contained herein.

Cover image: "Enlarged and hypertrophied ciliary processes associated with lens coloboma and cataract" by Susmita Paul, DNB, Fellow, Department of Glaucoma (Photographer) and Shahinur Tayab, MS, Associate Consultant, Department of Glaucoma (Clinician), Sri Sankaradeva Nethralaya, Guwahati, Assam. Equipment: Slit-lamp camera (Topcon, SLD2, Japan). This image originally appeared in *Ophthalmology*, August 2020, Volume 127, Issue 8.

Library of Congress Cataloging-in-Publication Data
Practical ophthalmology : a manual for beginning residents / Preston H. Blomquist, executive editor.—Eighth edition.
  p.; cm.
Includes bibliographical references and index.
ISBN 978-1-68104-405-7
Blomquist, Preston H., editor. II. American Academy of Ophthalmology, issuing body.
[DNLM: 1. Eye Diseases—diagnosis. 2. Diagnostic Techniques, Ophthalmological. 3. Ophthalmology—methods. WW141]
RE75
617.7'15—dc23

0230013

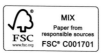

Printed in China.

19 18 17 16 15 14 13 12 11   1 2 3 4 5 6 7 8 9 10

Contents

Activities

Clinical Protocols

Tables

Videos

Preface

This eighth edition of *Practical Ophthalmology: A Manual for Beginning Residents* is being published at a historic time for ophthalmologic education. Traditionally, ophthalmology residents in the United States were required to have completed an internship in a broad field of medicine or surgery before starting their residency training. However, new program requirements from the Accreditation Council for Graduate Medical Education (ACGME) call for the incorporation of 3 months of ophthalmology training in the internship year. The new requirements also allow for true integration of the internship year with the residency. Programs will have the opportunity to design more meaningful internships to better prepare residents. These may include experiences in rheumatology, endocrinology, neurology, otolaryngology, emergency medicine, or other direct patient-care disciplines that will be of use to the future ophthalmologist. The introduction of ophthalmology training into the internship year has multiple benefits, not the least of which is the diminution of the "July effect." It is our hope that this manual can ease the transition of the intern into the study and practice of ophthalmology.

This manual covers practical principles and techniques essential or useful for providing a variety of ophthalmic examinations and tests and for interpreting their results. Some clinical and background information is included to help the novice understand the context of the information presented.

- The chapters that cover each element of a thorough ophthalmic examination are organized by the order in which those elements are usually performed.
- *Clinical Protocols* include stepwise instructions for some of the most important clinical procedures.
- *Pitfalls and Pointers* present practical tips for avoiding or resolving common problems.
- *Suggested Resources* list relevant and useful sources of more detailed information. Preferred Practice Patterns, Advisory Opinions, Information Statements, and Clinical Statements can be found on the American Academy of Ophthalmology (AAO) web site, www.aao.org.
- New in this edition are links to instructive videos and interactive simulators related to topics covered in the book. These are available to readers of the electronic and print versions of *Practical Ophthalmology* at www.aao.org /PracticalOphthalmologyvideo and www.aao.org/PracticalOphthalmologyactivity.

Mobile device–users can scan the QR codes below (a QR-code reader must already be installed on the device) to access this content.

Videos   Activities

This manual is not meant to cover every procedural topic that needs to be learned by new ophthalmology trainees. As interns become more facile with the ophthalmologic exam, they will benefit from expanding their base of knowledge by reading about their patients' conditions in the *Basic and Clinical Science Course* (BCSC) published by the AAO, in major ophthalmologic textbooks, and in current journals. This manual will have fulfilled its goals if it helps ease the stressful transition of the novice into the exciting and fulfilling field of ophthalmology.

Acknowledgments

This work evolved from an earlier AAO publication, *A Manual for the Beginning Ophthalmologist* (which was published in 3 editions). It represents a body of work over the years from ophthalmologists dedicated to training residents, and the contributions of previous authors can still be seen in this edition. The contributing ophthalmologists to this eighth edition are similarly talented educators: Andrew Barkmeier (Mayo Clinic College of Medicine and Science), Charlene Boente (Indiana University School of Medicine), Todd Mondzelewski (Naval Medical Center San Diego), Misha Syed (University of Texas Medical Branch), and Fasika Woreta (Wilmer Eye Institute). In addition, I want to thank the ophthalmologists who helped review the previous edition for currency and the chapter drafts for this edition: Gabriela Espinoza, Christopher Gappy, Denise John, Eleanore Kim, Ajay Kuriyan, Gary Legault, Jennifer Lindsey, Shannon Lynch, Daniel Moore, Andrew Reynolds, Jamie Rosenberg, Erin Seefeldt, Andrea Stahulak, Robert Swan, Anna Wishna, and Alice Zhang.

Preston Howard Blomquist, M.D.
Dallas, Texas

1

Introduction to the Practice of Ophthalmology

Like most important new endeavors, beginning an ophthalmology residency is both exciting and intimidating. This chapter offers some insights regarding what it means to become an ophthalmologist and to practice ophthalmology ethically, responsibly, and competently. It also describes ways in which this book can help you in your first few months of residency (and beyond, if you wish) and offers practical tips on dealing with some of the challenges you will face.

In this chapter you will find some general guidelines about how to approach the task of assimilating the large body of knowledge, the skills, and the attitudes needed to practice ophthalmology, your chosen specialty. You successfully addressed similar challenges before, when you embarked on your medical training, and you have undoubtedly developed your own system of acquisition and assimilation of knowledge along the way. The material in this chapter might be familiar to many beginning residents, but it is certainly fundamental enough to warrant emphasis.

Practicing Ophthalmology

Congratulations on your decision to study ophthalmology, a discipline with roots that date back 2000 years. The remarkable success of ophthalmology as a discipline is based on 2 main intertwined elements: ophthalmology's intrinsic strength as a medical and surgical specialty, and the perpetual flow of talented individuals into the field. Ophthalmology has attracted some of the brightest minds throughout history, and several Nobel laureates have been named for their work in vision research. Ophthalmology can claim several firsts in medicine. For example, in 1916, the first medical specialty examining board in the world was established; originally called the American Board for Ophthalmic Examinations, it was renamed the American Board of Ophthalmology in 1935. Ophthalmology was the first medical discipline in which randomized clinical trials were performed, the first to use lasers, the first to use antiviral agents, the first to perform successful allografts (corneal transplants), and, more recently, the first with an FDA-approved gene therapy (for Leber congenital amaurosis).

Practicing ophthalmology is a privilege, and ophthalmologists are intimately familiar with the rewards and personal satisfaction their efforts bring. The broad scope of ophthalmology practice combines medicine and surgery, and the treatment of pediatric as well as adult patients. The nature of ophthalmic practice permits the establishment of durable and satisfying doctor–patient relationships, which often last a lifetime. The subject matter of ophthalmology is intellectually challenging and fulfilling as well as sufficiently broad to ensure that everyone can find an intellectual niche in its vast array of topics. The intrinsic strengths of our chosen specialty and the love that it inspires in its practitioners will ensure the continued progress of ophthalmology.

Ophthalmologic services are regarded with respect by patients. Sight is so valued among Americans that, according to a survey by the National Society to Prevent Blindness, blindness is ranked second only to cancer in the fear it evokes in individuals. This fear emanates from the feeling that blindness has a catastrophic effect on one's social, economic, and personal life. It is particularly important for a new resident to understand this perception, because ophthalmic practice involves the care of patients with vision-threatening disorders. Some such patients believe, correctly or otherwise, that they will go blind. The treatment of these patients draws not only on the technical skills of the physician but also on the physician's compassion, understanding, and counseling ability.

Much of the practice of medicine, including ophthalmology, requires communication as a key skill. Communication might be with the patient, with the patient's family, with other health care providers, or with various sectors of society. Such communication should always be clear, forthright, timely, and free of jargon.

Communication with patients in general, but especially with patients or parents of children diagnosed with serious ophthalmic disease, is an art acquired over many years of experience. However, some general guidelines are helpful for the beginning resident. You might want to defer breaking the news of a serious ocular condition or the interpretation of a difficult clinical circumstance, leaving these tasks to the attending physician, who should have more experience in this area and possibly a different interpretation of the patient's condition. It is awkward to have to rescind your earlier message, as well as confusing to the patient who hears conflicting messages with different implications. In situations in which you do break the news, approach the situation truthfully, with clarity, empathy, compassion, and professional kindness. The communication should take place in private, and should be conducted in an unrushed manner. Try to strike a balance between being too exhaustive, on the one hand, and too brief, on the other. Finally, most children with blinding conditions still have some visual function, although it might be as poor as mere light perception. It is legally correct to label a person with only light perception as blind, but it might not be a suitable description to use when counseling parents who build hope on the scenario the physician describes. Most patients interpret the word "blindness" to mean no light perception. The terms "visual impairment," "low vision," or "limited vision" are usually preferable.

Consultation reports to other physicians should be written in clear language with few, if any, abbreviations. A poorly written consultation report, replete with abbreviations and jargon, carries little value if patients and other medical professionals cannot understand it; instead, it can create barriers between ophthalmology and other medical fields.

Responsibilities of the Resident

As a beginning resident, you will be a new member in an academic health care facility. Your goal is to acquire the knowledge, skills, attitudes, and behaviors needed to practice ophthalmology. It is helpful to be familiar with the general goals of the residency program and with the forces that affect the academic missions of medical schools and residency programs. Goals of the residency program are generally patient care, education, and research. Patient care is listed first because the primary goal of education and research is ultimately to enhance patient care.

Patient care is a fundamental component of clinical education, but beginning residents must be able to recognize the limits of their abilities in order to ensure the continued delivery of high-quality care to all patients. As you gain clinical experience, often while serving on the front line of ophthalmic care, be aware of the gaps in your knowledge and abilities as well as that you may be unaware of what you do not know. Be willing to accept supervision freely, because it is the ethical and professional responsibility of the supervising ophthalmologist to ensure that the quality of medical care does not suffer as a consequence of resident education.

Ophthalmologists are physicians. Because of the close interrelationship between ophthalmic and systemic health and disease, the modern practice of ophthalmology requires a wide base of medical knowledge. You must thoughtfully integrate new ophthalmic knowledge into the general medical knowledge you have already acquired.

Residents should strive to maintain a balance between responsibilities to home and family, and responsibilities to their health care team. A well-developed support system should help in this respect, and you should not hesitate to convey to the appropriate supervisors any concerns you might have about situations or events that interfere with your effectiveness or well-being. Pace your activities as a resident for the duration of your residency and beyond. Display your spirit of cooperation and helpfulness with your fellow residents. Take the opportunity to build lasting relationships with faculty, fellow residents, and other coworkers. Such relationships are usually as rewarding as anything else you acquire (ie, knowledge, experience) during your residency.

Stress During Residency Training

The formal literature that addresses the topic of stress during residency training has increased dramatically since the Libby Zion case, which involved the unexpected death in 1984 of an 18-year-old patient, allegedly caused in part by overworked and under-supervised medical trainees. The cost that stress during residency training can exact on society has since been extensively analyzed, and various steps have been undertaken to reduce pressures on trainees. Numerous factors can contribute to stress during residency training; here are a few:

- *Sleep deprivation.* Sleep deprivation is considered one of the most significant sources of stress during residency training. Night duty can subject residents to a level of repetitive sleep loss unsurpassed by many other work groups. The Accreditation Council for Graduate Medical Education (ACGME) has established work-hour rules to minimize sleep deprivation. These rules include: (1) a maximum of 80 hours of clinical duties per week and (2) a minimum of 1 day in 7 without clinical duties, both averaged over a 4-week period; (3) a minimum of 8 hours off between clinical shifts; and (4) no more than 24 hours of continuous patient care duties (followed by up to 4 hours of activities related to patient safety and care transition).
- *Role conflict and role ambiguity.* Role conflict arises when the resident's perceived image of the physician as a kind of "superhero" clashes with the reality of life as a resident. Role ambiguity is produced by the resident's status as both practicing physician and student. The resident can occupy the important and dignified role of the primary physician for very ill patients. At the same time, the resident can be expected to perform less exalted work, such as transporting patients or materials and answering to nurses and others whom the resident may perceive as lower

in status and knowledge. Ambiguity of the job role creates an unfixed and expandable workload. This wide discrepancy between the various roles is often the basis of resident stress and discontent.

- *Newer stresses.* Most research to date has focused on the stresses that arise from residents' work environment. Other evolving factors may also be influencing residents' attitudes and feelings about their profession and their patients. The rapid evolution of health care, societal attitudes about physicians, the rising cost of training, and the uncertainties of job availability and future income are stress factors that are assuming increasing significance.

Recognizing Stress and Its Sources

The consequences of stress in residency adversely affect the resident, the resident's family, the resident's patients, and society. Addictive behaviors (alcohol and drug abuse), divorce and broken relationships, psychopathologic behavior and disorders (anxiety, depression, and suicide), and professional dysfunction can result. The symptoms and signs can be subtle or overt. Residents and medical educators must learn to identify the signals of stress and to establish effective methods to cope with it. These signals can be divided into 4 categories:

- *Physical problems*: sleep and eating disorders, deteriorating personal hygiene and appearance, inability to concentrate, multiple physical complaints, and proneness to accidents
- *Family problems*: disrupted spousal relationships (separation and divorce, impotence, and extramarital affairs)
- *Social problems*: isolation from peers, withdrawal from nonmedical activities, unreliable and unpredictable behaviors at work, and inappropriate behavior at social functions
- *Work-related problems*: tardiness, absence without explanation, loss of interest in work, giving inappropriate orders or responses to telephone calls regarding patient care, spending excessive time at the hospital, and demonstrating marked mood changes, such as moroseness, irritability, anger, hostility, and difficulty getting along with others

Given all the adverse effects of residency stress, it might come as a surprise that there is no unanimity among medical educators and trainees about the effect of stress. Some view stress as necessary and beneficial, and others see it as harmful. Most agree, however, that stress becomes pathologic beyond a certain point.

Stress harms the doctor–patient relationship. Patients can be perceived as unwanted impositions during times of stress. The ability to empathize with patients is extremely important for delivery of health care with compassion. It can be argued that a stressed, sleep-deprived physician could be ill prepared to have or to show empathy, and might find the patient's complaints frivolous and trivial in comparison to their own. Because of the sacrifices they make, trainees can become egocentric and feel that "the world owes them something."

Recognizing the potential sources of stress and its deleterious effects is essential in the devising of effective coping strategies. Circumstances can evolve that are beyond the ability of an individual resident to resolve and for which the resident should consider seeking external help. Residents occasionally fall victim to the common misconception that a physician must have an answer for everything and must be able to cope independently with every problem. This misconception is exemplified by the adage "Physician, heal thyself," which might imply to some that asking for help is an admission of unworthiness and might deter residents and trained physicians from seeking help, admitting fault, and accepting guidance. Familiarize yourself with the expanding pool of resources and trainee assistance services provided by your institution, many of which offer discretion and anonymity.

Dealing with Early Discouragement

Discouragement early in residency is common. It stems largely from the psychological impact of having to assimilate a novel body of knowledge that deals with unfamiliar regional anatomy and physiology, and using special terminology, equipment, instrumentation, and procedures. The typically variable knowledge base among residents at the beginning of the residency can discourage those who feel they are starting behind their peers. Discouragement can be compounded by any of the types of stress described earlier. Throughout the history of medical education, residents have found that such discouragement is nearly always self-limited. It generally resolves within a few months as its sources are addressed and overcome.

The most effective method of dealing with early discouragement is a mature, methodical, long-term approach to the process of learning. Comparing and sharing experiences and feelings with colleagues at various levels of experience and training is helpful. The fact remains that the task of mastering ophthalmology can appear daunting to the beginning resident. There are no good substitutes for hard work combined with effective time management. A disciplined approach to knowledge acquisition, patient care, and ethical practice will lead to a professional life with continually increasing rewards.

Ethical Considerations

Ethics are reflections of our moral values. Your ethical standing is a reflection of your actions and attitudes. The ethical practice of ophthalmology must at all times be borne in mind by the physician-in-training; it safeguards the healthy foundations of the doctor–patient relationship. The principles involved, formalized in the Code of Ethics of the American Academy of Ophthalmology, are designed to ensure that the best interest of the patient is paramount. These principles can be summarized as the following:

- Provide care with compassion, honesty, integrity, and respect for human dignity.
- Do not refer to a patient as, for example, "the retinal detachment." Instead, always refer to patients by their names, except in public situations where patient confidentiality must be maintained.
- Seek a healthy personal lifestyle. An ill, problem-ridden physician is less likely to empathize genuinely with the minor ailments of patients.
- Understand the psychology of illness. Patients or family members might appear frightened, angry, or hostile. Learn to recognize and to deal effectively with these emotions without ever becoming defensive or hostile yourself.

- Maintain clinical and moral competence to avoid doing harm (Hippocrates: *primum non nocere*) and to ensure provision of excellent care. Clinical competence is accomplished by continued study and by appropriate consultation. Moral competence calls upon the physician to practice moral discernment (understanding and resolving the ethical implications of clinical encounters), moral agency (acting faithfully and respectfully on behalf of the patient), and caring in the doctor–patient relationship.

- Communicate openly and honestly with patients. Never misrepresent your status. Introduce yourself by name and identify yourself as a resident. Provide complete and accurate information about treatment options.

- Safeguard the patient's right to privacy within the constraints of the law, and maintain patient confidentiality in accordance with the policies of the Health Insurance Portability and Accountability Act (HIPAA) of 1996.

- Do not allow fees for ophthalmologic services to exploit patients or third-party payers.

- Always strive to preserve, to protect, and to advance the best interests of the patient. Reflect this in your actions and attitude by placing your patient's welfare ahead of your personal ambitions and desires.

- Take thoughtful measures to effect corrective action if colleagues deviate from professionally or ethically accepted standards.

Education and Training

The physician-in-training must strive to achieve a balance between education and training. Training connotes learning to perform specific tasks, such as examination steps and surgical procedures. The meaning of education is much broader, and entails the thoughtful integration of new knowledge into one's own personal experiences, insights, and actions. Residency training must be supplemented by self-driven education. It can be argued that the single most important factor that determines an excellent residency training outcome is the individual's own input into the education and training. A well-balanced education can be obtained by diversifying sources of learning to encompass a thoughtful mixture of reading books and journals, attending lectures and conferences, and participating in informal discussions. One time-honored approach to continuing education is to read about the disorders you find in your own patients as you encounter them. Your knowledge will be tested annually with the Academy's Ophthalmic Knowledge Assessment Program (OKAP) examination. This exam will help you identify your areas of strength and areas in which further study is needed.

All residents should strive to obtain certification by the American Board of Ophthalmology (ABO). Such certification is based on continuing education, licensure, verification of credentials by the chairperson of the residency program, the Written Qualifying Examination, and the Oral Examination. To ensure continued learning after residency, the ABO has instituted a maintenance of certification (MOC) process. The MOC process requires proof of state licensure, documentation of continued medical education, ongoing clinical knowledge, and medical practice improvement activities. The process is repeated every 10 years.

Active pursuit of education and training must continue beyond residency. The beginning resident must make a commitment to sharpen medical skills and knowledge through continual study, instruction, and experience. Maintaining competence is essential to the ethical practice of ophthalmology and to the promotion of intellectual and professional growth. Keeping up with medical and surgical discoveries and inventions, which seem to change the practice of medicine almost daily, is necessary to remain competitive in a marketplace that demands excellent outcomes.

The demands of health care reform will affect the challenge of becoming an excellent ophthalmologist. Increasing constraints on the time and economic resources available for education are further strained by the need to remain current and fully competent in an ever-evolving field. The American Academy of Ophthalmology (AAO) offers a framework of Academy resources that can help members accomplish their continuing educational goals in the face of new challenges and imperatives. For a listing of Academy products and services, visit the AAO web site at www.aao.org.

Pitfalls and Pointers

- Avoid cutting corners or taking shortcuts in your practice as a new resident. Learn your examination techniques and management protocols right the first time.

- Do not compromise patient care for the sake of training or for any other personal benefit. Always consult a more knowledgeable or experienced physician if you are uncertain about how to proceed in a clinical situation.

- Do not be embarrassed to use this (or any) introductory manual. Adopt a lifelong approach to learning.

- Do not hide your own limitations in skill and knowledge as you begin your residency. Strive to improve upon them and be receptive to criticism.

- Remember that professional success involves more than learning the medical facts and the surgical techniques. The art of practicing medicine is best achieved by a well-rounded, mature, and compassionate physician who also knows the medical facts well.

- Do not publicly denounce or belittle the care given by previous practitioners by saying such things as, "Your doctor did not know what they were doing," or "That was malpractice." Avail yourself of the facts before passing any judgments, but remember that you are a medical resident, not a judge.

Suggested Resources

Appropriate Examination and Treatment Procedures [Advisory Opinion]. American Academy of Ophthalmology; 2016. Accessed September 15, 2020. https://www.aao.org/ethics-detail/advisory-opinion-appropriate-examination -treatment-2

Basic and Clinical Science Course. San Francisco: American Academy of Ophthalmology; published annually.

Code of Ethics. American Academy of Ophthalmology; 2020. Accessed September 14, 2020. https://www.aao.org/ethics-detail/code-of-ethics

Common Program Requirements. Accreditation Council for Graduate Medical Education (ACGME) web site. Accessed September 14, 2020. https://acgme.org/What-We-Do/Accreditation/Common-Program-Requirements.

Durfee DA, ed. *The Profession of Ophthalmology: Practice Management, Ethics, and Advocacy,* 2nd ed. American Academy of Ophthalmology; 2010.

Learning New Techniques Following Residency [Advisory Opinion]. American Academy of Ophthalmology; 2020. Accessed September 14, 2020. https://www.aao.org/ethics-detail/advisory-opinion--learning-new-techniques-followin

The Ethical and Technical Competence of the Ophthalmologist [Information Statement]. American Academy of Ophthalmology; 2018. Accessed September 14, 2020.

2 Overview of the Ophthalmic Evaluation

The purpose of the ophthalmic evaluation is to assess visual function and ocular health. The specific objectives of the comprehensive ophthalmic evaluation include the following:

- Obtain an ocular and a systemic history.
- Determine the optical and health status of the eye, visual system, and related structures.
- Identify risk factors for ocular and systemic disease.
- Detect and diagnose ocular abnormalities and disease.
- Establish and document the presence or absence of ocular signs or symptoms of systemic disease.
- Discuss with the patient the nature of the findings and their implications.
- Initiate an appropriate response, such as diagnostic tests, treatment, or referral, when indicated. Often the patient needs only explanation and reassurance.

The physician accomplishes these objectives by obtaining the patient's history and performing the necessary examinations, using specific equipment as needed. A successful encounter requires a professional demeanor and begins with a clear introduction and description of one's role within the health care team (ie, trainee, attending). Patient privacy is protected by closing examination room doors, covering patients' charts and tests, and ensuring that open electronic medical record screens do not have information related to other patients. Finally, the evaluation must be documented clearly, accurately, and in a timely manner.

History

Obtaining a thorough history from the patient is the important first step in an ophthalmic evaluation (see Chapter 3). In general, the history includes the following information:

- demographic data, including name, date of birth, sex, race/ethnicity, and occupation
- the identity of other pertinent health care providers utilized by the patient, including the name of the physician requesting consultation, if applicable
- chief concern, or the main problem that prompted the visit
- history of present illness, which is a more detailed description of the chief concern(s)

- present status of vision, including the patient's perception of their own visual status, visual needs, and any ocular symptoms
- past ocular history, including baseline visual status, prior eye diseases, injuries, diagnoses, treatments, surgeries, ocular medications, and use of glasses or contact lenses
- past systemic history, including allergies, adverse reactions to medications, medication use (including prescription and nonprescription medications and herbal and nutritional supplements), and pertinent medical problems, surgeries, and hospitalizations
- family history, including poor vision (and cause, if known), and other pertinent familial ocular and systemic diseases
- social history, including vocational and avocational visual requirements, and use of personal protective equipment (eg, safety glasses or goggles)

Examination

The comprehensive ophthalmic evaluation includes an analysis of the physiologic function and anatomical status of the eye, visual system, and related structures. Components of the evaluation and chapters in this book in which they are discussed are noted below:

- visual acuity examination (visual acuity is determined with and without the present correction, if any, at distance and at near; see Chapter 4)
- determination of corrected distance visual acuity, also called best-corrected visual acuity, with use of retinoscopy and refraction (see Chapter 5)
- ocular alignment and motility examination (see Chapter 6)
- pupillary examination (see Chapter 7)
- visual field examination (see Chapter 8)
- examination of the external eye and ocular adnexa (see Chapter 9)
- examination of the anterior segment (see Chapters 10 and 11)
- tonometry to determine intraocular pressure (see Chapter 12)
- posterior segment examination (see Chapter 13)

Ophthalmic Equipment

The ophthalmic examination room and its equipment are sometimes referred to as "a lane." Although the equipment in examining rooms varies widely, the components typically include the following:

- *Snellen acuity chart.* This printed hanging chart, projected chart, or video display is used in determining visual acuity and in refraction (see Chapter 4).
- *Near visual acuity chart.* This printed, handheld chart is used to determine near visual acuity and as an aid in refraction (see Chapter 4).

- *Pinhole occluder.* Improvement in visual acuity when one looks through a pinhole suggests the presence of uncorrected refractive error.

- *Penlight or Finnoff transilluminator (muscle light).* These instruments are used to check pupillary light reflexes and the corneal light reflex. Auxiliary uses include illumination for the external examination and transillumination of the globe (see Chapters 6, 7, and 9).

- *Slit-lamp biomicroscope.* This optical magnifying instrument is used primarily to perform anterior segment examinations. When combined with an auxiliary lens, such as a +90 or +78 diopter lens or a Goldmann 3-mirror lens, it can be used to examine the posterior segment. It is also used in conjunction with a gonioscopy lens to examine the anterior chamber angle (see Chapters 10, 11, and 13).

- *Goldmann applanation tonometer.* This device attaches to the slit-lamp biomicroscope and is used to measure intraocular pressure. Handheld devices (eg, the Tono-Pen or the iCare tonometer) can also be used to measure intraocular pressure (see Chapter 12).

- *Streak retinoscope.* This handheld instrument is used to perform retinoscopy, which provides an objective measurement of a patient's refractive state (see Chapter 5).

- *Phoropter.* This device (also called a refractor) stores a range of trial lenses. It is used when retinoscopy and refraction are performed (see Chapter 5).

- *Trial frame and loose trial lenses.* This equipment is used when retinoscopy and refraction are performed and to confirm refractive findings (see Chapter 5). It is also useful in tests that evaluate ocular alignment of patients without their glasses.

- *Direct ophthalmoscope.* This handheld instrument is used for posterior segment examinations and also to assess the red reflex (see Chapter 13).

- *Indirect ophthalmoscope.* This device, worn on the head, is used for the posterior segment examination in conjunction with auxiliary handheld diagnostic condensing lenses (see Chapter 13).

- *Keratometer.* This device measures corneal curvature and is typically used in the fitting of contact lenses and to diagnose disorders such as keratoconus.

- *Prisms.* These optical devices, available individually or held together in a prism bar, are used to measure strabismus (see Chapter 6).

- *Sensory testing equipment.* The Worth 4-dot testing equipment consists of red-green eyeglasses (with a red lens for one eye, usually the right, and a green lens for the other/left eye) and a flashlight that illuminates 4 colored dots. The Titmus test utilizes a stereoscopic test booklet and a pair of polarized spectacles. Both of these tests are used to assess binocular vision as a part of the motility examination (see Chapter 6).

- *Color vision testing equipment.* Standardized books of colored plates, such as the Ishihara pseudoisochromatic color tests, are used when congenital or acquired color vision defects are suspected (see Chapter 4).

- *Exophthalmometer.* This instrument is used to assess the anterior-posterior position of the globes by measuring the distance from the lateral orbital rim to the corneal apex (see Chapter 9).

Ancillary Equipment

Other equipment is commonly used to measure visual function or to assess ocular structures:

- *Visual field analyzer (perimeter)*. This device is usually automated, but it may be manual. It is used to assess the central and peripheral field of vision (see Chapter 8).
- *Corneal topography system*. This automated system is used to measure corneal curvature. It is most useful in refractive surgery, after corneal transplant surgery, and to evaluate patients with keratoconus.
- *Optical coherence tomography (OCT)*. This system provides a high-resolution cross-sectional image of the optic nerve and retina. It is useful for evaluation of retinal disease such as macular edema, and in the monitoring of glaucomatous nerve disc changes. OCT can also be used to visualize anterior segment structures.
- *Ultrasonography*. This imaging modality provides 1-dimensional ("A-scan") or 2-dimensional ("B-scan") cross-sectional views of the eye. It is often used to evaluate the posterior segment when direct visualization is obscured by opacities in the cornea, lens, and/or vitreous (see Chapter 13).
- *Specular microscope*. This device is used to evaluate the corneal endothelium. It demonstrates cell morphology and calculates endothelial cell density (see Chapter 11).
- *Pachymeter*. This instrument is used to measure corneal thickness. It may be found as a slit-lamp attachment or as a handheld device.

Physician Demeanor and Approach to the Patient

When performing the ophthalmic evaluation, the ophthalmologist should listen to patients' concerns carefully and with undivided attention. Patients' descriptions of ocular problems, in their own words, are of vital importance. After completion of the ophthalmic evaluation and counseling of the patient, it is advisable that the ophthalmologist ask if the patient has any additional questions or concerns and address them at that time.

Certain situations may create barriers to proper care and effective patient–physician communication. The ophthalmologist should proactively look for potential obstacles to each patient's adherence to care, including specific work schedules, travel distance and transportation, lack of insurance, and so on. Compassionate and nonjudgmental efforts to address barriers to care will also build trust and ultimately improve patient outcomes. Familiarity with local and institutional resources will help the physician optimize care when potential obstacles arise.

When the patient and the ophthalmologist do not speak the same language, the physician is ethically and legally obligated to provide access to qualified translator services. Bilingual family members or staff may be used to bridge minor communication gaps; however, this should be avoided if informed consent is required for a procedure, particularly if the family member is a minor.

In some situations, the mental status of the patient limits the extent of first-person history taking. In these cases, the family members, guardians, or attendants of the patient can usually provide additional important information. Some patients have a deep-seated fear of the health care environment, which inhibits their ability to communicate; other patients have an unspoken fear of blindness that can cause them to minimize or exaggerate ocular complaints. By creating an atmosphere of trust, respect, and openness, the ophthalmologist can encourage the patient to communicate freely, and effective patient–physician communication can be achieved.

Pediatric Patients

Pediatric patients warrant special consideration. The parent or caretaker will be the primary source of information for preverbal children. Furthermore, the pediatric eye examination is nuanced and may involve specialized components; it is important to know when to ask for help from a more experienced practitioner. Some pediatric patients will not tolerate a comprehensive examination and may require an examination under anesthesia in order to identify or rule out pathology. Older children should be involved as much as possible in history taking and in discussions of the findings and treatment plans, depending on the child's age, comprehension, and ability to communicate.

Elderly Patients

With advancing age comes an increased prevalence of major causes of visual impairment (eg, diabetic retinopathy, glaucoma, cataract, and age-related macular degeneration). The ophthalmologist-in-training needs to give specific consideration to the relationship between vision loss and common comorbidities, as well as to the special needs and impact of visual loss in aged patients:

- *Hearing impairment.* Visual loss and hearing impairment often coexist, and the presence of both sensory deficits is more detrimental than either one alone. Ophthalmologists should recognize hearing-impaired patients and refer them as needed for management.

- *Mood disorders.* Visual loss is commonly associated with depression and anxiety, especially in elderly patients. Depression is a debilitating, yet treatable, condition that patients may not recognize and that is not commonly reported to the ophthalmologist. Asking patients with vision loss if they have recently felt down or depressed, or if they have less interest in activities they previously enjoyed can help identify those for whom formal evaluation may be beneficial.

- *Dementia.* Vision and cognitive function are interdependent. Decreasing vision can worsen symptoms of dementia and often disproportionately impacts global function in patients with cognitive dysfunction. Dementia also alters the perception and interpretation of visual information. Patients who have dementia might report visual complaints such as, "I get lost easily," or, "I can see but I can't read," or describe difficulties that appear inconsistent with objectively measured vision parameters. One rapid dementia screening technique is the "clock draw." The patient is asked to draw a clock face, including hour numbers (from 1 to 12) and clock hands, to represent a time of 10 minutes past 11 o'clock. Patients who fail this test may benefit from a formal cognitive evaluation.

- *Fall prevention.* Loss of visual function increases the incidence and severity of falls and fractures, which occur in up to 35% of the elderly per year. Fall prevention is a much more effective strategy than treating the injuries that result from falls. Ophthalmologists should reinforce for elderly patients the importance of reducing the risk of falling, which can be achieved by increasing lighting, decreasing glare, increasing contrast of steps and corners, reducing clutter and tripping hazards, and using and wearing appropriate walking aids and footwear.

- *Driving.* Ophthalmologists must recognize that driving often plays both an important practical and symbolic role in an individual's sense of independence. However, driving on public roads is a privilege rather than a right, and impaired drivers pose significant risk to themselves and others. Although there is general agreement that severe visual impairment (20/200 visual acuity or a 20° visual field) should preclude driving, there is no consensus regarding moderate visual impairment. Visual acuity is a poor standalone predictor of at-fault crash involvement. Safe driving requires the sensory ability to perceive information in the rapidly changing environment, the attentiveness to process multiple pieces of information, the cognitive ability to judge this information and make appropriate decisions, and the motor ability to react appropriately in a timely fashion. A history of at-fault crash involvement in the presence of motor, sensory, and/or cognitive defects may identify a driver-at-risk.

- *Terminology.* Although the word "senile," as in *senile cataract,* is well established in medical terminology, it has unpleasant connotations and should not be used in the presence of patients. *Involutional* or *age-related* are far preferable if an equivalent adjective is needed.

- *Evaluation of low vision.* Visual loss can have profound effects on many activities of daily living, such as walking, going outside, getting in and out of bed, grocery shopping, paying bills, cleaning, cooking, and driving. Many of these problems can be helped by evaluation of low vision and treatment with optical and nonoptical rehabilitative aids. One of the most simple, common, and useful aids is a high-plus reading prescription that serves to magnify reading material. Social, family, community, and other support services often improve the visually impaired patient's quality of life.

Medical Record Keeping and Communication

Timely, legible, and thorough documentation of the ophthalmic evaluation is of tremendous importance to patient care and will serve as an important future reference for the ophthalmologist and other caregivers. Although some abbreviations are widely employed, terminology that will be understandable to other healthcare providers should be used in ophthalmic medical records. Excessive use of jargon should be avoided. As a medicolegal document, the medical record must present sufficiently detailed findings and treatment recommendations. The record must be sufficiently complete to justify coding levels for charges and reimbursement. Many ophthalmologists now use an electronic medical record, and advantages of such a system include improved legibility, multisite accessibility, and reduced space requirements for storage.

Communication with referring physicians and other health care providers, whether written or verbal, is crucial in providing the patient with continuity and coordination of care. Such communication should be clear, timely, and informative. As in any medical setting, it is important to maintain the confidentiality of all patient information and interactions. Telephone and in-person communication with colleagues should be discreet and outside the earshot of those uninvolved in the patient's care. Electronic communications that include patient information should use appropriate encryption and adhere to all institutional protocols with respect to patient data use and sharing.

Some ocular conditions occur as manifestations of systemic diseases that constitute a threat to public health, such as gonococcal conjunctivitis and ocular infections related to human immunodeficiency virus. Some such diseases, by statutory guidelines, must be reported to the state health department. States also often want reports about patients who have recently become legally blind. Reporting guidelines vary from state to state; ophthalmologists should contact their state health departments for appropriate details.

Pitfalls and Pointers

- The beginning resident should strive to learn a systematic, comprehensive approach to the history and examination of each patient. In this way, key historic points or examination findings are much less likely to be omitted.

- New residents in ophthalmology might at first feel overwhelmed by unfamiliar diagnostic techniques, equipment, and nomenclature. This reaction is normal. With hard work, perseverance, and diligent study, what is unfamiliar now will seem like second nature in a relatively short time.

- As the beginning resident strives to master new ophthalmologic techniques and skills, they should not lose sight of the fact that a patient sits behind the refractor.

Suggested Resources

Comprehensive Adult Medical Eye Evaluation [Preferred Practice Pattern]. American Academy of Ophthalmology; 2015. Accessed September 14, 2020. https://www.aao.org/preferred-practice-pattern/comprehensive-adult-medical-eye -evaluation-2015

Durfee DA, ed. *The Profession of Ophthalmology: Practice Management, Ethics, and Advocacy,* 2nd ed. American Academy of Ophthalmology; 2010.

Miller AM. "Clinical Pearls for Pediatric Ophthalmology." *American Academy of Ophthalmology YO Info Newsletter*, July 2008. Accessed September 14, 2020. www.aao.org/young-ophthalmologists/yo-info/article/clinical-pearls-pediatric -ophthalmology

Pediatric Eye Evaluations [Preferred Practice Pattern]. American Academy of Ophthalmology; 2017. Accessed September 14, 2020. https://www.aao.org /preferred-practice-pattern/pediatric-eye-evaluations-ppp-2017

Pediatric Ophthalmology and Strabismus. Basic and Clinical Science Course, Section 6. American Academy of Ophthalmology; published annually.

3 History Taking

Although similar to the general medical history that you learned in medical school, the ophthalmic history emphasizes symptoms of ocular disease, present and past ocular problems, and ocular medications. The history is intended to elicit any information that might be useful in evaluating and managing the patient; it may be as brief or as extensive as required by the patient's particular problems. This chapter provides an overview of the ophthalmic history and its goals, recording methods, and components.

Goals of the History

The history should allow for the recording of important information that could affect the patient's diagnosis and treatment. The 5 most important objectives include the following:

1. *Identify the patient.* If it has not already been collected, record demographic information about the patient, such as name, date of birth, sex, race, medical record number, and updated contact information. Strict confidentiality of this information should be maintained, according to the Health Insurance Portability and Accountability Act (HIPAA) standards. If you are using an existing chart, use of two identifiers, such as name and date of birth, should be verified to ensure that you have the correct patient.

2. *Identify other practitioners who have cared for the patient or who may care for the patient in the future.* Such individuals might need to be contacted for additional information or be given information about the patient, especially if the patient was referred for consultation, in which case a written report is required. Reports also are often needed after referrals from attorneys, insurance companies, or governmental agencies.

3. *Develop a preliminary differential diagnosis.* The likely diagnosis, or at least a reasonable differential diagnosis, often can be supposed merely on the basis of a good history. This, in turn, allows for the planning and tailoring of a more useful and efficient examination.

4. *Select therapy.* Knowing and recording treatments that have already been tried, and whether (and in what ways) they were helpful, is invaluable in planning therapy. Insufficient knowledge of the results of prior therapeutic efforts can also lead to misdiagnosis.

    Where therapy is concerned, it is important also to try to ascertain what the patient wants and expects from the physician. This can be done directly, by questioning the patient as well as, in many cases, indirectly, by listening attentively to and interpreting what the patient says. Some patients require definitive therapy, whereas others need only explanation and reassurance, documentation of a problem, or periodic observation.

5. *Consider socioeconomic and medicolegal factors.* Insurance payments, workers' compensation payments, disability payments, and the like (on the patient's behalf), as well as legal proceedings, often depend on detailed, accurate reports (or even testimony) from the physician. Such reports can be inadequate and sometimes even detrimental to the patient if a thorough history has not been obtained. In addition, a well-taken history can save time and expense by obviating needless tests and examination procedures. Finally, the components and thoroughness of the history are considered and may be audited by payors (eg, Medicare) to determine the appropriateness of coding and charges for services.

Methods of Recording the History

The precise method of recording the history depends on the requirements of the practice or institution. The history may be handwritten on paper, dictated for later transcription, or entered into an electronic medical record. Clinical photographs or videos can be of value in documenting the presence or absence of particular problems (eg, ptosis, abnormal ocular motility, proptosis, facial nerve palsy, etc.), but it is of utmost importance to follow correct protocols and procedures. These includes obtaining proper informed consent; de-identifying images; maintaining patient privacy; and properly storing, and responsibly presenting, publishing, or distributing patient information.

Components of the History

As described below, the components of the ophthalmic history are essentially the same as the components of any general medical history, except that ophthalmic aspects are emphasized. The components of the history are the following:

- chief concern
- history of the present illness
- past ocular history
- ocular medications
- general medical and surgical history
- systemic medications
- allergies
- social history
- family history
- review of systems

Chief Concern

The patient's main concern(s), also commonly referred to as "chief complaint(s)," should be recorded *in the patient's own words* or in a nontechnical paraphrasing of the patient's words. It is not advisable in this early phase of the history for the ophthalmologist to draw hasty conclusions by employing medical terms that suggest premature diagnoses. For example, chief concerns should be listed as *redness, burning,* and *mattering,* or *light flashes,* instead of *conjunctivitis* or *photopsia.* The patient's own words are important for knowing and being able to document the patient's point of view as distinct from that of the physician. The physician's impression is appropriate only later, after a proper history has been taken and a suitably thorough examination has been performed.

Of course, patients are sometimes troubled by more than 1 symptom or problem and so might have more than 1 chief concern. Problems that are of lesser importance should be cited along with the chief concern. Here are some examples of the kinds of questions that can help to elicit the patient's main concerns:

- What are the main problems that you are having with your eyes?
- What other problems are you having with your eyes?
- Why did you come (or why were you sent) here?
- In what way are you hoping that we might help you?
- What is it about your eyes that worries or concerns you? (This type of question sometimes reveals entirely unfounded fears, such as blindness or cancer.)
- What is the main problem that you would like me to address?

History of the Present Illness

Evaluation of the patient's present illness consists mainly of an effort to record additional information and details about the chief concern(s). The patient's own words may be used here when desired, although the physician's words, including medical terminology and abbreviations, are more often used to represent what the patient said. Information elicited about the present illness allows the ophthalmologist to begin developing a preliminary diagnostic impression.

The following eight general areas of inquiry are important components for developing information about the present illness, and are also necessary for accurate coding and billing.

1. *Location.* What is the site of the problem? Is the problem unilateral or bilateral?
2. *Quality.* What is the nature of the discomfort? Is it constant, intermittent, acute, chronic, improving, or worsening?
3. *Severity.* How bad is the problem? For example, on a scale of 1 to 10, how bad is the pain?
4. *Duration.* How long has this problem been going on?
5. *Timing.* Has the problem been intermittent or seasonal, or does it worsen at a particular time of day?
6. *Context.* Is the problem associated with any activity or location? For example, is the problem worse at school or work?
7. *Modifying factors.* What might have precipitated the condition, made it better or worse, or made no difference? Asking about prior therapeutic efforts is especially important, including when the patient's refractive prescription was last changed.

8. *Associated signs and symptoms.* Is the problem causing other problems, such as blurry vision, headache, or tearing?

It is sometimes necessary to clarify what the patient means by certain concerns. For example, does "mattering" of the eye mean sealing of the eyelids by sticky discharge, the mere presence of strands of mucus at times, or simply tiny granules on the eyelids (as from dried mucus or the drying and crystallization of eyedrops)? Countless other situations exist in which it is important to clarify what the patient means, so it is vital to question the patient thoroughly.

Specific ocular concerns that might be recorded under "history of the present illness" are too numerous to list here in their entirety. Nevertheless, one needs to keep in mind certain general categories of ocular concerns, which are listed below together with examples of accompanying specific concerns.

Disturbances of vision
- blurred or decreased central vision (distance, near, or both)
- decreased peripheral vision
- altered image size (micropsia, macropsia)
- distortion of images (metamorphopsia)
- diplopia (monocular, binocular, horizontal, vertical, oblique)
- floaters (moving lines or specks in the field of vision)
- photopsia (flashes of light)
- iridescent vision (halos, rainbows)
- dark adaptation problems (nyctalopia)
- dyslexia (difficulty processing the written word)
- color vision abnormalities
- blindness (ocular, cortical, perceptual)
- oscillopsia (movement or shaking of images)

Ocular pain or discomfort
- foreign-body sensation (a feeling of scratchiness, as though a particle is present on the surface of the eye)
- ciliary (deep) pain (an aching, often severe, pain within and around the eye, sometimes radiating to the ipsilateral temple, forehead, malar area, and even the occiput, secondary to spasm of the ciliary muscles)
- photophobia (a less severe form of ciliary pain that is present only upon exposure to light)
- headache
- burning
- dryness
- itching; true itching, which compels the patient to rub the eye(s) vigorously (and which usually indicates allergy), must be differentiated from burning, dryness, and foreign-body sensation
- asthenopia (eyestrain)

Abnormal ocular secretions
- lacrimation (tearing/welling up of tears on the ocular surface)
- epiphora (actual spilling of tears over the margin of the eyelid onto the face)
- dryness
- discharge (purulent, mucopurulent, mucoid, serous, or watery; the first 2 kinds of discharge are associated with neutrophils and can cause true sealing of the eyelids overnight)

Abnormal appearances
- ptosis (drooping of the eyelid)
- proptosis or exophthalmos (protrusion of the eye or eyes)
- enophthalmos (the opposite of proptosis)
- blepharitis
- misalignment of the eyes
- redness, other discolorations, opacities, masses
- anisocoria (asymmetric pupil size)

Other concerns
- "something my doctor wanted to be checked"
- the need for a second opinion regarding diagnosis, surgery, or other management

Trauma
Cases of ocular trauma in particular can require very detailed reports based on a thorough history and examination, and important issues such as workers' compensation, disability, and medicolegal factors must be kept in mind.

- the date, time, and place (including the precise address) of the injury
- what happened, in the patient's own words (particularly in the case of trauma, the patient's words are useful in the history of the present illness as well as in the chief concern)
- what safety precautions were taken, if any, including the wearing of safety glasses
- what measures were taken for emergency treatment (treatment takes priority over obtaining a history in a true emergency [see chapter 14], although the history remains important)
- the size, type, material composition, and roughly estimated speed of any foreign body, and whether part or all of the object was recovered after the injury
- whether the vision has been affected
- tetanus immunity status
- time the patient last ate (in case the patient needs to be taken to the operating room for surgical repair)

Some patients with ocular trauma may have suffered from intimate partner violence. Screening questions are asked when the patient's spouse is not at the bedside; referral to a social worker or alerting the emergency department physician may be lifesaving.

Past Ocular History

Prior ocular problems can have a bearing on a patient's diagnosis and management. You should ask the patient about the existence of any such problems so that their possible role in the present illness can be evaluated, and so that they can be managed, if necessary.

To begin this line of query, the physician usually asks if the patient has experienced any eye problems in the past, but it is often useful to ask specifically about the following:

- use of eyeglasses or contact lenses (the date of the most recent prescription may be recorded here or with the present illness)
- past use of ocular medications
- ocular surgery (including laser surgery)
- ocular trauma
- history of amblyopia (lazy eye) or of ocular patching in childhood

If the patient responds positively to any of the above, it might be valuable to ask why, when, how, where, and by whom, as applicable.

Ocular Medications

Knowledge of the patient's use of ocular medications is essential. It is necessary to know how the patient responded to prior therapy. In addition, recent therapy can affect the patient's present status, because toxic and allergic reactions to topical medications and preservatives sometimes resolve slowly.

All current and prior ocular medications used for the present illness should be recorded, including dosages, frequency, and duration of use. Also ask about the use of any over-the-counter (nonprescription) medications, home remedies, herbal medicines, and dietary supplements.

Patients sometimes do not know the names of their medications. In such cases, the physician might learn the general classes of medications being used by asking the color of the cap on the container, because some containers for eyedrops have caps of different colors to facilitate identification:

- green: cholinergic (miotic) drugs such as pilocarpine, carbachol, echothiophate iodide (phospholine iodide)
- red: anticholinergic (dilating cycloplegic or mydriatic) drugs such as atropine, homatropine, scopolamine, cyclopentolate, tropicamide, phenylephrine
- yellow: beta-adrenergic blocking agents (timolol 0.5%, levobunolol 0.5%)
- blue: timolol 0.25%, betaxolol (a β_1-adrenergic blocking agent), levobunolol 0.25%, timolol/brimonidine combination (Combigan), timolol/dorzolamide combination (Cosopt)
- white: many medications, including certain antibiotics, artificial tears, corticosteroids, and anti-allergy eyedrops
- purple: α-adrenergic agonists such as brimonidine
- teal: prostaglandin analogues (latanoprost, travoprost, bimatoprost, unoprostone)
- orange: topical carbonic anhydrase inhibitors (dorzolamide, brinzolamide)

- tan: fluoroquinolone antibiotics (ciprofloxacin, levofloxacin, gatifloxacin, moxifloxacin)
- gray: nonsteroidal anti-inflammatory medications (ketorolac, nepafenac, diclofenac)
- pink: corticosteroid-containing eyedrops

General Medical and Surgical History

The patient's present and past general medical history is important for several reasons. First, many ocular diseases are manifestations of or are associated with systemic diseases. Second, treatment choice may depend on the patient's medical status. And third, the general medical status must be known for the physician to perform a proper preoperative evaluation.

All medical and surgical problems should be recorded, along with the approximate dates of onset, medical treatments, and surgeries, when possible. The duration and adequacy of control of diabetes should be determined, including the results of the patient's most recent HbA1c test. The history of and treatment for sexually transmitted diseases can be pertinent in certain situations.

The evaluation of a pediatric patient might require obtaining historic information from the parents about pregnancy, such as prenatal care, medications used, substance abuse during pregnancy, complications during labor, prematurity, delivery, birth weight, and the neonatal period.

Systemic Medications

Systemic medications can cause ocular, preoperative, intraoperative, and postoperative problems and can provide clues to systemic disorders the patient might have. Particular attention should be given to the use of alpha-antagonists, such as tamsulosin, as these medications can cause intraoperative floppy iris syndrome (IFIS) during cataract surgery, or aspirin and other anticoagulant agents, as these can cause intraoperative and postoperative bleeding. The patient's use of systemic medications (eg, acetazolamide, vitamins) that are taken for ocular problems may be recorded here or, preferably, under "Ocular Medications."

It is sometimes sufficient merely to ask what systemic medications the patient takes, but it can be useful in selected cases to inquire specifically about antibiotics, tranquilizers, narcotics, sleeping pills, anticonvulsants, anti-inflammatory agents, oral contraceptives, vitamins, herbal compounds, or alternative medications, especially when the patient is unsure about medications being used. Certain medicines, such as antimalarial drugs, phenothiazines, amiodarone, tamoxifen, and systemic steroids, can have ocular toxicity.

Allergies

The patient's history of allergies to medications is important. However, patients often have difficulty differentiating true allergic reactions from side effects or other nonallergenic adverse effects of medications, so it is important to ask about (and record) the nature of any claimed reaction. Itching, hives, rashes, wheezing, or frank cardiorespiratory collapse clearly suggest true allergy, whereas statements such as "the eyedrops burned" or "the pills upset my stomach" do not.

In addition to inquiries about allergic reactions to topical and systemic medications, the physician should ask about allergies to environmental agents (atopy) that result in any of the following:

- atopic dermatitis
- allergic asthma
- allergic rhinitis, conjunctivitis (hay fever)
- urticaria (hives)
- vernal conjunctivitis

Social History

A social history should be taken; included in it are tobacco and alcohol use, drug abuse, sexual history (including sexually transmitted diseases), tattoos, body piercing, and environmental factors. A detailed occupational history should be taken to include the visual requirements of the patient's job and hobbies. Because many jobs have specific visual requirements (eg, commercial truck driver, law enforcement officer, pilot), this information is vital. The questioning should be pursued in a nonjudgmental way, with sensitivity and due respect for privacy. Except as might be required by law, or with the patient's permission, such information should not be revealed to third parties. When you obtain a sexual history or drug use history, you may ask members of the family to leave the room so that you can speak alone with the patient.

Family History

The family history of ocular and nonocular diseases is important when genetically transmitted disorders are under consideration. The physician might begin by asking a general question such as, "Are there any eye problems, other than just needing glasses, in your family history?" before asking specifically about corneal disease, glaucoma, cataract, retinal disease, or other heritable ocular conditions.

Knowledge of familial systemic diseases can be helpful in ophthalmic evaluation and diagnosis. Examples include atopy, thyroid disease, diabetes mellitus, certain malignancies, various hereditary syndromes, and many others. Inability of the patient to provide information about the family medical background should not be construed or recorded as a negative family history. Rather, the chart should reflect the fact that the patient's knowledge was incomplete or lacking. Examination of family members can be useful when patients present with possible heritable disorders.

Review of Systems

A pertinent review of systems, tailored to the patient's concerns, should be conducted, including questions related to dermatologic, cardiac, renal, hepatic, pulmonary, gastrointestinal, central nervous system, and autoimmune collagen vascular (including arthritic) diseases.

Pitfalls and Pointers

- Avoid taking an insufficiently detailed history. The history need not be of great length, but it should contain all the details that are pertinent to the patient's concerns and problems.
- Although sufficient detail in a history is important, it is also important not to emphasize minutiae to the detriment of the main sources of concern (ie, why the patient is here and what they need and want from the ophthalmologist).

- Parents, guardians, other relatives, or friends are sometimes needed to give histories for patients who are unable to speak for themselves. An interpreter is required for any patient who does not speak the physician's language.

- Avoid phrasing your questions in a way that would elicit feelings of guilt or imply a causal relationship, such as when asking about prenatal and gestational history for a patient with a congenital eye disorder. Doing so may lead the parents to think that their child's condition is due to something they might or might not have done.

- Good history taking involves communication skills on the part of the physician not only to guide the discussion, but also to bring out useful information, convey empathy, and allow the patient to feel heard and understood.

- A good history may be brief or lengthy, as long as it is thorough, relative to the ultimate goal of helping the patient. The ability to take a complete, yet efficient, history is an important aspect of the art of medicine. Nevertheless, the beginning ophthalmology resident whose histories fall short of ideal should not be dismayed; the skill improves greatly with practice.

Suggested Resources

Fundamentals and Principles of Ophthalmology. Basic and Clinical Science Course, Section 2. American Academy of Ophthalmology; published annually.

Intraocular Inflammation and Uveitis. Basic and Clinical Science Course, Section 9. American Academy of Ophthalmology; published annually.

Pediatric Ophthalmology and Strabismus. Basic and Clinical Science Course, Section 6. American Academy of Ophthalmology; published annually.

4 Visual Acuity Examination

▶ *This chapter includes a related video, which can be accessed by scanning the QR codes provided in the text or going to aao.org/PracticalOphthalmologyvideo.*

Vision is a complex human sense with many facets that cannot be measured. Ophthalmologists rely on a variety of psychophysical assessments and express vision as a measure of visual acuity, although acuity is only 1 component of vision. Vision consists of, but is not limited to, visual acuity, visual field, and contrast sensitivity. This chapter deals mainly with measuring distance and near visual acuity, near points of accommodation and convergence, and stereopsis.

Testing Conventions and Materials

The term *visual acuity* refers to an angular measurement that relates testing distance to the minimal object size resolvable at that distance. Ophthalmologists typically use Snellen acuity as a measure of the resolving ability of the eye. The traditional Snellen measurement of distance acuity utilizes targets, or *optotypes,* that subtend a visual angle on the retina of 5 minutes of arc. Each smaller component of the optotype, such as the individual bars and spaces of the letter "E," subtends a visual angle of 1 minute on the retina. One minute is the smallest angle discernible for normal human vision. In Snellen notation, 20/20 is considered normal visual acuity. If the vision is tested at a distance other than 20 feet, the target size must be adjusted to maintain the correct visual angle. Larger targets are designated by a larger number in the denominator. This number represents the distance at which that target subtends a visual angle of 5 minutes. For example, a 20/60 optotype is 3 times as big as the 20/20 optotype and subtends the standard 5 minutes of arc at a distance of 60 feet.

Varieties of measurement and notation methods, test targets, and abbreviations have been developed for the purpose of performing visual acuity and visual function testing and for documenting the results. This chapter presents an overview of the standard conventions and steps used in performing these tests.

Measurement Notation

The Snellen notation is the most common method of expressing visual acuity measurement. By convention, this expression is written as a fraction, but it is not a mathematical fraction or expression. The optical meaning of the fraction is described above, but a more practical way to think of it is that the number in the numerator position is the equivalent of the testing distance from the eye to the chart being used, in either feet or meters, while the number in the denominator position is the distance at which a subject with unimpaired vision can read the same figure. This notation quantifies visual discrimination of fine detail.

Other types of visual acuity notations are used besides the Snellen notation. A decimal notation converts the Snellen fraction to a decimal; for example, Snellen 20/20 equals decimal 1.0, Snellen 20/30 equals decimal 0.7, Snellen 20/40 equals decimal 0.5, and so forth. Other expressions of acuity are the M, or metric, and the logMAR notations. The latter expresses visual acuity as the logarithm of the minimum angle of resolution (logMAR). The minimum angle of resolution is the inverse of the Snellen fraction. Acuity of 20/20 has a logMAR value of 0 ($\log_{10} 1 = 0$), 20/50 a value of 0.4 ($\log_{10} 2.5 = 0.4$), and 20/200 a value of 1.0 ($\log_{10} 10 = 1.0$). The Jaeger (J) notation, which assigns arbitrary numbers to Snellen equivalent figures, is used by many practitioners to express near visual acuity. Methods of calculating these acuities and detailed comparisons with Snellen acuity can be found in textbooks that are more comprehensive.

Test Targets

Various test targets are used in visual acuity testing (Figure 4-1). Each individual letter, number, or picture on a testing chart is referred to as an optotype. Charts with such optotypes have achieved almost universal acceptance in the United States. Some optotypes are more difficult to recognize than others. For example, B (a relatively complex

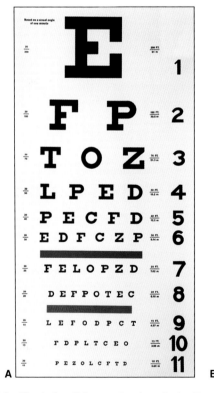
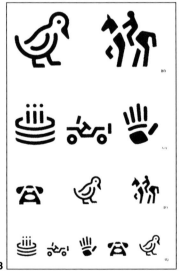

Figure 4-1 Charts for distance visual acuity testing. **A,** Snellen letter chart. **B,** Allen picture chart.

letterform) is the hardest for patients to recognize and can easily be interpreted as an E or the number 8. The letters C, D, and O are often confused because their shapes are similar. The easiest letter to recognize is L, which can be mistaken for few letters other than the letter I. This means that the examiner can consider a patient's misinterpreting a B during visual acuity testing to be less significant than missing an L.

Most letter and number charts require some degree of literacy and some verbalization skills. The tumbling E and Landolt C tests can be done by matching, but both involve some degree of laterality and therefore test psychophysical components other than vision. Picture charts are nonthreatening for young children but can result in overestimation of visual acuity because, as with certain letters, the optotypes are not equally recognizable. Children easily learn the limited number of optotypes used, which can result in inaccurate acuity measurements due to educated guessing. A test that involves a chart and matching cards that employ the 4 letters H, O, T, and V is particularly useful with young children. These letters were chosen because they are symmetric, can be used for matching, and are useful with nonverbal or illiterate patients.

A procedure for testing visual acuity that uses isolated HOTV optotypes surrounded by bars is the Amblyopia Treatment Study (ATS) visual acuity testing protocol, and it is gaining widespread acceptance for use with young children. Studies have demonstrated that this protocol has a high level of testability in 3- to 7-year-olds and excellent test-retest reliability.

Most charts have a notation either to the side or below each line of optotypes. This notation compares the size of the optotype with that of the standard 20/20 line. When the patient can read at least one-half of the letters correctly in any given line, the size of that optotype becomes the denominator of the Snellen acuity expression for that patient. The distance at which the patient is placed in reference to the chart is the numerator of the Snellen expression. For example, if a patient is 20 feet from the test chart and reads one-half of the optotypes on the 20/40 line correctly, the vision may be recorded as 20/40, but if the patient is only 15 feet from the chart and reads the same line, the vision should be recorded as 15/40. The examiner should also record whether the patient missed some letters on that line by adding the number of letters missed as a superscript notation to the acuity measurement. For example, if 2 letters are missed on the 20/40 line, the acuity may be expressed $20/40^{-2}$. If the patient misses 2 letters on that same line but was only 15 feet away from the chart, the expression is modified to $15/40^{-2}$. If the patient reads several letters on the next smaller line, the examiner may modify the superscript notation with a plus sign instead of a minus sign and denote the number of letters read correctly.

Standard Abbreviations

In addition to Snellen or other numeric notation, certain conventional abbreviations and notations are used in the patient record to indicate the type, circumstances, and results of visual acuity or visual function testing. The most common of these are shown in Table 4-1. The use of these abbreviations in recording the results of patient testing is described throughout this chapter where individual tests are detailed. Other abbreviations, such as C, S, M (central, steady, maintained fixation), and F & F (fixes and follows), are used for preverbal or nonverbal children.

Table 4-1   Visual Acuity Notations and Abbreviations

Abbreviation	Stands for	Abbreviation	Stands for
VA	Visual acuity	CF or FC	Count fingers or finger counting
$\overline{cc}$	With correction	HM	Hand motion
$\overline{sc}$	Without correction	LP $\overline{c}$ proj	Light perception with projection (specify quadrants)
N	Near	LP $\overline{s}$ proj	Light perception without projection
D	Distance	NLP	No light perception
PH	Pinhole	C	Central
OD or RE	Right eye	S	Steady
OS or LE	Left eye	M	Maintained
OU	Both eyes (together)	F/F	Fixes/follows
J	Jaeger notation	NPA	Near point of accommodation
HOTV	HOTV chart	$20/40^{-2}$	Missed 2 letters on the 20/40 line
E	Tumbling E chart or E game	$20/50^{+2}$	Read 2 letters on the line following the 20/50 line

Testing Procedures

The most basic types of vision testing are the distance and near visual acuity tests. Even though they test 2 different aspects of fine-detail central vision, these tests share some conventions, such as the use of corrective lenses and an established order for testing each eye. This section presents general background and specific steps for performing distance, pinhole, and near visual acuity testing and for measuring near points of accommodation and convergence.

Distance Acuity Test

On an initial visit, a patient should be tested both with and without corrective lenses. When recording visual acuity test results in the patient's record, the abbreviation *cc* indicates that corrective lenses were worn for the test.

When vision is measured without the use of corrective lenses, the abbreviation *sc* is used. On subsequent tests, a patient who habitually wears eyeglasses or contact lenses should wear them for the test, and this should be documented in the record. Distance correction should be used to test distance vision. To avoid confusion in the recording of information, a testing routine should be established. By convention, the right eye is tested first. Clinical Protocol 4-1 presents instructions for performing a distance visual acuity test.

A variety of occluders, held by either the patient or the examiner, can be used to cover the eye that is not being tested. These include a tissue, a paddle, or an eye patch. The palm of the patient's or the examiner's hand can also be used to occlude the eye not being tested. If a standard occluder is not used, it is important to ensure that the patient cannot see through or around the object that covers the eye. Any occluder that is used for more than 1 patient should be cleaned before reuse.

Before the test begins, determine if the patient is familiar with the optotypes being used. This is particularly important for children. If the patient is comfortable with letters, use that chart, if it is available. If the patient prefers numbers, use that chart. Because people tend to memorize the sequence of images that they have seen numerous times, present different charts or optotype sequences whenever possible. If only 1 type of chart is available, a patient can quickly memorize the order of the optotypes, whether intentionally or not. In this case, it is useful to ask the patient to read the letters in reverse order with the second eye. Newer computerized charts are particularly useful, as the letters can be changed as often as desired. The type of chart and the method of presentation used should be noted in the patient's record, for example, "isolated numbers," "linear letters," or "pictures."

Pinhole Acuity Test

Below-normal visual acuity can be the result of a refractive error. This possibility can be inferred by having the patient read the testing chart through a pinhole occluder. The pinhole admits only central rays of light, which do not require refraction by the cornea or the lens. If the pinhole improves the patient's acuity by 2 lines or more, it is likely that the patient has a refractive error. If poor uncorrected visual acuity is not improved with the pinhole, the patient's reduced visual acuity is likely due either to an extreme refractive error or to nonrefractive causes (eg, optic neuropathy). However, lack of improvement on pinhole testing does not rule out refractive error, as some patients simply do not perform the test well.

A pinhole no more than 2.4 mm in diameter should be used, and either a single or multiple pinhole design is acceptable. One commonly used multiple pinhole design has a central opening surrounded by 2 rings of small perforations.

Clinical Protocol 4-2 describes the pinhole acuity test. Patients should be positioned as for the distance acuity test, and they should wear their habitual optical correction. The test is done for each eye separately and is not repeated under binocular viewing conditions.

Near Acuity Test

Near acuity testing assesses the ability of a patient to see clearly at a normal reading distance. Keep in mind, however, that a patient's preferred reading distance can vary from the standard distance used for near testing and will be affected by the types of near activities in which the patient engages. The examiner should determine whether the patient uses near spectacles and, if so, the patient should use them during near vision testing. Occasionally, as with patients who are bedridden or who are examined in the emergency department, near-vision testing might be the only available method of measuring visual acuity.

The test is usually performed at 16 inches (40 cm) with a printed, handheld card (Figure 4-2). If the distance is not accurate, the near visual acuity measurements will not be equivalent to the distance acuity. Most test cards specify the distance at which they are to be held to correlate properly the measurements with those obtained for distance acuity. Some near reading cards come equipped with a chain that is 40 cm long to facilitate obtaining an accurate testing distance.

Figure 4-2 For near vision testing, the patient can hold the small near vision card at a normal reading distance (or the distance recommended on the near card). (Photo by Dan McGarrah.)

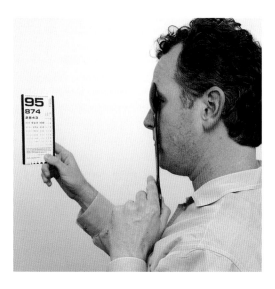

A Rosenbaum pocket vision screener, a Lebensohn chart, or the equivalent should be used to test near visual acuity. Clinical Protocol 4-3 presents instructions for testing near vision in adults. For children, near visual acuity can be tested with Allen reduced picture cards, the Lighthouse picture card, the HOTV equivalent cards, or the Lea figure set.

As with the Snellen chart, the near test card shows numeric notations alongside each line of optotypes. Most cards should have an equivalent Snellen acuity fraction next to each line. Other notations might also be present, the most common being the Jaeger notation, also referred to as *number acuity*.

Other Tests of Near Vision

Near vision depends not only on the eye's focusing ability, but on the near point of accommodation (NPA), a monocular attribute, and the near point of convergence (NPC), a binocular characteristic. The NPA is the nearest point at which the eye can focus so that a clear image is formed on the retina. As people age, their NPA recedes, a condition referred to as *presbyopia*. Clinical Protocol 4-4 describes the procedures for measuring NPA and NPC. The distance noted for measurement of the NPA, if expressed in meters, can be converted into diopters. A Prince or RAF (Royal Air Force) rule that has distance and diopters noted on the side is attached between the eyepieces of some phoropters and can be used for the conversion. This information is useful in determining the add power that will be needed for corrective lenses and for assessing residual accommodative capacity. The NPC is the nearest point to which both eyes can move nasally (converge) and still maintain a single image. The normal NPC is between 6 cm and 10 cm, irrespective of a person's age.

Acuity Tests for Patients with Special Needs

Patients with extremely low vision need special testing. Infants and toddlers as well as illiterate adults and nonverbal patients also need special testing methods and attention.

Low-Vision Testing

If a patient is unable to read the largest line of the visual acuity testing chart at the standard distance, repeat the acuity test at successively shorter distances. For example, repeatedly halve the distance between the patient and the chart. In this situation, note the distance at which the acuity measurement is successfully taken. This distance is used as the numerator of the Snellen fraction. For example, the notation 5/200 indicates that the patient read the 20/200 line successfully while standing 5 feet in front of the chart.

If the patient is unable to read the standard chart even at extremely close distances, the examiner can hold up fingers and ask the patient to count them. The patient with extremely low vision can also be asked to recognize the examiner's hand movements or identify the position of a penlight. Accepted abbreviations for recording low-vision test results are noted in Table 4-1. Clinical Protocol 4-5 describes the specific steps in a visual acuity examination for patients with low vision.

Testing Children and Special Adults

Many toddlers are uncomfortable with strangers, and most do not want to actively participate in an examination with someone they do not know. For these reasons, the examiner should allow these children to sit with a parent or other familiar caretaker and approach them thoughtfully. Ask the parents questions regarding their child's visual behavior, such as whether their child recognizes their faces from a distance, responds to their smiles, or uses visual or auditory clues to identify objects or people. Having pictures, toys, or items of interest around the room can allow observation of what a child attends to visually, which can provide clues to vision.

Newborns should show a consistent blink response to a bright light, even through closed eyelids while they are sleeping. With infants and preverbal children, an estimation of visual function can be made based on their ability to look directly at (fixate on) an object, follow the object, and maintain steady fixation. Infants with normal visual function are able to maintain steady fixation and follow an object by the age of 3 months. Clinical Protocol 4-6 describes standard procedures for testing an infant's vision.

In infants and preverbal children, vision should be assessed by testing each eye separately, with the other eye covered with a hand, occluder, or patch. If 1 eye fixes or follows better than the other eye, amblyopia or another cause of reduced vision should be suspected. If the infant or child objects when only 1 eye is covered, a difference in vision between both eyes should be strongly suspected. For example, if they consistently object to occlusion over the right eye only, suboptimal vision should be suspected in the left eye. Fixation preference testing, usually with the induced tropia test, is a useful adjunct for detection of amblyopia in preverbal children. Clinical Protocol 4-7 describes the induced tropia test.

Teller acuity cards, if available, can be used to estimate acuity (Figure 4-3). These cards are large photographic plates (approximately 3 feet×1 foot) with line gratings printed at 1 end. Cards with progressively smaller line gratings are presented to the infant. The examiner looks through a central pinhole to determine the baby's direction of gaze. The baby will look preferentially toward the side of the card that has a discernible image. Once the resolving ability of the eye has been surpassed, the baby's gaze will be random. These cards are reliable until a child is approximately 1 year. For reliable acuity measurements to be obtained, the examiner must be experienced, the lighting must be

Figure 4-3 Teller acuity cards.

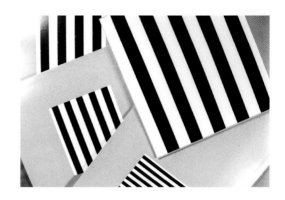

Figure 4-4 An OKN drum (*top*) and a homemade striped OKN target used to test nonverbal or preverbal patients.

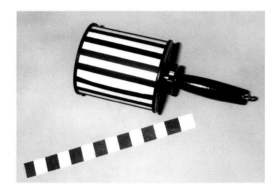

good, and the cards must be kept meticulously clean. Detailed testing and interpretation instructions are included with the test kits.

As an alternative testing method, optokinetic nystagmus (OKN) can be elicited with the use of any regularly striped object. This object can be as simple as a paper with lines drawn on it or a standard tape measure, or as formal as a commercially produced OKN drum (Figure 4-4). In all cases, the stripes are passed slowly and steadily in front of the baby while the examiner observes the movement of the baby's eyes. Fine oscillatory movements, with the slow phase going in the direction that the stripes rotate, indicate that the baby has a potential for discriminating detail of at least the width of the stripe. Neurologic implications in the interpretation of the OKN response are covered in greater detail in more advanced texts. Horizontal OKN should be present by 3 months of age, whereas vertical OKN might not be elicited until a child is approximately 6 months of age.

Toddlers and preliterate children as well as illiterate or nonverbal adult patients might be tested with a picture chart, Lea symbols, the Landolt C or tumbling E test, or the HOTV chart. Matching these letters or objects to a key held near the patient may improve willingness and accuracy of these tests. Crowding bars may also be used to induce the crowding phenomenon, which makes the test more sensitive for amblyopia.

Young children often become bored very quickly with vision testing. Some children do better with numbers; others prefer letters. If a child seems bored or hesitant with 1 kind of chart, try another. If you are using the tumbling E chart, position yourself on 1 side of the chart and the parent on the other and ask the child, "Which direction are the legs pointing—to the ceiling, to the floor, to me, or to Mommy/Daddy?" Alternatively, you can ask the child to point a hand or finger in the same direction that the legs of the letter point. When you use the Landolt ring chart, you can position yourself and the parent as with the tumbling E chart and ask the child to indicate, for example, which side of the "cookie" has a bite in it. Some very shy children will not talk but can be coaxed into whispering the answer to a parent. Positive reinforcement, such as cheering for correct answers, can encourage a child to complete the test.

Variables in Acuity Measurements

Falsely high or low acuity measurements can be obtained under a variety of circumstances. In general, the near and distance acuities should be comparable unless myopia is present. Possible causes of near acuity being poorer than distance acuity include the following:

- presbyopia/premature presbyopia
- undercorrected or high hyperopia
- overcorrected myopia
- small, centrally located cataracts
- accommodative insufficiency
- systemic or topical drugs with an anticholinergic effect
- convergence insufficiency (applies to binocular visual acuity)
- Adie pupil (see Chapter 7)
- functional visual loss

Other conditions can cause variability in acuity measurements for both near and distance. Examples of external variables include the following:

- Lighting conditions must remain equivalent for acuity tests to be comparable.
- Charts with higher contrast will be seen more easily than those with lower contrast.
- If a chart is not kept clean, smaller letters become more difficult to identify. When a projector chart is used, the cleanliness of the projector bulb and lens and the condition of the projecting screen will affect the contrast of the letters viewed by the patient.
- The distance between the projector and the chart will affect the size of the letters. The sharpness of the focus of a projected chart and the incidental glare on the screen can also influence the patient's ability to read the optotypes.
- Charts that have the letters crowded together might be more difficult to read.
- Patient fatigue or boredom are difficult variables to assess but will also affect acuity measurements and may be noted in the chart at the examiner's discretion.

Optical considerations also influence the ability of the patient to discern detail. They include the following:

- If a patient is wearing eyeglasses, the lenses need to be clean. Dirty lenses of any kind, whether trial lenses, phoropter lenses, eyeglass lenses, or contact lenses, will decrease acuity, and the measurements obtained will be falsely low.
- Effects of tear film abnormalities, such as dry eye syndromes, can be minimized by the generous use of artificial tear preparations.
- Corneal surface abnormalities can produce distortions.
- Corneal or lenticular astigmatism might necessitate the use of special spectacle or contact lenses. Discussions regarding the prescribing of these lenses can be found in specialized clinical texts.
- Other interferences from media opacities might have to be addressed either medically or surgically.
- Patients with neurologic impairments might have motility problems or central nervous system abnormalities that can influence the measurement of acuity, as described here.
- A visual or an expressive agnosia will usually be identified while the physician obtains the history by the way questions are, or are not, answered.
- Motility defects such as nystagmus (the presence of spontaneous oscillatory movements of the eyes) or any other movement disorder that interferes with the ability to align the fovea on the object of regard will lower the acuity measurement.
- Nystagmus might be difficult to determine when the amplitude of the nystagmus is small. In latent nystagmus, a condition that occurs only when 1 eye is occluded, the unoccluded eye develops nystagmus, and the measured visual acuity will be lower than expected and significantly lower than the binocular acuity.

Other neurologic considerations that can influence visual acuity testing include the following:

- visual field defects
- optic nerve lesions
- pupillary abnormalities
- impairment by drugs, legal or illicit

If latent nystagmus is suspected or diagnosed, the fellow eye may be blurred with use of a +10.00 to +20.00 diopter lens instead of a standard occluder. "Fogging" the fellow eye in this manner does not induce latent nystagmus because it allows light to enter both eyes; therefore, the best possible monocular visual acuity is obtained. As an alternative, vectographic projection slides of polarized images, with a different polarized image presented to each eye, can be used to conduct visual acuity examinations.

When nystagmus is present, the patient might have a null position. In this situation, the patient maintains a head position to decrease the amplitude of the nystagmus. Visual acuity will improve when the head is held in that position. If the patient assumes a head position when they look at objects, determine if this improves acuity by allowing them to maintain that head position while you measure binocular visual acuity for distance and near. The anomalous head position may also be allowed for monocular visual acuity testing, as long as it does not cause the patient to see around the occluder or fogging lens. Frequently patients with congenital nystagmus will have significantly better visual acuity for near than for distance. This occurs if the nystagmus dampens with convergence.

Psychological factors, whether conscious or unconscious, affect visual acuity measurement results. In an attempt to please the examiner or parent(s) or to "score" better on the test, children might try to peek around the occluder. Familiarity with the test can also lead to inadvertent memorization of the lines by the patient. External variables such as patient distraction, fatigue, and age should be considered when an unexplained poor acuity measurement is obtained.

Uncorrectable Visual Acuity

The Snellen standard of 20/20 is considered normal vision. Sometimes this acuity cannot be achieved with optical correction such as eyeglasses or contact lenses. The terms "visual impairment" and "visual acuity impairment" are used to describe this situation. Visual impairment is not the same as a visual disability, which implies a subjective judgment by the examiner. The World Health Organization divides low vision into 3 categories based on visual acuity (VA) and visual field. The criteria for the categories based on VA are as follows:

- moderate visual impairment: corrected distance VA (also called best-corrected VA) is less than 20/60 (including 20/70–20/160).
- severe visual impairment: corrected distance VA is less than 20/160 (including 20/200–20/400).
- profound visual impairment: corrected distance VA is less than 20/400 (including 20/500–20/1000).

Visual acuity is an important factor that the examiner may use to make estimates regarding a patient's potential disability. The acuity level is considered in determination of reading aids and reading distances. These factors are summarized in Table 4-2. Severe visual impairment in both eyes is required for inclusion in the category "legal blindness" and is the criterion usually used to determine eligibility for disability benefits.

The disabling effect, if any, of a visual impairment depends upon the individual and might or might not be perceived by the patient as a disability. Table 4-2 also summarizes levels of visual impairment and visual disability, which are important for evaluating legal or physical limitations for a patient. Definitions of legal blindness differ from state to state, especially regarding eligibility for a driver's license. In most states, the visual acuity must be correctable to 20/40 or better in at least one eye for an unrestricted license, which was the level of acuity proposed by the Low Vision Rehabilitation Committee of the American Academy of Ophthalmology in a policy statement regarding vision requirements for driving. The guidelines for issuing noncommercial driving licenses also include the recommendation that an uninterrupted visual field of 140° horizontal diameter be present for individuals with 20/40 or better visual acuity.

Table 4-2   Visual Impairment and Estimates of Visual Disability

Visual Impairment	Visual Disability	Comment	Reading Distance: Reading Aids
20/12 to 20/25	Normal vision at normal reading distance	Healthy young adults average better than 20/20.	*>33 cm:* Regular bifocals (up to 3 D)
20/80 to 20/160	Moderate low vision; (near) normal per-formance with magnifiers	Strong reading glasses or vision magnifiers usually provide adequate reading ability; this level is usually insufficient for a driving license.	*16–10 cm:* Half-eye glasses (6–10 D), with prisms for binocularity Stronger magnifiers (>8 D)
20/200 to 20/400	Severe low vision: legal blindness by US definition	Gross orientation and mobility generally adequate, but difficulty with traffic signs, bus numbers, etc. Reading requires high-power magnifiers; reading speed is reduced, even with reading aids.	*8–5 cm (cannot be binocular):* High-power reading lenses (12–20 D) High-power magnifiers (>16 D)
20/500 to 20/1000	Profound visual impairment	Limited spot reading with visual aids.	*4–2 cm (cannot be binocular):* High-power reading lenses (24–28 D) High-power magnifiers (>28 D) Video magnifier Talking devices and vision substitutes
CF 8 ft to 4 ft	Unreliable vision	Increasing problems with visual orientation and mobility. Long cane is useful to explore environment. Talking devices and vision substitutes are useful.	
Less than CF 4 ft	Nearly total blindness	Vision unreliable, except under ideal circumstances; must rely on nonvisual devices.	
NLP	Total blindness	No light perception; must rely on talking devices and vision substitutes.	

Amblyopia

Amblyopia, when unilateral, is a visual disorder defined as a difference in optically cor-rectable acuity of more than 2 lines between both eyes that results from abnormal visual input in early childhood. The lay term for amblyopia is "lazy eye." Normal development of vision occurs early in life through ongoing stimulation of vision-receptive cells in the brain. Amblyopia results when there is an interruption of this process. A patient with amblyopia demonstrates impaired vision due to structural and functional damage in the lateral geniculate nucleus and visual cortex, which do not receive proper visual input from the affected eye.

Causes of unilateral amblyopia include anisometropia, strabismus, and unilateral media opacities such as monocular congenital cataracts. Amblyopia can also be bilateral and can be associated with a variety of other conditions, including long-standing uncorrected refractive errors and nystagmus. (Causes of amblyopia are dealt with in greater detail in other clinical ophthalmology textbooks.) In general, the younger the patient, the more successful the amblyopia treatment is. Many patients with amblyopia exhibit the "crowding phenomenon," in which smaller optotypes can be correctly identified when they are viewed singly rather than in a line with figures on both sides. As a result, many amblyopic patients correctly identify the first and last letters of a line more easily than those in the middle. If visual acuity is checked with use of isolated figures, this should be recorded in the medical record. The crowding phenomenon is not specific to amblyopia.

Although many practitioners end treatment when a patient is between ages 8 and 10, evidence indicates that some improvement in vision can be achieved in older children and teenagers. Therefore, a trial of amblyopia therapy may be attempted in an older child after a thorough discussion with the parents and the child of the benefits and drawbacks of such treatment.

Other Tests of Sensory Visual Function

Contrast sensitivity refers to the ability to discern relative darkness and brightness and the ability to see details, edges, and borders of images. Contrast sensitivity can be impaired even in the presence of excellent Snellen acuity. Alterations in contrast sensitivity imply abnormalities in the anterior visual receptive systems, from the tear film to the optic nerve. (Specific patterns of alteration of contrast sensitivity function are discussed in more advanced textbooks.)

In the simplest contrast sensitivity tests, patients are shown printed charts with contrasting lines, referred to as *gratings,* which are presented in varying orientations. The difference in the intensity between the background of the chart and the printed lines is gradually decreased, and the patient is asked to identify the direction of the lines. The end point is reached when the patient can no longer correctly identify either the presence of any lines or the direction of their orientation. Testing methods that are more technical involve presentation of grating patterns or letters on an oscilloscope screen. The end points and reporting methods are similar in both techniques.

Glare occurs when light from a single bright source scatters across the visual field, and so reduces the quality of the visual image. The perception of troublesome glare, which causes distorted vision and, in some cases, mild pain, can be a symptom of cataract. As with contrast sensitivity testing, glare testing (by exposing the patient to bright light under controlled circumstances) can suggest the presence of cataract or other opacity.

Color vision differences between two eyes may indicate optic nerve or retinal disease. The most commonly recognized color vision abnormalities are the X-linked congenital red-green deficiencies, but many other color vision anomalies exist. Color vision defects can be acquired or asymmetric. Most patients with inherited color vision defects see red as less bright than individuals with normal vision see it and, according to a standard established by testing individuals with normal vision, fail to identify color mixtures that include red. Although not disabling, color vision anomalies can impair performance in some careers or activities. However, colors can often be altered to accommodate those who have difficulty discriminating certain shades, for instance, in some computer graphics applications.

Evaluation of color vision is often performed with a book that displays multicolored dot patterns, called *pseudoisochromatic color plates*. Patients with normal color vision easily detect specific numbers and figures composed of and embedded in the dot pattern, but patients with impaired color vision do not detect the same numbers or may not detect any numbers. Various combinations of colors are used to identify the nature of the color vision deficit.

Another test of color vision, the 15-hue test (Farnsworth-Munsell D-15 test), consists of 15 pastel-colored chips, which the patient must arrange in a related color sequence. The sequence is obvious to patients with normal color vision, but patients with color deficits arrange the chips differently.

Principles and performance of contrast sensitivity, glare, and color vision testing are covered more thoroughly in other, more detailed textbooks and in manufacturers' instructions that accompany testing materials.

Pitfalls and Pointers

- Be aware of the variables possible in visual acuity measurement. Ensure that all lenses, projectors, and charts are clean.
- Pay special attention to distances and calibrations that are associated with each type of near and distance acuity screen. Ensure that the patient is properly positioned for each screen.
- Avoid glare on the viewing chart or screen.
- Avoid glare in patients' eyes from overhead lights or outside windows.
- Learn appropriate ways of interacting with patients who have low vision or are blind. Alert the patient to your movements beforehand, particularly if there is severe visual impairment. Offer an arm to patients, but do not attempt to grab their hands or arms.
- Ensure that you are using the appropriate tests for the patient's abilities.
- Refrain from using the term "blindness" when you counsel patients or parents of children with severe visual impairment. Most of these patients have some useful vision, and many of them will amaze you with their resourcefulness.
- Use a demeanor and a test of visual function that is appropriate for the patient's age. Infants and young toddlers will respond best to a gentle, gradual approach and to the use of interesting toys to assess their fixing and following behaviors.

Suggested Resources

Amblyopia [Preferred Practice Pattern]. American Academy of Ophthalmology; 2017. Accessed September 15, 2020. https://www.aao.org/preferred-practice-pattern/amblyopia-ppp-2017

Clinical Optics. Basic and Clinical Science Course, Section 3. American Academy of Ophthalmology; published annually.

Pediatric Ophthalmology and Strabismus. Basic and Clinical Science Course, Section 6. American Academy of Ophthalmology; published annually.

Vision Rehabilitation [Preferred Practice Pattern]. American Academy of Ophthalmology; 2017. Accessed September 15, 2020. https://www.aao.org /preferred-practice-pattern/vision-rehabilitation-ppp-2017

CLINICAL PROTOCOL 4-1

Testing Distance Visual Acuity

1. Ask the patient to stand or sit at a designated testing distance (20 feet from a well-illuminated wall chart is ideal). If a projected chart is used, distance may vary; the projected optotype size must be focused and adjusted to be equivalent to the corresponding Snellen acuity for the distance used.

2. Occlude the left eye. Be sure that the occluder does not touch or press against the eye. Observe the patient during the test to make sure there is no conscious or inadvertent peeking with the eye not being tested.

3. Ask the patient to say aloud each letter or number, or name the picture object, on the lines of successively smaller optotypes, from left to right or, alternatively, as you point to each character in any order, until the patient correctly identifies at least one-half of the optotypes on a line. If a patient is hesitant (at times for fear of being wrong), tell them that it is all right to guess.

4. Note the corresponding acuity measurement shown at that line of the chart. Record the acuity value for each eye separately, with correction and without correction, as illustrated below. If the patient misses half or fewer than half the letters on the smallest readable line, record how many letters were missed; for example, $20/40^{-2}$.

5. Repeat steps 1–4 for the left eye, with the right eye covered.

6. If desired, retest acuity with the patient using both eyes simultaneously, and record acuity OU (see the following example).

$$D \bigvee \overline{sc} \quad \begin{array}{l} \text{OD 20/200} \\ \text{OS 20/100} \end{array} \quad \text{OU 20/80}$$

$$D \bigvee \overline{cc} \quad \begin{array}{l} \text{OD 20/20} \\ \text{OS 20/25} \end{array} \quad \text{OU 20/20}$$

7. Record the power of the corrective lenses worn for the distance acuity determination (see Clinical Protocol 5-1).

8. If visual acuity is worse than 20/20, recheck with a pinhole (see Clinical Protocol 4-2).

Video 1 demonstrates visual acuity testing.

VIDEO 1　Visual Acuity
Courtesy of Lindreth G. DuBois, MEd, MMSc, CO, COMT.
Access all *Practical Ophthalmology* videos at www.aao.org /PracticalOphthalmologyvideo.

CLINICAL PROTOCOL 4-2

Testing Pinhole Visual Acuity

1. Position the patient and occlude the eye not being tested, as was done for the distance acuity test.
2. Ask the patient to hold the pinhole occluder in front of the eye that is to be tested. The patient's habitual correction may be worn for the test.
3. Instruct the patient to look at the distance chart through the single pinhole or through any one of the multiple pinholes.
4. Instruct the patient to use small hand or eye movements to align the pinhole to resolve the sharpest image on the chart.
5. Ask the patient to begin to read the line with the smallest letters that are legible as determined on the previous vision test without the use of the pinhole.
6. Record the Snellen acuity obtained and precede or follow it with the abbreviation *PH*.

CLINICAL PROTOCOL 4-3

Testing Near Visual Acuity

1. With the patient wearing the habitual corrective lens for near and the near card evenly illuminated, instruct the patient to hold the test card at the distance specified on the card.
2. Ask the patient to occlude the left eye.
3. Ask the patient to say each letter or read each word on the line with the smallest characters that are legible.
4. Record the acuity value for each eye separately in the patient's chart according to the accepted notation method (see the example below).
5. Repeat the procedure with the right eye occluded and the left eye viewing the test chart.
6. Repeat the procedure with both eyes viewing the test card.
7. Record the binocular acuity achieved (see the following example).

$$N \bigvee \overline{sc} \quad \begin{matrix} \text{OD } 20/200 \\ \text{OS } 20/100 \end{matrix} \quad \text{OU } 20/80$$

$$N \bigvee \overline{cc} \quad \begin{matrix} \text{OD } 20/20 \\ \text{OS } 20/25 \end{matrix} \quad \text{OU } 20/20$$

CLINICAL PROTOCOL 4-4

Testing for NPA and NPC

Testing for Near Point of Accommodation (NPA)

1. With the patient wearing full distance correction and with the left eye occluded, place the near testing card at a distance of 16 inches (40 cm) from the patient and ask the patient to read the 20/40 line with the unoccluded eye.
2. Move the test card slowly toward the patient as you ask the patient to state when the letters have become blurred.
3. Record this distance in centimeters or inches (whichever you are using).
4. Repeat steps 1–3 for the other eye and record the results as described above.
5. The NPA is that point (in centimeters or inches) where the patient can no longer bring the image into clear focus.

Testing for Near Point of Convergence (NPC)

1. With the patient wearing appropriate correction and with neither eye occluded, hold a target, such as a pencil tip, at a distance of approximately 16 inches (40 cm) from the patient and ask the patient to fixate on it.
2. Slowly move the object closer to the patient and ask the patient to tell you when the image doubles.
3. Observe whether both eyes are converging.
4. Note the position at which the image doubles or 1 eye deviates away from the fixation target. The NPC is that point where a single image can no longer be maintained. Record the distance (in centimeters or inches) between that point and the upper bridge of the nose at the midpoint between the eyes.

CLINICAL PROTOCOL 4-5

Testing Acuity for Patients with Low Vision

1. If the patient is unable to resolve the largest optotype on the distance acuity chart from the standard testing distance, ask the patient to stand or sit 10 feet from the well-illuminated test chart. A projected chart is less desirable to use in this situation than a printed wall chart. A low-vision test chart, if available, is preferable for these patients.
2. Occlude the eye not being tested.
3. Repeatedly halve the testing distance (up to 2.5 feet) and retest the distance visual acuity at each stage until the patient successfully identifies half the optotypes on a line.

4. Note the corresponding acuity measurement shown at that line of the chart. Record the acuity value for each eye separately, with correction and without correction, as would be done for standard distance acuity testing, recording the distance at which the patient successfully reads the chart as the numerator of the Snellen acuity designation; for example, *5/80*.

5. If the patient is unable to resolve the largest optotypes on the chart from a distance of 2.5 feet, display 2 or more fingers of 1 hand and ask the patient to count the number of fingers displayed. Record the longest distance at which counting is done accurately; for example, *CF at 2 ft*.

6. If the patient cannot count fingers, move your hand horizontally or vertically before the patient at a distance of approximately 2 feet. Record the distance at which the patient reports seeing your hand move; for example, *HM at 2 ft*.

7. If the patient cannot detect your hand motion, shine a penlight toward the patient's face from approximately 1 foot and turn it on and off to determine if light perception is present. If the patient cannot see the light, dim the room lights and shine the brightest light available (usually the indirect ophthalmoscope) toward the patient's eye again. If the patient cannot see even the brightest light, record the response as *NLP* (no light perception). If the patient can see the light, record the response as *LP* (light perception). No record of distance is required.

8. If light is perceived from straight ahead, move the light sequentially into each of the 4 quadrants of the visual field. Turn the penlight on and off in each field, and ask the patient to identify when the light comes on.

9. If the patient correctly identifies the direction from which the light is coming, record the response as *LP with projection*. Specify the quadrant(s) in which light projection is present. If the patient is unable to identify any direction but is able to discern light in the straight-ahead position, record the response as *LP without projection*.

10. If the light can be seen from straight ahead, colored filters can be placed in front of the light and the patient asked to identify the color of the light. Record whether color perception is present.

11. Repeat steps 1–10 for the fellow eye, as appropriate.

CLINICAL PROTOCOL 4-6

Testing an Infant's Fixing and Following Behavior

1. Seat the infant on a familiar adult's lap, so that the infant is comfortable.

2. Select a small toy or other attention-attracting object that stimulates sight only; do not use a sound-producing object. Hold the object about 1–2 feet from the infant's face and move it horizontally to either side.

3. Watch the infant's eyes for fixation and following movements.

4. Cover 1 eye and repeat the test. Cover the other eye and repeat again. Observe for any difference between the eyes in the quality of fixation and smooth pursuit or in the amount of objection to occlusion. If you suspect

a difference but are unsure, repeat these tests, using a different toy, if available, to maintain the infant's interest.

5. When tested monocularly, very young infants will respond with better following movements for objects moved from the temporal to the nasal field; this preference decreases after an infant is approximately 6 months old.

CLINICAL PROTOCOL 4-7

Performing the Induced Tropia Test in Nonstrabismic Infants

1. This test is used to detect a fixation preference (and amblyopia) in an infant without strabismus or with a very small strabismic angle. Position the infant and select a toy as you would to elicit fixing and following, and present an interesting target at near fixation.

2. Place a 15 or 20 prism diopter (PD) base-down prism in front of the right eye. Determine if the infant looks upward through the prism to view the target (maintains right eye fixation), views the target without an upward shift of fixation (maintains left eye fixation), or shifts fixation upward and downward spontaneously (alternates fixation).

3. Repeat the test with the prism placed before the left eye.

4. Combine the results from both eyes, and record as:

   a. alternates fixation (amblyopia unlikely)

   b. alternates, but prefers fixation with OD/OS (amblyopia suspected)

   c. fixes only with OD/OS (amblyopia likely)

5 Refraction

▶ *This chapter includes related videos, which can be accessed by scanning the QR codes provided in the text or going to aao.org/PracticalOphthalmologyvideo.*

👆 *This chapter includes a related activity, which can be accessed by scanning the QR code provided in the text or going to aao.org/PracticalOphthalmologyactivity.*

Refraction is the process by which the patient is guided through the use of a variety of lenses so as to achieve the best possible acuity on distance and near vision tests. Refraction can be performed with both objective and subjective measurements. This chapter offers instruction in these basic techniques of refraction, including guidelines for spectacle lens prescription. Because refraction requires an understanding of basic refractive states of the eye and the basic characteristics of lenses used for optical correction, this chapter briefly reviews those topics and provides instruction for determining the prescription of existing corrective lenses.

Overview of Refraction

In physics, the term "refraction" is defined as the bending of light rays as they encounter interfaces between materials with differing refractive indices. In clinical ophthalmology, the term "refraction" is employed to describe the process to measure a patient's refractive error, determine the optical correction needed to focus light rays from distant and near objects onto the retina, and provide the patient with clear and comfortable vision. The clinical process of refraction comprises several activities, which are discussed in greater detail later in this chapter.

1. *Retinoscopy* (or *objective refraction*) is a clinical test used to determine the nature and extent of a patient's refractive error (ie, nearsightedness, farsightedness, or astigmatism). It is sometimes called *objective refraction* because it does not require subjective responses from the patient. Retinoscopy is performed primarily with a retinoscope, which is a handheld instrument that consists of a light source and a viewing component, and correcting lenses (either loose lenses or a phoropter). Another method to obtain an objective refraction is with the use of an automatic refractor. This rapid method uses infrared light and provides a good estimate of the refractive error and correction for it prior to refinement of the final prescription.

2. *Refinement* (or *subjective refraction*) utilizes patient participation and reaction ("I can see better with this lens than with that one") to obtain the refractive

correction that gives the best visual acuity. Tools used in refinement include the phoropter (also called a *refractor*), or trial lenses and a trial frame, and a visual acuity chart. Because refinement requires subjective participation from the patient, it is not possible to perform this part of refraction with infants, most toddlers, and other patients who are unable to adequately communicate or comprehend the test.

Both retinoscopy and refinement can be done in the presence or absence of *cycloplegia*. Cycloplegic refraction uses eyedrops to paralyze accommodation temporarily in order to allow the refractionist to determine the patient's baseline nonaccommodative refractive error. If cycloplegic eyedrops are not used, then the refraction is called "manifest" (or "dry").

3. *Binocular balancing* is the final step in subjective refraction; it determines whether accommodation has been equally relaxed in both eyes.

4. *Prescription of spectacle lenses* is the outcome of the clinical process of refraction. The patient is given an optical prescription based on the results of steps 1–3.

Overview of Ophthalmic Optics

Performing accurate retinoscopy and refinement, and prescribing appropriate optical correction, requires a fundamental understanding of the properties of light rays, the types and properties of optical lenses, and the interaction between them. This chapter touches on the principles of ophthalmic optics only briefly; more detailed information is available in Section 3, *Clinical Optics,* of the Basic and Clinical Science Course, published by the American Academy of Ophthalmology.

Principles of Vergence

Vergence is a measure of the spreading (or coming together) of a bundle of light rays that come from (or head toward) a single point. Vergence is the reciprocal of the distance from a lens to the point of convergence of the light. Light rays that are moving away from each other are termed *divergent*. Light rays that are moving toward each other are termed *convergent*. Parallel light rays have zero vergence (ie, they do not move toward or away from each other). Figure 5-1 illustrates these 3 types of rays.

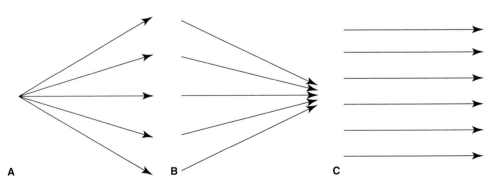

A   B   C

Figure 5-1 Light rays can be divergent **(A)**, convergent **(B)**, or parallel (0 vergence) **(C)**.

Light rays that emanate from a point source of light are divergent. Convergent light rays do not usually occur in nature but are the result of the action of an optical system (eg, a convex lens). Light rays that emanate from the sun are essentially parallel and have zero vergence.

Power (or *vergence power*) describes the ability of a curved lens to converge or diverge light rays. By convention, divergence is expressed in minus power; convergence is expressed in plus power. A *diopter* (abbreviated "D") is the unit of measurement of the refractive power of a lens. The *focal length* of a lens is the distance between the lens and the image formed by an object at infinity:

$$f = 1/D$$

where f = focal length (in meters) and D = lens power (in diopters).

Types of Lenses

Lenses may be spheres, cylinders, or spherocylinders. A *spherical lens* has the same curvature over its entire surface, and thus the same refractive power in all meridians. Convex spherical lenses converge light rays and are called *plus lenses;* concave spherical lenses diverge light rays and are called *minus lenses* (Figure 5-2). Examples of plus and minus lenses that illustrate the relationship of lens power to focal length are shown in Figure 5-3. In the case of convex, or plus, lenses, and using the mathematical formula $D = 1/f$, 1 diopter of plus power converges parallel rays of light to focus at 1 m from the lens. A +0.25 D lens focuses parallel light rays 1/0.25 m, or 4 m, from the lens. A +4.00 D lens converges parallel light rays to a focus at 1/4.00 m, or 0.25 m from the lens. In the case of concave, or minus, lenses, parallel light rays that enter the lens diverge; a virtual image is considered to appear at a focal point in front of the lens. A minus lens with a focal length of 1 m has a power of −1.00 D; a minus lens with a focal length of −0.25 m has a power of 1/(−0.25) D or −4.00 D.

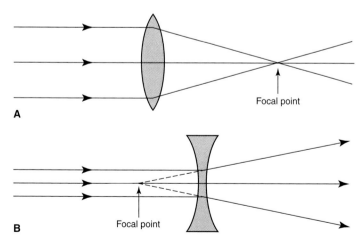

Figure 5-2   Types of lenses include **(A)** converging (convex or plus) lenses, and **(B)** diverging (concave or minus) lenses. The focal point of a plus lens occurs where parallel light rays that have passed through the lens converge to form an image. The focal point of a minus lens occurs where parallel light rays entering the lens appear to diverge.

Figure 5-3 Relationship of lens power to focal length for plus lenses **(A, B, C)** and minus lenses **(D, E, F)**. *F* = focal point.

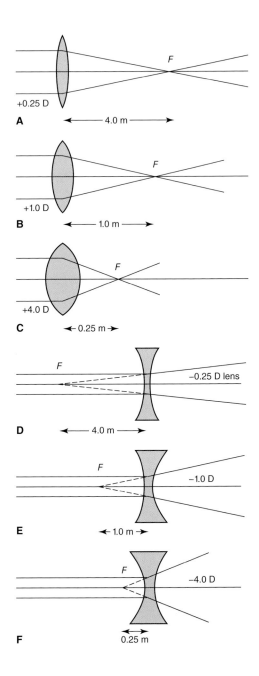

Cylindrical lenses have vergence power in only 1 meridian, which is perpendicular to the axis of the cylinder. They have no power in the meridian parallel to the axis (Figure 5-4). Cylindrical lenses focus light rays to a line (Figure 5-5). From the perspective of the physician, who is facing the patient, the orientation of the axis of cylindrical lenses is assigned by convention, as noted in Figure 5-6. The orientation of corrective cylindrical lenses is the same for the right and left eyes; ie, 0°–90° is to the patient's left, whereas 90°–180° is to the patient's right.

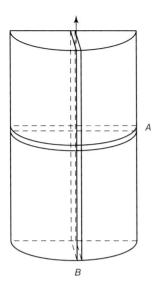

Figure 5-4 Refracting (vergence) power of a cylindrical lens. Maximum refractive power occurs in the meridian perpendicular to the axis of the cylinder (curved undotted line *A*). The cylinder has no refractive power in the meridian that corresponds to the axis of the cylinder (vertical undotted lines *B*).

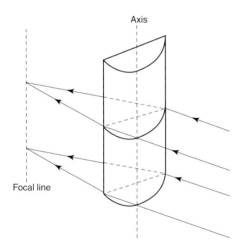

Figure 5-5 Because a cylindrical lens has refracting power in only 1 meridian (which is perpendicular to its axis), it focuses light rays to a focal line.

Spherical and cylindrical lenses can be combined in 1 lens to form a *spherocylindrical lens,* also known as a *compound lens* or *toric lens.* Unlike a spherical lens, which has the same curvature (and thus refracting power) in all meridians, the curvature of a spherocylindrical lens varies from a minimum value to a maximum value, with the extreme values located in meridians 90° apart. Because the refracting power varies from 1 meridian to the next, a spherocylindrical lens cannot bring a beam of light rays to a point focus. Instead, the light rays are focused over a range bounded by 2 focal lines, each parallel to 1 of the principal meridians of the spherocylindrical lens. The shape of the light rays as focused by the spherocylindrical lens is called the *conoid of Sturm* (Figure 5-7). Between the 2-line foci produced by the conoid of Sturm is a point called the *circle of least confusion,* which represents the point of best overall focus for a spherocylindrical lens.

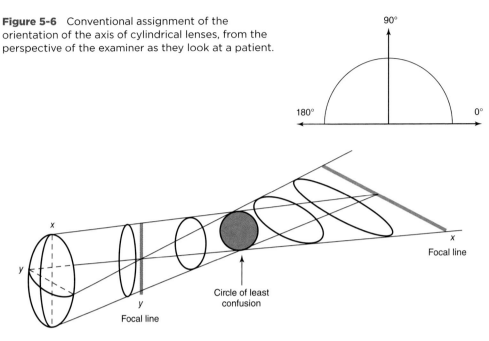

Figure 5-6 Conventional assignment of the orientation of the axis of cylindrical lenses, from the perspective of the examiner as they look at a patient.

Figure 5-7 Because its 2 radii of curvature (*x, y*) are not equal, a spherocylinder lens does not focus light to a point, but to 2 lines (*y* focal line, *x* focal line) in different places. The clearest image is formed between the 2 lines, at the circle of least confusion. The conoid of Sturm is the name given to the shape the light rays take as they are focused by a spherocylindrical lens.

Prisms are technically not lenses, but prismatic effects are inherent characteristics of lenses. A *prism* is a wedge of refracting material with a triangular cross section that deviates light toward its base. Objects viewed through a prism appear to be displaced toward the apex of the prism (Figure 5-8). Spherical lenses can be thought of as paired prisms, with convergent (plus) lenses made of prisms that are base to base, and divergent (minus) lenses made of prisms that are apex to apex. Thus, a spherical lens has prismatic power at every point on its surface except at the optical center of the lens.

The power of a prism to deviate light rays is expressed in *prism diopters* (abbreviated PD or with a superscript delta: ᐃ). A prism diopter is the deviation, in centimeters, from the optical axis when measured at a distance of 100 cm (1 m) from the prism (Figure 5-9).

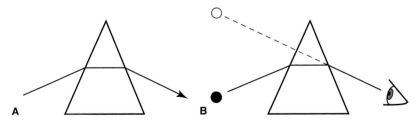

Figure 5-8 Prism. **A,** Because of its shape, a prism refracts light rays toward its base. **B,** If an object is viewed through a prism, the object appears in space as if it were displaced toward the prism apex.

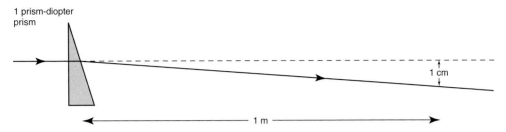

Figure 5-9 Measurement of prism power. A prism that measures 1 PD (1 △) deflects a light ray 1 cm at a distance of 1 m.

Refractive States of the Eye

In the normal eye, parallel light rays are focused sharply on the retina, a condition known as *emmetropia*. When the relaxed, or *nonaccommodating,* eye is unable to bring parallel light rays from a distant object into focus, the condition is referred to as *ametropia*. The 3 basic conditions that may produce ametropia are:

- myopia (nearsightedness)
- hyperopia (farsightedness, also called *hypermetropia*)
- astigmatism

A *myopic* (nearsighted) eye has excessive convergent power; the light rays focus anterior to the retina. A minus (divergent) lens is used to correct myopia (Figure 5-10 A, B). A *hyperopic* (farsighted) eye has insufficient convergence power to focus light rays on the retina; the rays focus posterior to the retina. A plus (convergent) lens is used to correct hyperopia (Figure 5-10 C, D).

The cornea (and sometimes the eye's crystalline lens) might not have the same radius of curvature in all meridians. Aberration of the corneal or lenticular surfaces that produce differing radii of curvature is called *astigmatism*. A cylindrical lens is used to neutralize astigmatism (Figure 5-10 E, F). In most patients, the axis of plus cylinder needed to correct the astigmatism is either close to 90° (with-the-rule astigmatism) or close to 180° (against-the-rule astigmatism). In clinical practice, many myopic patients and hyperopic patients also have astigmatism. A spherocylindrical lens is used to correct myopic and hyperopic astigmatism.

Accommodation is the mechanism by which the eye changes refractive power by altering the shape of its crystalline lens. The point of focus moves forward in the eye during accommodation and allows one to focus on objects at near. *Presbyopia* is a progressive loss of accommodative ability of the crystalline lens caused by the natural process of aging. It generally manifests itself after the age of 40 years as difficulty with near visual work, such as reading. Presbyopia occurs in the presence of myopia, hyperopia, and astigmatism. It can be remedied optically with use of plus lenses for near work.

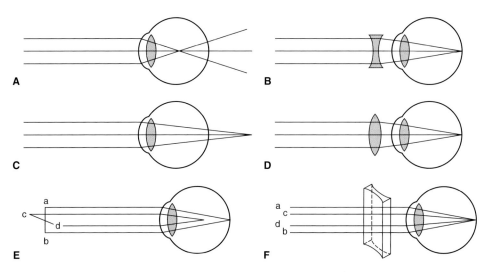

Figure 5-10   Concave, convex, and cylindrical lenses. **A, B,** A concave (minus) lens is used to correct myopia, in which parallel rays are focused anterior to the macula. **C, D,** A convex (plus) lens is used to correct hyperopia, in which parallel rays are focused posterior to the macula. **E, F,** A cylindrical (or spherocylindrical) lens is used to correct astigmatism, in which parallel rays are not focused uniformly in all meridians.

Lens Notation

A written spectacle lens prescription follows a standard format. The power of the sphere (abbreviated *sph*) is recorded first, along with its sign (+ or −). This is followed by the power of the cylinder, if a cylinder is required, with its sign and axis. The axis of the cylinder is designated by ×, followed by the degree of the orientation of the cylinder axis. The degree symbol is commonly omitted and only the numbers written. A prescription is recorded for each eye, with the abbreviation OD (*oculus dexter*) used for the right eye and OS (*oculus sinister*) for the left eye. Table 5-1 displays examples of typical spectacle prescriptions.

Lens Transposition

In a written spectacle lens prescription, cylinder power can be recorded in either plus form or minus form. Many ophthalmologists customarily record cylinder with plus notation,

Table 5-1   Typical Spectacle Prescription Notations

Hyperopia	OD	+2.00 sph
	OS	+2.25 sph
Myopia	OD	−2.50 sph
	OS	−3.00 sph
Hyperopic astigmatism	OD + 1.00. +1.00 × 90 *or* +2.00 − 1.00 × 180	
	OS plano +1.50 × 180 *or* +1.50 − 1.50 × 90	
Myopic astigmatism	OD − 0.75 + 0.50 × 150 *or* −0.25 − 0.50 × 60	
	OS − 1.00 + 0.50 × 120 *or* −0.50 − 0.50 × 30	

except for contact lenses, whereas opticians and optometrists generally use minus notation. A plus cylinder is ground onto the anterior surface of a lens, and the minus cylinder is ground onto the posterior surface of the lens. Unless specifically stated by the practitioner, the lenses will be filled as minus cylinders, even if the prescription was written in plus-cylinder form. This generally allows for a more cosmetically acceptable lens, because plus cylinders produce more magnification than the equivalent minus-cylinder form. A conversion of a prescription from one form to the other is called *lens transposition* and is achieved in 3 steps:

1. Add, algebraically, the cylinder power to the sphere power.
2. Reverse the sign of the cylinder.
3. Add 90° to the cylinder axis. If the resulting number exceeds 180°, then subtract 180.

Examples of lens transposition:

$-1.00 + 1.50 \times 95$ is equivalent to $+0.50 - 1.50 \times 05$

$+3.00 + 2.00 \times 20$ is equivalent to $+5.00 - 2.00 \times 110$

$-2.00 + 1.00 \times 160$ is equivalent to $-1.00 - 1.00 \times 70$

Spherical Equivalent

The average power of a spherocylindrical lens is called the *spherical equivalent*. It represents the dioptric position of the circle of least confusion of the conoid of Sturm. Spherical equivalent is useful when one compares or tries to balance both eyes, and when one tries to reduce an excessive cylindrical correction. The spherical equivalent is frequently used in the prescription of contact lenses. It is calculated as follows:

Spherical equivalent = power of the sphere + (cylinder power/2)

Lensmeter

The *lensmeter* is an instrument used to measure the power of a patient's present spectacle lenses. Both manual and automated lensmeters are available. Figure 5-11 shows a commonly used manual lensmeter. The lensmeter measures 4 principal properties of spectacle lenses:

- spherical and cylindrical *power*
- cylindrical *axis* if cylinder is present
- presence and orientation of *prism*
- optical *centration*

Clinical Protocol 5-1 describes the steps for using a standard manual lensmeter for single-vision spectacles. Clinical Protocol 5-2 describes measurement of bifocal spectacles. Clinical Protocol 5-3 lists steps for measuring prism power and orientation, and Clinical Protocol 5-4 describes measurement of optical centration of lenses.

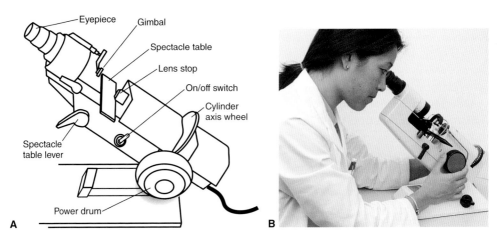

Figure 5-11   Lensmeter. **A,** Parts of the manual lensmeter. **B,** Lensmeter in use. (Photo by Dan McGarrah.)

Retinoscopy and Refinement

The goal of retinoscopy (objective refraction) is to determine the nature of the patient's refractive error (if any) and the approximate lens power that will diminish (neutralize) that error and achieve clear vision. In the process of refinement (subjective refraction), the examiner determines the patient's final refractive correction by presenting various lenses to the patient until the patient responds that a best-corrected, and balanced (if the patient has binocular vision), visual acuity has been reached.

Retinoscopy and refinement, perhaps more than most other ophthalmologic examination techniques, require artistry and experience to perform successfully. They demand fine motor skills, ambidextrousness, clinical observation skills, knowledge of optical principles, and subjective judgment. Retinoscopy and refinement are best learned through hands-on, guided training with an experienced practitioner. This text can only present an overview of the instrumentation and steps in these processes. A list of recommended books and resources that treat these topics in greater detail appears at the end of this chapter.

Instrumentation

The examiner must become familiar with and skilled in the use of the variety of specialized instruments that are used in retinoscopy and refinement, namely, the retinoscope, trial lenses and frames, phoropter (or refractor), Jackson cross cylinder, and distometer. Automated refractors combine many of the individual refraction instruments or duplicate their functions automatically.

Retinoscope

The handheld *streak retinoscope* comprises a viewer (peephole), a mirror assembly, and a light bulb with a delicate filament that can be rotated and focused by manipulating a sleeve on the instrument's handle (Figure 5-12). It produces a streak of light, as differentiated from the round dot of light produced by a *spot retinoscope*, which is used less frequently. The vergence of the slit (ie, the focus of the beam) on the streak retinoscope is adjusted by moving the sleeve up or down on the instrument's handle. To perform

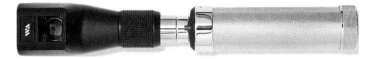

Figure 5-12 A standard streak retinoscope. (Photo by Dan McGarrah.)

retinoscopy, the examiner looks through the retinoscope peephole viewer and aligns the retinoscope streak with the patient's visual axis. By shifting the position of the instrument, manipulating its light characteristics in specific ways, and observing the movement of the light reflex from the patient's eye, the examiner can determine the patient's refractive state and accurately estimate their corrective needs.

Trial lenses and frames

During retinoscopy (and subsequent refinement), the examiner has the patient look through a variety of lenses until an appropriate optical correction is determined. One way to do this is with the use of trial frames—eyeglasses that can hold a variety of lenses from a trial set of spheres, cylinders, and prisms (Figure 5-13). Trial frames have adjustable eyepieces, temple pieces, and nosepieces, and the examiner should become proficient in adjusting these elements to align the frame properly on the patient's face. For some patients, especially infants and small children, the examiner holds loose lenses or retinoscopy paddles (or "racks") directly in front of the eye instead of using a trial frame.

Halberg clips, which can be affixed onto the patient's own eyeglasses, also hold trial lenses and can be used to allow for modification of the patient's glasses with them in place, a procedure referred to as *overrefraction*. This term is also used to refer to the refraction, with a trial frame or phoropter, of a patient who is wearing contact lenses.

Phoropter

The phoropter, or refractor, provides an alternative to a trial frame and loose lenses. It consists of a faceplate that can be suspended before the patient's eyes. The plate contains a wide range of spherical and cylindrical lenses that the examiner can dial into position (Figure 5-14). Most phoropters have a variable setting for the interpupillary distance and have a convergence lever feature to allow the eyes to converge for determination of near vision correction. Other accessories vary widely among makes and models. Table 5-2 lists the major phoropter controls and their uses.

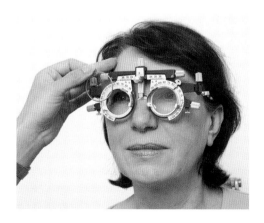

Figure 5-13 A trial frame can be adjusted to conform to the patient's anatomy and allows manual insertion of multiple lenses selected from a trial set. (Photo by Dan McGarrah.)

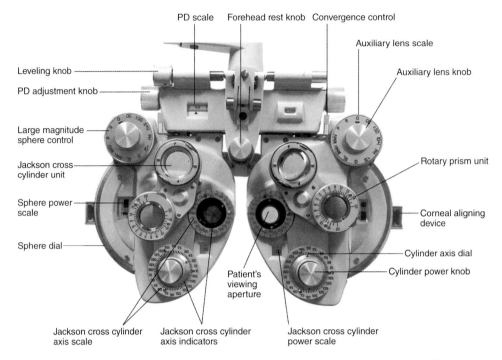

PD scale   Forehead rest knob   Convergence control

Auxiliary lens scale

Leveling knob

PD adjustment knob

Auxiliary lens knob

Large magnitude sphere control

Jackson cross cylinder unit

Sphere power scale

Rotary prism unit

Sphere dial

Corneal aligning device

Cylinder axis dial

Cylinder power knob

Patient's viewing aperture

Jackson cross cylinder axis scale

Jackson cross cylinder axis indicators

Jackson cross cylinder power scale

Figure 5-14   The examiner's view of the phoropter, or refractor. The most frequently used controls are listed and described in Table 5-2.

Jackson cross cylinder

This instrument is a special lens used as part of the refinement process to confirm first the axis and then the power of a correcting cylindrical lens for astigmatism (Figure 5-15). The Jackson cross cylinder is composed of 2 cylinders of equal power, 1 minus and 1 plus, set at right angles to each other. The 2 principal meridians of the Jackson cross cylinder are indicated with small white and red dots. The white dots identify the axis of the plus cylinder, and the red dots identify the axis of the minus cylinder. A cross cylinder is usually built into the phoropter, but handheld Jackson cross cylinders are available for use with trial frames.

Distometer

A distometer is a small handheld device used to determine *vertex distance,* the distance between the patient's eye and the back of the corrective lens. A distometer is illustrated in Figure 5-16. The vertex distance can vary among patients, but is usually between 12 mm and 14 mm. It is important to keep the vertex distance for the patient's eyeglasses constant during refractometry. If the vertex distances used for both eyes differ, the effective power of the patient's corrective lenses will be different and, potentially, intolerable. When the prescription is filled, unless the optician has been informed of a specific measurement, a distance of 13.5 mm is often assumed for each eye. Vertex distance is especially critical in patients with high refractive errors (more than 5.00 D of plus or minus sphere), as changing the vertex distance changes the effective power of the corrective lens. Clinical Protocol 5-5 details the method of using the distometer to measure vertex distance.

Table 5-2   Frequently Used Refractor Controls

Control	Purpose
PD adjustment knob	Adjusts viewing apertures to fit patient's interpupillary distance
Leveling knob	Tilts front face plate if eyes are not at same level
Forehead rest knob	Maintains constant distance from back surface of phoropter lenses to the patient's eyes
Convergence control levers	Adjusts angle of viewing apertures to about 150° for near-vision measurements (not present on all models)
Sphere dial	Adjusts sphere in 0.25 D increments
Sphere power scale	Displays power of sphere
Cylinder dial	Adjusts power of cylinder in 0.25 D increments
Cylinder power scale	Displays power of cylinder
Cylinder axis dial	Adjusts axis of cylinder
Cylinder axis scale	Displays axis of cylinder
Large magnitude sphere control	Adjusts sphere in 3.00 D increments
Auxiliary lens knob and scale (select examples)	**O** = Open (to test the eye) **OC** = Occlude (to occlude the eye) **R** = Retinoscopic lens (usually +1.50 D sph) **P** = Polarizing lens **PH** = Pinhole **RL** = Red lens (right eye) **GL** = Green lens (left eye) **RMV/WMV** = Maddox rod vertical: red (right), white (left) **RMH/WMH** = Maddox rod horizontal: red (right), white (left)

Retinoscopy Technique

For retinoscopy, the examining room lights are dimmed. The relative positions of the patient and the examiner are very important. While sitting in the examining chair, the patient is instructed to look directly into the light (if cycloplegia is used) or past the examiner's ear at a fixation light, letter, or object located at effective optical infinity (20 feet or more). The examiner sits facing the patient with eyes on the same level as the patient, at a standard distance, usually about arm's length. In most cases, situate yourself as follows:

- *To examine the right eye:* Seat yourself slightly to the patient's right; hold the retinoscope in your right hand and look through it with your right eye. Use your left hand to manipulate the phoropter or trial lenses.
- *To examine the left eye:* Seat yourself slightly to the patient's left, in front of the patient's left shoulder; hold the retinoscope in your left hand and look through it with your left eye. Use your right hand to manipulate the phoropter or trial lenses.

It is critical to know that the eye being examined is the fixating eye, especially if the patient has strabismus. When the patient is unable to control alignment, as in the case

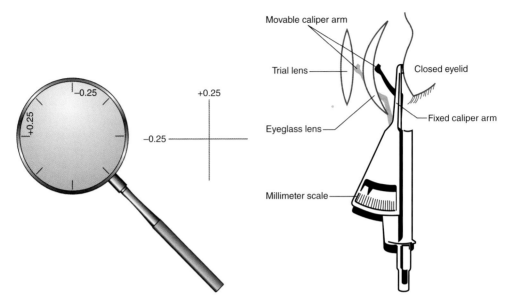

Figure 5-15 The Jackson cross cylinder with axes marked on the lens, and the corresponding power cross representation. The handle of the cross cylinder is attached 45° to the principal meridians, which allows quick twirling from 1 orientation of the cross cylinder to the exact opposite orientation.

Figure 5-16 A distometer is used to measure vertex distance accurately. The separation distance between the patient's eye and the back surface of the refracting lens is the vertex distance. The distometer scale takes into account the thickness of the average eyelid.

of manifest strabismus, the retinoscopic reflex will not be in the visual axis but rather in the axis of the deviation. The measurement of the eye's refractive error made in this axis will not be accurate. If the eye is not aligned with the retinoscopic reflex, the examiner can occlude the eye not being examined, with either a hand or an occluding device. If cycloplegia is used, the patient is instructed to look directly into the light. Video 5-1 demonstrates the retinoscopy technique.

 VIDEO 5-1 Retinoscopy: Basics
Courtesy of Thomas F. Mauger, MD.
Access all *Practical Ophthalmology* videos at www.aao.org
/PracticalOphthalmologyvideo.

Working distance

The distance between the examiner and the patient's eye must be measured and converted into diopters. For convenience in changing lenses in the phoropter or trial frame, most examiners use a working distance of arm's length, usually about 66 cm (26 inches), and assign the patient a corresponding working lens of +1.50 D. A working distance of 50 cm would require a +2.00 D working lens, and a working distance of 1 m would require a working lens of +1.00 D. The working distance must remain constant throughout the examination, although the examiner may move forward and backward slightly from this position to evaluate the movement of the patient's light reflex. How to account for your working distance when determining a final prescription is discussed later in this chapter.

Neutralization with a Retinoscope

Neutralization refers to the achievement of the point at which a lens placed before the patient's eye effectively "neutralizes" the retinoscopic reflex and the patient's pupil fills with reflected light. Because of its subtleties and complexities, retinoscopy is best learned by hands-on instruction. Nevertheless, the basic steps in retinoscopic neutralization are outlined below.

1. Set the retinoscope so that the emanating light rays are parallel. This can be ensured if the streak cannot be focused (ie, looks broad instead of thin and sharp) on a surface of any sort, such as a wall or the palm of your hand.

2. Position the patient and yourself for comfort and appropriate testing positions and distance (as discussed earlier in this section). Position the trial frame or phoropter as necessary.

3. Direct the patient to look at a specific distance target, such as an optotype on a vision test chart. If you are using cycloplegia, you may direct the patient to look into your light.

4. Look through the examiner's eyepiece of the retinoscope and direct the light into the patient's pupil. If the reflection from the patient's pupil is not easy to see, consider the following possible reasons:

   a. The retinoscope bulb is dim, dirty, or turned off.

   b. The patient has a very high refractive error.

   c. The room lights are not sufficiently dimmed.

   d. The patient has a cataract or other media opacity.

   If you see several reflections, the "extra" ones may be coming from other surfaces, such as the cornea or the trial lens that you are using. Try moving slightly to either side, tilting the trial lens slightly, ascertaining that the trial lens surface is clean, or adjusting room lights to make sure you are not seeing reflections of lights in the examining room.

5. Because the 2 principal meridians of the eye are most commonly at or near 90° and 180°, first orient the streak of the retinoscope horizontally and then move it up and down. Alternatively, you may start by orienting the streak vertically and then moving it right and left. Do this first without any lenses in place.

6. Note if the motion of the reflex in the pupil is the same as ("with") or opposite ("against") the direction of your sweeping movement. If the light reflex moves in the direction opposite your movement, add minus lenses in front of the eye in half-diopter (0.50 D) increments until you no longer see "against" movement. If the movement of the light reflex is in the same direction that you are sweeping the retinoscope light, the exiting rays are too divergent, so plus (converging) lenses must be added. Increments of 0.50 D are added until it becomes difficult to tell if the movement of the reflex is "with" or "against," at which time increments of 0.25 D may be more helpful. Figure 5-17 illustrates the reflexes produced by the streak of the retinoscope.

7. Smaller sweeps are useful as the reflex band appears to widen. When the reflex fills the pupil and movement cannot be ascertained, the reflected light rays coming from the eye are parallel, and the lens combination that you have used to reach this point

Figure 5-17   Reflexes produced by the streak retinoscope. **A,** Normal starting position, before sweeping movements are made. **B,** "With" motion: The reflex moves in the same direction as the streak of light, which indicates the need for a stronger converging (plus) lens. The eye is relatively more hyperopic than the lenses are correcting. **C,** "Against" motion: The reflex moves in the direction opposite that of the streak, which indicates the need for a stronger diverging (minus) lens. The eye is relatively more myopic than the lenses are correcting. **D,** Neutralization point: There is no apparent movement of the reflex, and the pupil is filled with a red glow.

(minus the dioptric equivalent of your working distance) is the objective measurement of the refractive error of the eye. This is referred to as *neutrality*.

8. To confirm that you have achieved neutrality, you can move your eye/retinoscope several inches closer to the patient. At this point, "with" movement of the reflex band should occur as you continue to sweep. Return to your original working distance, while continuing the sweeping motion, and note that the reflex again fills the pupil and has no apparent motion. Additional confirmation of neutrality can be made by moving several inches farther away from the eye, repeating the sweeping movements, and noting that the reflex is now "against" your direction of movement.

9. Note the power of the lens or lenses that you have used to reach neutrality. Subtract the dioptric equivalent of your working distance. This gives you the refractive error in the axis that you were sweeping. For example, if you were sitting 66 cm in front of a patient and needed a −1.00 D lens to obtain a neutral reflex with your streak in either the horizontal or the vertical direction, the patient's refractive error is −2.50 sphere. If you obtained different reflexes from the horizontal and the vertical orientation of the streak, an astigmatic refractive error is present, which will need to be neutralized with cylinders in the final eyeglass prescription.

Video 5-2 demonstrates the plus-cylinder technique for retinoscopy.

 VIDEO 5-2   Retinoscopy: Plus-Cylinder Technique
Courtesy of Thomas F. Mauger, MD.

Determining Cylinder

The following steps are taken to determine the presence of astigmatism:

1. Position yourself and the patient and illuminate the patient's pupil with the retinoscope as outlined in steps 1–4 above. Orient the streak horizontally and sweep it up and down. Change the orientation to vertical, and sweep it right and left.

2. Compare the intensity and the direction of the reflex. If both are comparable in intensity and direction, an insignificant astigmatism is present.

3. If the streak is brighter in 1 direction than it is in the other, or if the reflexes move in opposite directions, a cylindrical, or astigmatic, refractive error is present.

4. Rotate the sleeve of the retinoscope so that the streak is oriented perpendicular to the direction of the initial orientation. In other words, if you first achieved neutrality with the streak oriented horizontally, now orient it vertically.

   a. If you are using cylinders for retinoscopy, the axis of the cylinder should be placed so that it is aligned with the direction that you are moving the retinoscope reflex. With plus cylinders, you should achieve neutrality in 1 direction and still note "with" movement when the streak of the retinoscope is rotated 90°. If you are working with minus cylinders, "against" movement will be noted after you have neutralized all the "with" movement and then rotated the streak 90°.

   b. If you are using only spheres for retinoscopy, neutralize the reflex in 1 orientation and note the power of the sphere used in that axis. Change the orientation of the streak by 90°, repeat the neutralization procedure as outlined above, and note the power of the sphere used in this orientation. The difference between the 2 sphere powers is used to calculate the cylinder power as outlined below.

5. If you cannot achieve neutrality with the streak oriented horizontally and vertically, an oblique astigmatism might be present. The principal meridians can be determined by observing the characteristics of the streak reflex.

   a. A *break* is seen when the streak is not parallel to a principal meridian. The break disappears when the streak is rotated onto the correct axis.

   b. The *width* of the streak appears narrowest when the streak aligns with the correct axis.

   c. The *intensity* of the streak is brightest when it is aligned on the correct axis (this is a subtle finding, and useful only with small cylinders).

   d. *Skew*, oblique motion of the streak reflex, occurs when the streak is off-axis. The reflex and the streak move in the same direction (perpendicular to the orientation of the streak) when the streak is aligned with 1 of the principal meridians.

   Methods of neutralization for oblique astigmatism, which take more time and practice to acquire than the usual techniques, are further detailed in textbooks and video presentations on retinoscopy.

6. Note the power of the lens combination(s) that you used at each axis. If you are writing the eyeglass prescription in plus-cylinder form, write the power and the axis of the least-plus lens that you used to neutralize the reflex. For example, when using spherical lenses for retinoscopy, if you were sitting 66 cm in front of a patient and needed a −1.00 D lens to obtain a neutral reflex with your streak in the horizontal direction (ie, as you moved it up and down), the patient's refractive error at 180° is −2.50 D, which accounts for your working distance. Then, if you needed a −0.50 D lens to neutralize the reflex when your streak was oriented vertically, the patient's refractive error at 90° is −2.00 D. The resultant prescription is written −2.50 + 0.50 × 90. In other words, the cylinder is the difference between the 2 lens powers used to neutralize each axis.

If you are using cylindrical lenses for retinoscopy, first determine the power of the sphere in 1 principal meridian and then add a correcting cylindrical lens. The direction of the sweeping movement is the meridian, and it is at right angles to the axis of the cylinder. In the example above you would have used a −1.00 D sphere together with a +0.50 D cylinder with the axis line oriented vertically to achieve neutralization. Once the dioptric equivalent of the working distance (in this case, 1.50 D) was subtracted from the sphere, the resultant prescription would again be written as −2.50 + 0.50 × 90.

Summary of Retinoscopy Steps

1. Establish alignment in front of the patient's pupil.
2. Shine the retinoscope light into the patient's eye while maintaining a constant distance between yourself and the patient.
3. Rotate the streak to determine the meridian that you wish to neutralize first. This will depend on whether you are using plus cylinders, minus cylinders, or spheres only. As you move a horizontal streak up and down, you are neutralizing the vertical meridian with the axis at 180°. As you move a vertical streak to the right and the left, you are neutralizing the horizontal meridian, for which the axis is 90°.
4. Neutralize the reflex at the chosen axis.
5. Orient the streak 90° to the original orientation and neutralize the reflex at that axis.
6. Note the power of the lenses needed to achieve neutrality at both orientations.
7. Calculate the power of the resultant eyeglass prescription (remember to subtract the dioptric equivalent of the working distance).

Residents should review videos about retinoscopy, read more detailed textbooks, and gain hands-on training in order to master the finer details of neutralization, estimation of cylinder axis and power, and interpretation of aberrations. Activity 5-1 is helpful for learning and putting into practice the principles of retinoscopy.

 ACTIVITY 5-1   Retinoscopy Simulator
Access all *Practical Ophthalmology* activities at www.aao.org/Practical Ophthalmologyactivity.

Refinement

Refinement, or subjective refraction, can be performed either with or without the use of cycloplegic eyedrops. Refinement performed without the use of cycloplegic eyedrops is often referred to as the "manifest" refraction or "dry" refraction. A cycloplegic (or "wet") refraction may be performed in addition to (or instead of) a manifest refraction. Because cycloplegia suspends accommodation, the examiner can make an accurate measurement of the nonaccommodative refractive state of the eye during the time that the cycloplegic eyedrops have full effect. Some of the indications for performing a cycloplegic refraction are discussed later in this chapter in the sections "Cycloplegic Refraction" and "Guidelines for Prescribing Glasses."

Several methods are used to perform subjective refraction. Some of them, such as the Lancaster astigmatic clock and the stenopeic slit, are rarely used. One of the more common methods involves the use of the phoropter and the Jackson cross cylinder to adjust and refine the sphere and refine cylinder axis and power. The refinement instructions that follow apply to the use of a phoropter, but refinement can be performed with the trial frame and trial lenses as well. As with retinoscopy, this text can provide only a basic outline of the procedure; residents should consult more detailed textbooks and videos and gain sufficient hands-on training with an experienced practitioner to become proficient.

Adjust sphere

1. Place 1 of the following lens prescriptions in the phoropter:

    a. Retinoscopic findings

    b. Previous eyeglass prescription

    c. Previous manifest refraction

    d. Prescription from an automatic refractor

2. Occlude the eye not being tested by dialing in *OC* (occluding lens) on the auxiliary dial of the phoropter. Adjust the auxiliary lens knob to position *O* (open) for the eye being tested.

3. Measure visual acuity for the eye to be tested, using the standard Snellen chart and technique. Use optotypes 1 or 2 lines larger than the patient's best visual acuity for testing, because introduction of the cross cylinder produces blur, and the patient will be more aware of changes at this already slightly blurred level of acuity.

4. Adjust the sphere dial on the phoropter to the most-plus or the least-minus setting that gives the patient the best visual acuity. Ask the patient, "Which lens makes the letters clearer, number 1 or number 2, or are they the same?" and dial 2 "clicks," or +0.50 D sphere. The patient is presented with 2 choices and will select either the original lens (choice number 1) or an addition of +0.50 D sphere (choice number 2).

    a. If the patient prefers choice number 2, repeat the process, adding another 2 clicks of plus (+0.50 D) and ask the patient, "Which is better, number 3 or number 4, or are they the same?" Continue adding increments of +0.50 D sphere until the patient notes that the 2 choices are equivalent.

    b. If the patient prefers choice number 1, subtract 2 clicks of sphere (that is, subtract –0.50 D sphere) and ask, "Which is clearer, number 3 or number 4, or are they the same?" Continue subtracting in increments of –0.50 D sphere until the patient notes that the 2 choices are equivalent. You might need to advise many myopic patients to choose the lens that lets them actually see the letters more clearly, not the one that just makes the letters smaller and darker. If the patient describes the change in the letters as just smaller and darker, too much minus power has been added.

    c. Avoid confusion with previous choices by giving the patient different numbers for subsequent choices, such as, "Which is better, 1 or 2, 3, or 4," and so on. If the patient persists in always choosing either the first or the second lens presented, reverse the order of presentation to check for consistency. Present the 2 choices quickly; give the patient adequate time to view the testing letters, then briskly present the second lens choice.

d. If cycloplegia is not in effect and the patient tends to accommodate (as is the case with young patients or hyperopic patients), it can be helpful to start with more plus power than is needed and then slowly to decrease plus power until the best sphere is found. This technique, called fogging, encourages the patient to relax accommodation.

Refine cylinder axis

1. Position the Jackson cross cylinder in front of the eye to be tested, with the axis 45° to the principal meridians of the cylinder axis (this is referred to as "straddling the axis"). In the example in Figure 5-18A, the 90° axis is straddled.

2. Flip the cross cylinder (turn it over and then back) and ask the patient, "Which is better, number 1 or number 2, or are they the same?"

3. For the plus-cylinder method, rotate the cross cylinder 5°–10° toward the plus axis (white dot) of the preferred choice. If minus cylinders are being used, the cylinder axis is rotated toward the minus axis (red dot) of the preferred choice.

4. Continue the process until the patient reports that the 2 choices look the same and are equally blurred.

Refine cylinder power

1. Align the cylinder axis with the Jackson cross cylinder axis. This alignment is sometimes referred to as "on axis." In Figure 5-18 B and C, the cross cylinder axis is aligned "on axis" with the 90° axis of the refracting lens.

2. Flip the cross cylinder and ask the patient, "Which is better, choice 1 or choice 2, or are they the same?"

3. If the patient prefers the plus cylinder (white-dot axis), add 1 click of cylinder power (+0.25 D). If the patient prefers the minus cylinder (red-dot axis), subtract 1 click of cylinder power (−0.25 D). If minus cylinders are being used, add more minus cylinder power if the minus cylinder (red-dot axis) is preferred, and subtract minus cylinder if the plus cylinder (white-dot axis) is preferred.

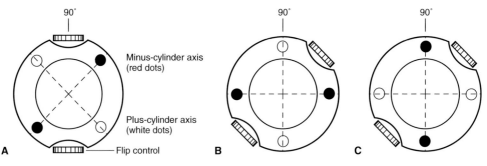

Figure 5-18   The phoropter's Jackson cross cylinder. **A,** The cross cylinder "straddling" the 90° axis. An imaginary line is drawn on the cross cylinder to indicate the position of the minus-cylinder and plus-cylinder axes. **B,** The cross cylinder "on axis" with the 90° axis, showing the white dots of the plus-cylinder axis aligned with the 90° axis. **C,** The red dots of the minus-cylinder axis aligned with the 90° axis.

4. For each 2 clicks (+0.50 D) of cylinder power added, subtract 1 click (−0.25 D) of sphere power, using the sphere dial on the phoropter to maintain the same spherical equivalent. If minus cylinders are used, for each 2 clicks (−0.50 D) of cylinder power subtracted, 1 click of "plus" (+0.25 D) must be added to the sphere power. Adding or subtracting significant cylinder power requires modifying the sphere to avoid final inaccuracy.

5. The end point has been reached when the patient notes that the choices presented appear equal.

If the patient does not have a cylinder in the current spectacles or in the retinoscopic findings, it is a good idea to check for the presence of astigmatism during the refinement to see if visual acuity can be improved by adding cylinder. The Jackson cross cylinder is placed arbitrarily at 90° and 180°, the cylinder is flipped, and the patient is asked to make a choice. If a preferred flipped position is found, cylinder is added with the axis parallel to the respective plus or minus axis of the cross cylinder until the 2 flip choices are equal. If no preference is found with cross cylinder axes at 90° and 180°, check again with axes at 45° and 135° before assuming that no astigmatism is present. If cylinder power is found, refinement of both power and axis is performed in the usual manner (the axis of astigmatism is defined first, followed by power). After the power of the cylinder has been determined, the axis may be rechecked and adjusted if necessary.

Refine sphere
After refinement of the axis and power of the cylinder, another refinement of sphere is performed by repeating the same method used initially to refine sphere.

1. Ask the patient, "Which lens makes the letters clearer, number 1 or number 2, or are they the same?" and dial 1 to 2 clicks, or +0.25 to +0.50 D sphere, on the sphere dial of the phoropter. The patient is presented with 2 choices and will select either the original lens (choice 1) or an additional spherical power (choice 2).

2. If the patient prefers choice number 2, repeat the process, adding another 1 to 2 clicks of plus (+0.25 to +0.50 D), and ask the patient, "Which is better, number 2 or number 1, or are they the same?" Continue adding increments of +0.25 to +0.50 D sphere until the patient notes that the 2 choices are equivalent.

3. If the patient prefers choice number 1, subtract 1 to 2 clicks of sphere (that is, subtract −0.25 to −0.50 D sphere) and ask, "Which is clearer, number 1 or number 2, or are they the same?" Continue subtracting in increments of −0.25 to −0.50 D sphere until the patient notes that the 2 choices are equivalent.

Summary of refinement
1. Adjust sphere.
2. Refine cylinder axis.
3. Refine cylinder power.
4. Refine sphere.

Cycloplegic Refraction

Cycloplegia can be useful as an adjunct to refraction for almost any patient, but it is especially helpful for a patient who has active accommodation. A cycloplegic refraction should be done at least once for every patient, preferably during an initial evaluation. Cycloplegia achieved at the time of dilation for retinal examination can be used to verify noncycloplegic refraction measurements in adults, and it is the ideal time to do retinoscopy for children.

Cycloplegic refraction is indicated:

- in patients younger than age 15 before they are prescribed glasses (manifest refraction is unreliable in children under 10 years and usually does not need to be performed)
- in hyperopic patients up to age 35, especially if they are symptomatic
- in pre- and early presbyopia, especially when glasses have not previously been worn
- whenever refraction yields variable or inconsistent results, especially in patients under age 50
- whenever the patient's symptoms are disproportionate to the manifest refractive error, or if symptoms suggest an accommodative problem
- for patients who tend to accommodate during refraction
- for suspected or known *accommodative esotropia*
- whenever the refractionist is forced to rely on retinoscopy to provide all of the refractive information
- in bilateral refractive asymmetry, or whenever a good binocular balance cannot be achieved

As with the use of any medication, the patient should be asked about allergies before cycloplegic drugs are given. Ascertaining the use of other medications and the existence of other medical conditions is also important because the side effects of cycloplegic drugs, especially cyclopentolate (Cyclogyl), can include exacerbation of seizures, cardiac arrhythmias, and precipitation of angle-closure glaucoma. Table 5-3 outlines the systemic effects of common cycloplegic drugs. Although these signs and symptoms are seldom experienced after use of topical eyedrops, it is important to be aware of all potential systemic side effects of these medications. Cycloplegic drugs that are commonly used include tropicamide, cyclopentolate, atropine, and a combination eyedrop marketed as Cyclomydril, which is used for young infants (typically six months and under).

Duochrome Test

The duochrome test (Figure 5-19) is a quick method of determining if a patient has too much minus or too much plus in a spectacle correction. The test uses a projected red light and green light, which are each superimposed over half of the visual acuity test targets. This test is based on the principle that shorter wavelengths of light are refracted more than longer wavelengths as both enter more optically dense media, which would be the case for light traveling through the cornea toward the retina. Therefore, relative to the macula, the letters seen in the green light are refracted more and thus are more anterior than the letters on the red side. If one sees the black letters on the green background as

Table 5-3   Systemic Effects of Topical Cycloplegic Medications

Drug Name	Symptoms and Signs
Atropine	Dryness of mouth and skin Fever Delirium Urinary retention Tachycardia Flushed face Respiratory depression **Note:** If ingested, induce emesis and treat as emergency.
Cyclopentolate	CNS disturbance (particularly hypersensitivity) reported in infants, young children, and children with spastic paralysis or brain damage Psychotic reaction (particularly with 2%), ataxia, incoherent speech, restlessness, seizures, hallucinations, hyperactivity Disorientation; failure to recognize familiar people Feeding intolerance (vomiting is more frequent for several hours after administration in neonates) Abdominal distention in infants from paralytic ileus Other similar to atropine
Tropicamide	Similar to cyclopentolate but less frequent and less severe
Phenylephrine	Caution with use within 21 days of monoamine oxidase (MAO) inhibitor use due to risk of hypertensive crisis Tachycardia Rebound miosis Hypertension, systemic vasopressor response (especially 10% solution)

being darker, these letters are focused closer to the macula than are the letters on the red background, which in this case are actually imaged posterior to the macula.

Each eye is tested separately, and the patient is asked, "Which are sharper (or darker), the letters on the green side or the letters on the red side, or are they the same?" If the patient answers that the letters on the green side are sharper, too much minus power has probably been added, so the examiner should add plus sphere. If the answer is that the red side is blacker or sharper, then the overall power is probably too plus, and minus sphere should be added. The mnemonic RAM-GAP (Red Add Minus—Green Add Plus) is often used in performance of the duochrome test. The end point of the duochrome test is achieved when the red and the green letters are equidistant from the macula.

Because this test is based on chromatic aberration and not color discrimination, it can be used even with colorblind patients. The test may be inaccurate if the patient is exercising accommodation. The duochrome test is most reliable when conducted after the patient has been given cycloplegic eyedrops.

Binocular Balancing

The final steps in subjective refraction, known as *binocular balancing*, ensure that accommodation has been relaxed equally in both eyes. Several methods of binocular balancing are commonly used. Most balancing methods require that correctable vision be essentially equal in both eyes.

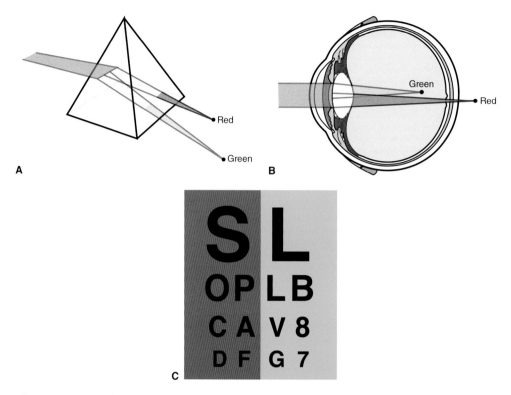

Figure 5-19   Duochrome test. **A,** Green light is refracted more than red light as both enter optically dense media. **B,** The end point of the duochrome test is achieved when the letters on the red background and the letters on the green background are imaged equidistant from the macula. (Illustration by Mark M. Miller.) **C,** Example of duochrome test as seen by the patient. (Part C courtesy of Tommy Korn, MD.)

Fogging

Subtle differences in clarity between the 2 eyes are often easier for the patient to detect when both eyes are intentionally blurred. By fogging (blurring) the end-point refraction with use of +2.00 D spheres for each eye, the visual acuity should be reduced to approximately 20/100. Placing a −0.25 D sphere first before 1 eye, and then the other, and rapidly alternating occlusion of the eyes will enable the patient to identify clearly the eye with the −0.25 D sphere as having the clearer image. If the eyes are not in balance, sphere should be added or subtracted in steps of 0.25 D until balance is achieved.

Prism dissociation

The most sensitive method of binocular balance is achieved by fogging both eyes with use of +1.00 D spheres and then placing vertical prism of 4^Δ or 5^Δ before 1 eye. A single line, usually 20/40, is projected on the chart. The patient is then able to see 2 lines vertically displaced, 1 above the other. The 2 images should be comparable in size and clarity. Differences between the fogged images in both eyes of 0.25 D sphere, or even less, can be identified readily by the patient. The sphere power is adjusted until both eyes are equally blurred. Once a balance between both eyes has been established, the prism is removed. The power of the fogging lenses is then gradually reduced simultaneously in front of both eyes in 0.25 D increments. The desired end point is reached when the patient achieves maximum vision with the lowest minus or the highest plus spheres.

Cycloplegia

Binocular balance is achieved simply by applying the monocular findings when full cycloplegia has been used. It is important to ascertain that cycloplegia is complete in both eyes if this method is to be used. Residual accommodation can be determined by asking the patient to look at a distance target while you neutralize the reflex (the standard way of performing retinoscopy), and then asking the patient to look directly at the retinoscope light while you note if the reflex is moving more "with" your sweep. If additional "with" movement is noted, accommodation has not been fully reduced.

Near Point and Reading Add

As fine print is moved closer to the patient, the print eventually becomes blurred at a certain point. This point is called the *near point of accommodation* (NPA). Because of presbyopia, patients over the age of 40 or 45 typically require a plus-lens "reading add" in addition to their distance spectacle prescription to see near objects well. The binocular near point is usually closer than the monocular near point and can be estimated in a simple, practical way by asking the patient to fixate on small print and to state when the print blurs as it is moved closer to the eye.

To measure the NPA, place the patient's distance prescription in the phoropter. Most phoropters have a convergence control lever on the front that allows the examiner to adjust the front tilt so that the eyes can still view near reading material as they converge (see Figure 5-14). Either adjust this lever to converge the eyes, or decrease the interpupillary distance by at least 5 mm to account for the convergence that naturally accompanies any accommodation. Begin with the near vision test card about 50 cm in front of the patient's eye. Ask the patient to fixate on the small print (5-point type), and move the test card toward the eye until the patient states that the print is blurred. This position, measured in meters, is the NPA and can be converted into diopters using the formula $D = 1/f$. For example, a patient who reports blur at 25 cm (0.25 m) has an NPA of 1/0.25, or 4 diopters.

Most phoropters are equipped with an accommodation ruler, such as the Prince rule. This combination of a near-vision card with a ruler calibrated in centimeters and diopters provides a convenient method of measuring the NPA. The ruler can be attached to the front of the phoropter or used separately.

To select the appropriate reading add, follow these steps:

1. Determine the accommodation requirements for the near-vision task. For example, reading at 40 cm would require 2.50 diopters of accommodation (1/0.4 m = +2.50 D).

2. Measure the accommodative amplitude for each eye. A simple way to do this is to have the patient fixate on a reading target (eg, a 20/25 line of print held at 40 cm) with each eye. Stimulate accommodation by placing successively stronger minus spheres until the print blurs. Then relax accommodation by using successively stronger plus lenses. The print will clear, but as successively stronger plus lenses are added, the onset of blurring will again be noted. The sum of the 2 lenses used to reach the blur points is a measure of accommodative amplitude. For example,

if the patient accepted −3.00 D to blur (stimulate accommodation) and +2.50 D to blur (relax accommodation), the amplitude would be 5.50 D.

3. From the measured accommodative amplitude, allow one-half to be held in reserve and consider one-half to be the available accommodation. Other techniques for more precise measurement of accommodative amplitudes and for measurements of binocular amplitude of accommodation are beyond the scope of this text, but in general a consideration of both the NPA and the patient's age will give a good prediction of the add that will be needed. Average accommodative amplitudes for different ages are summarized in Table 5-4.

4. Subtract the patient's available accommodation (step 3) from the total amount of accommodation required for the task at hand (step 1) for the tentative power of the add that will be needed.

5. Add this extra plus power (the reading add) to the sphere of the distance refractive correction already in the phoropter and again determine the patient's near visual acuity. If you are using a trial frame, make sure you have placed the distance sphere lens in the appropriate slot on the back of the frame, and the cylindrical lens in the front, as you would normally do for determining the distance correction. Put the appropriate plus lens as an additional lens in front of the lens combination already in place.

6. By moving the reading material closer to and then farther away from the patient, you can determine that the add allows the patient an adequate range for seeing near work clearly.

Guidelines for Prescribing Glasses

To help you avoid many common problems and establish proper prescribing habits, this section presents general guidelines and tips on determining prescriptions for myopia, hyperopia, and astigmatism as well as for presbyopia. Consult the detailed textbooks on this topic that are listed at the end of this chapter for more complete discussions than are supplied here.

General Prescribing Guidelines

- If the patient has good vision and is asymptomatic, do not prescribe new glasses or change old ones (it is hard to improve the asymptomatic, happy patient).
- Don't prescribe minor changes (less than 0.50 D) unless the patient can definitely appreciate an improvement over the old spectacle correction.
- Specify the testing vertex distance for lenses with power of 5.00 D or more.
- Try to avoid changing cylinder axis more than 10°. If a greater change must be made, let the patient walk around wearing the prescription in a trial frame for 20–30 minutes, and warn the patient that an adjustment period probably will be necessary.
- Check the final eyeglass prescription with the duochrome test.
- Put the prescription in a trial frame and let the patient walk around in the waiting room if you think the prescription might be questionable, if this is a first prescription, or if there is a change from the previous prescription of more than 0.50 D.

Table 5-4   **Average Accommodation Amplitudes for Different Ages**

Age	Average Accommodative Amplitude[a]
8	14.0 (±2 D)
12	13.0 (±2 D)
16	12.0 (±2 D)
20	11.0 (±2 D)
24	10.0 (±2 D)
28	9.0 (±2 D)
32	8.0 (±2 D)
36	7.0 (±2 D)
40	6.0 (±2 D)
44	4.5 (±2 D)
48	3.0 (±2 D)
52	2.5 (±2 D)
56	2.0 (±2 D)
60	1.5 (±2 D)
64	1.0 (±2 D)
68	0.5 (±2 D)

[a]Continuing back from age 40, accommodation increases by 1 D for every 4 years. Beyond age 40, the decrease in accommodation is somewhat more rapid. From age 48 on, 0.5 D is lost every 4 years. Thus, one can recall the entire table by remembering the amplitudes at age 40 and age 48.

- Double-check the written prescription for accuracy. Errors are often made when copying the prescription from the phoropter or trial frame into the medical record and onto a prescription pad.
- If a patient returns to you dissatisfied with the new prescription, use a lensmeter to verify that the glasses were made correctly.

Prescriptions for Myopia

The typical presentation of uncorrected myopia is blurred distance vision with good near vision. Patients often state that they need to squint to see objects far away.

- In general, give the manifest refraction for best acuity and do not overcorrect. Young myopic patients will often prefer more minus power in the manifest refraction than they need for best acuity, because the additional minus enhances the contrast of the dark test letters on the light chart background. During the subjective refraction, to help prevent overcorrection, ask the patient if the letters are actually clearer and if detail is more easily seen, or if the letters are just darker and smaller. Overcorrection causes the patient to accommodate, which often leads to asthenopia (eyestrain).

- Use the results of cycloplegic retinoscopy and cycloplegic refraction to avoid overcorrection.
- For myopic patients older than 40, make sure that increasing the minus power does not induce presbyopic symptoms. Check that all patients can read comfortably with their new distance prescriptions.

Prescriptions for Hyperopia

Most young children are hyperopic, but they can easily compensate for this ametropia without a glasses prescription by accommodating. Consider reducing the plus power for the cycloplegic refractive prescription of a child by 1.00 to 2.00 D to account for this accommodation. If the child is cooperative, a manifest refraction can be useful, because the full hyperopic prescription can cause blur at distance. Correcting hyperopia in children is dependent on many factors, including age and presence of strabismus, but general indications include:

- moderate to high hyperopia (eg, greater than 3.50 D in children between the ages of 3 and 4 years, or greater than 5.00 D in those between the ages of 1 and 2 years), or lesser degrees of hyperopia if the child is symptomatic (with asthenopia, or vague eye discomfort such as intermittent blurring or trouble reading)
- decreased uncorrected acuity with improvement in acuity with use of hyperopic spectacles
- anisometropia (prescribe glasses if a hyperopic error of 1.50 D or greater in 1 eye, compared with the fellow eye, is noted during the amblyogenic period—before the child is 6 or 7 years—especially if there is any difference in measurable acuity)
- esotropia

Hyperopic adults can partially compensate for their hyperopia by accommodating. The manifest hyperopia is the amount of plus power needed for sharp distance vision. After cycloplegia, an additional latent component of the hyperopia can be detected by both retinoscopy and refinement. This is the portion of the hyperopia that the patient overcomes by accommodating. Symptoms can occur because of the inability to maintain the accommodation necessary to overcome hyperopia. Symptoms include decreased distance vision or intermittent blurring of distance vision as latent hyperopia becomes manifest; difficulty with near work as part of the loss of accommodation that accompanies the normal aging process; early presbyopia in young, hyperopic adults with uncorrected vision; asthenopia or visual discomfort, including burning and tearing, and even bifrontal headaches exacerbated by near work; and fatigue after reading for short periods.

For adults, give the manifest refraction. If the refraction was performed with cycloplegia, a postcycloplegic refraction prior to prescribing may be necessary because young and middle-aged adults may not accept the full hyperopic correction when not cyclopleged. To correct for infinity rather than the 20-foot examination-room length, reduce the manifest refraction by –0.25 D.

Prescriptions for Astigmatism

Symptoms of uncorrected astigmatism include blur at both distance and near. Uncorrected astigmatic patients often report the need to squint for both distance and near to improve vision. The patient with uncorrected astigmatism might also complain of a bifrontal headache with prolonged near work. Observe the following prescribing guidelines in cases of astigmatism:

- For children older than 3 or 4 years, if more than 1.50 D of cylinder is detected, glasses are indicated. For children younger than 3 or 4, glasses are indicated for higher amounts of astigmatism. Prescribe the full astigmatic correction and advise full-time wear.
- Be cautious about changing the axis of the astigmatic correction, especially in adults, because such changes are often poorly tolerated. Asking the patient to walk around for several minutes while wearing the prescription in a trial frame is helpful in this situation.
- Ascertain that any new astigmatic correction produces significant improvement in both distance acuity and near acuity.
- Be wary of introducing new astigmatic correction in adults, as it can produce intolerable distortions for the patient even if measurable acuity is improved.
- Advise patients that a period of adjustment to the new correction may be needed.

Prescriptions for Presbyopia

The predominant symptom of uncorrected presbyopia is difficulty reading at near. Patients with early presbyopia also sometimes report that they need more light to read and that they can read well in the morning, but not at night, after a long day of accommodative effort (close work). Patients experience difficulty reading fine print, such as that used in newspapers, and threading a needle. Very early in presbyopia, patients note that their eyes are slow to focus on near print, and are then slow to change focus as they look at more remote objects. The usual onset of presbyopia is approximately between ages 40 and 45, but presentation can be earlier in those with undercorrected hyperopia and later in those with undercorrected myopia.

The following guidelines can be useful in determining presbyopic correction:

- Myopic patients with refractive errors under −3.00 D might not complain of difficulty with near tasks because they routinely remove their glasses for reading. Remember to ask about this habit, because these patients might have symptoms with accommodative effort if they wear their correction full time.
- Various medications can exacerbate presbyopic symptoms. Some of these are barbiturates, tricyclic antidepressants, antihistamines, and decongestants (including nonprescription medications).
- Bifocals with adds of +0.75 D or less are rarely necessary, although they might be required for specific tasks, such as reading sheet music on a music stand.
- Alternatives for the presbyopic emmetropic patient are single-vision readers, bifocals with plano tops, and half glasses.

- Alternatives for presbyopic myopic and presbyopic hyperopic patients are separate glasses for reading and distance, and bifocals. Myopic patients also can remove their glasses or use half glasses when reading.

Several bifocal and trifocal styles are illustrated in Figure 5-20. In general, the type and the placement of the bifocal or trifocal segment is best left up to the optician, who will discuss the various options with the patient. The patient should be encouraged to tell the optician about specific near-vision requirements, such as the need to view a computer screen at a particular distance.

Most patients have heard about "bifocals without a line," by which they usually mean one of a number of the *progressive addition lenses* (see Figure 5-20H) (also known as *variable focus lenses* or *lineless bifocals*). These lens styles have no visible demarcation line and not only are more cosmetically acceptable for many patients, but also eliminate much of the image jump and displacement that can occur as gaze is shifted from the distance to the near segment. Because the correct fitting of these lenses is crucial to successful use, the fitter's personal expertise can be as important as the choice of the add power itself. *Blended bifocals* (see Figure 5-20G) also lack a sharp demarcation line and are less expensive than progressive addition lenses, but they have an area of blur where the near and distance segments join. This is at approximately the same position that the patient might experience an image jump as fixation shifts from 1 segment of the bifocal to the other.

Trifocals can be useful for patients who have intermediate distance needs, such as computer use (see Figure 5-20B, D, F). Other special-need adds are sometimes used for particular purposes, such as reading music, reading blueprints, or viewing museum exhibits. Try to duplicate the special-needs situation during testing. It is useful to ask the patient to measure the distances for the tasks for which the glasses will be worn. This will allow you to determine a more appropriate add.

When you prescribe a patient's first pair of bifocals, advise the patient that an adjustment period will probably be required, particularly when walking down stairs in unfamiliar surroundings. Viewing the ground through the bifocals while moving may initially cause difficulties with depth perception and visual disorientation.

Optical Fitting Considerations

Pantoscopic Tilt

Spectacle lenses in frames are tilted slightly to conform with the rotation of the eye on the optical axis of the spectacle lens. This minimizes the effect of oblique astigmatism, an aberration that would be induced with down gaze if the lens were fitted perpendicular to the distance visual axis. Vertex distance changes are also minimized with this adjustment. The tops of the spectacle lenses are intentionally tilted forward, which helps achieve a plane that allows a more constant distance between the back surface of the spectacle lens and the front surface of the cornea. *Pantoscopic tilt* is not an exact measurement, but because most opticians incorporate this tilt when they fit spectacle lenses, it should be taken into account when one uses either a phoropter or a trial frame. In general, most spectacles are fitted with a downward tilt of between 5°–10° to the visual axis. This means that the top of the spectacle lens is tilted slightly forward compared with the bottom of the spectacle lens.

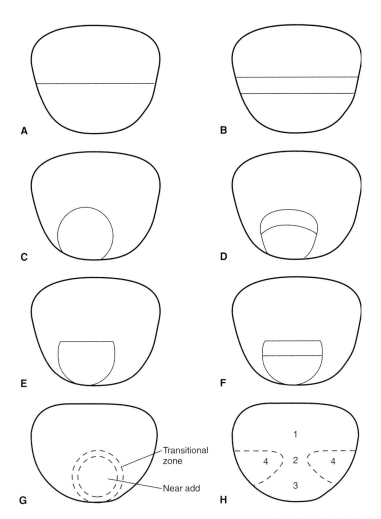

Figure 5-20 Common multifocal lens styles. **A, B,** Executive bifocal and trifocal. **C, D,** Round-top bifocal and trifocal. **E, F,** Flat-top ("D" segment) bifocal and trifocal. **G,** Invisible, or blended, bifocal. **H,** Progressive-addition multifocal lens showing (1) distance correction, (2) the corridor of increasing plus power, (3) maximum plus power of the near segment, and (4) the zone of significant distortion.

Interpupillary Distance

It is important to know the distance between the 2 pupils so as to align and center spectacle lenses properly. Make adjustments for the *interpupillary distance* (IPD) measurement when you use either a trial frame or a phoropter.

An effective and rapid method for measuring the IPD is to stand directly in front of the patient, hold a millimeter ruler (with the numbers facing you) at arm's length, and steady it on the base of the patient's nose. Instruct the patient to look directly into your left eye; you then close your right eye as you align the 0 mark of the ruler with the nasal border of the patient's right pupil. Next, without moving the ruler, instruct the patient to look into your right eye. Close your left eye and note the position of the temporal border of the patient's left pupil. The distance between the nasal border of 1 pupil and the temporal border of the other is a usable estimate of the IPD. Remember to align your left eye with the patient's right eye and your right eye with the patient's left eye. Do not stand close enough to the patient to induce excessive convergence, or you will under-estimate the IPD by several millimeters. The IPD should be adjusted on the phoropter or the trial lens frame before retinoscopy is performed. Most trial frames require each eyepiece to be adjusted separately, while most phoropters have a single knob that adjusts the 2 eyepieces simultaneously.

More than 90% of adults have IPDs between 60 mm and 68 mm. This measurement is not exactly the same as the geometric IPD, which is of importance only when high-power lenses are being fit. If lenses over 4.00 D are decentered, sufficient prism may be induced to affect binocular viewing. Usually the nose is midway between the 2 pupils, but occasionally there is significant facial asymmetry. If this is the case, special fitting adjustments must be made. More detailed discussion of IPD determination and optical centration measurements can be found in the reference books listed at the end of this chapter.

Pitfalls and Pointers

- The examiner's eyes and the patient's eyes must be properly aligned with each other for retinoscopy. If they are not, the prescription will be inaccurate, and aber-rations from the patient's lens, glare, and extraneous reflections will interfere with the accuracy of retinoscopic measurements. In addition, the examiner might de-velop back or neck strain after repeated examinations.

- Retinoscopy is easier to perform if cycloplegia is used and the patient's pupils are dilated.

- Remember that retinoscopic "with" motion indicates the need for plus-power lenses to be added, whereas "against" motion indicates the need for minus-power lenses to be added.

- If an irregular reflex or a very dull reflex is noted in retinoscopy, suspect high my-opia or hyperopia, keratoconus, other surface irregularities, cataract or other media opacity, a dirty lens, or a dim bulb in the retinoscope.

- *Manifest* means "without cycloplegia." This term is often incorrectly used as syn-onymous with subjective refraction. If the refraction is done under cycloplegia, this should be noted. Subjective refinement of all refractions is generally assumed unless the refraction is identified specifically as retinoscopy.

- When the patient is asked whether lens choice number 1 or number 2 is better or whether they are the same, the patient may say that it is impossible to choose. Encourage a preference until the patient states that the 2 choices are equal. Patients sometimes think that they have performed poorly because they cannot decide which lenses are preferable. Explain that you were specifically looking for the point at which they could see no difference and that therefore they actually per-formed very well.

- Although retinoscopy and subjective refraction seem to be difficult techniques to perform, with practice they become manageable and part of your everyday exam-ination skills. Don't be discouraged if they seem bewildering at first.

Suggested Resources

Clinical Optics. Basic and Clinical Science Course, Section 3. American Academy of Ophthalmology; published annually.

Corboy JM. *The Retinoscopy Book: An Introductory Manual for Eye Care Professionals*. 5th ed. Slack; 2003.

Hunter DG, West CE. *Last-Minute Optics: A Concise Review of Optics, Refraction, and Contact Lenses.* 2nd ed. Slack; 2010.

Kolker RJ, Kolker AF. *Subjective Refraction and Prescribing Glasses.* 3rd ed. Slack; 2018.

Orge FH, Epley KD. *Retinoscopy Simulator* [an online interactive simulator designed for students to learn and practice the principles of retinoscopy] Available on the American Academy of Ophthalmology web site at www.aao.org/interactive-tool/retinoscopy-simulator. Accessed September 15, 2020.

Pediatric Eye Evaluations [Preferred Practice Pattern]. American Academy of Ophthalmology; 2017. Accessed September 15, 2020. https://www.aao.org/preferred-practice-pattern/pediatric-eye-evaluations-ppp-2017

Refractive Errors and Refractive Surgery [Preferred Practice Pattern]. American Academy of Ophthalmology; 2017. Accessed September 15, 2020. https://www.aao.org/preferred-practice-pattern/refractive-errors-refractive-surgery-ppp-2017

CLINICAL PROTOCOL 5-1

Using the Manual Lensmeter

Focusing the Eyepiece

The focus of the lensmeter eyepiece must be verified each time the instrument is used.

1. Ensure that there is no lens in place in the lensmeter, and then look through the eyepiece of the instrument. Turn the power drum until the mires (perpendicular crossed lines) viewed through the eyepiece are grossly out of focus.
2. Turn the eyepiece in a plus direction, normally counterclockwise. This will fog (blur) the target seen through the eyepiece.
3. Slowly turn the eyepiece in the opposite direction until the target is clear, then stop turning. This procedure focuses the eyepiece.
4. Turn the power drum to focus the mires. The mires should focus at a power drum reading of 0 (plano). If this does not occur, repeat the procedure.

Positioning the Eyeglasses

1. Place the lower rim of the eyeglasses on the movable spectacle table, with the temple pieces facing away from you. You are now prepared to read

the back surface of the lens, normally the appropriate surface from which to measure.

2. Looking through the eyepiece, align the eyeglass lens so that the mires cross in the center of the target by moving the eyeglass lens on the spectacle table.

Measuring Sphere and Cylinder Power

The following steps describe the plus-cylinder technique:

1. Turn the power drum to read "high minus" (about −10.00 D).

2. Bring the closely spaced mires (often called "single lines") into sharp focus by rotating the power drum counterclockwise while at the same time rotating the cylinder wheel to straighten the single lines where they cross the widely spaced perpendicular set of mires (often called "triple lines").

3. If the single lines and the triple lines come into focus at the same time, the lens is a sphere (Figure 1). If only the single lines come into focus, you have identified the sphere portion of a spherocylinder. Record the power drum reading at this point as the power of the sphere.

4. If cylinder power is present, after noting the power drum reading for the sphere, measure cylinder power by moving the power drum further counterclockwise (less minus, or more plus), to bring the triple lines into sharp focus (Figure 2).

5. Calculate the difference between the first power drum reading for the focused single lines and the second power drum reading for the focused triple lines. Record this figure as the plus-cylinder power of the lens.

6. Read the axis of the cylinder from the cylinder axis wheel.

Video 1 demonstrates neutralization of spectacles.

 VIDEO 1   Neutralization of Spectacles
Courtesy of Lindreth G. DuBois, MEd, MMSc, CO, COMT.

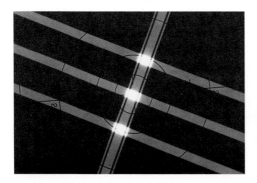

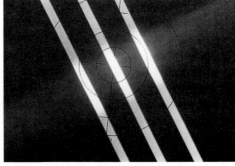

Figure 1 Measuring sphere.   **Figure 2** Measuring cylinder power.

CLINICAL PROTOCOL 5-2

Measuring Bifocal Power

1. After you measure the sphere and cylinder distance portion of a bifocal eyeglass lens, center the bifocal add at the bottom of the lens in the lensmeter gimbal (the ringlike frame) and refocus on the triple lines.
2. The difference between the distance reading of the triple-line focus and the new triple-line focus is the add, or bifocal power.
3. If the distance portion of the eyeglass lens is a sphere, refocus the bifocal segment and calculate the algebraic difference between the power in the top segment and the power in the bifocal.
4. For a trifocal lens, follow the same procedure as for the bifocal segment to measure the trifocal segment directly. Customarily, a trifocal is one-half the power of the bifocal.

Note: This method is applicable to standard bifocals. Progressive-addition lenses (also known as variable focus lenses or "lineless bifocals") are read according to the manufacturer's directions. Many have the power of the add imprinted on the lens itself.

CLINICAL PROTOCOL 5-3

Measuring Prism Power and Orientation

The existence of prescribed prism power in a spectacle lens generally is revealed when the lensmeter mires cannot be centered in the central portion of the lensmeter target. Once you have determined the presence of a prism, measure prism power and determine orientation as follows:

1. With a nonpermanent marker, mark the position on the lens through which the patient is viewing while they are looking straight ahead. Center this mark in the lensmeter target.
2. Count the number of black concentric circles from the central cross of the lensmeter target to the center of the vertical and/or horizontal crossed mires (Figure 1). Each circle represents 1 prism diopter.
3. Record the direction of the thick portion (base) of the prism by determining the direction of the displacement of the mires. For example, if the mires are displaced upward, the prism base is base up. Downward displacement indicates base-down prism, displacement toward the nose indicates base-in prism, and displacement toward the temples indicates base-out prism.

Prism-compensating devices are incorporated into some lensmeters. Such devices permit the measurement of prism without use of the concentric circles. To avoid recording prism power that is not actually present when you use these devices, be sure that the prism-compensating device is set to 0. Auxiliary prisms are available for use with some lensmeters to assist in measuring lenses with prism power greater than the number of concentric circles.

Figure 1 Measuring prism power. In this figure of the right lens, the mires are displaced toward the nose and fall on the second concentric circle (labeled "2" and circled in red here). This lens has 2$^{\Delta}$ base in prism.

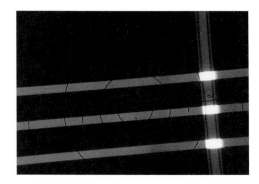

CLINICAL PROTOCOL 5-4

Measuring Optical Centration of Spectacle Lenses

At times, it is important to be able to note the proper position of the optical center of a spectacle lens in order to see if it lines up appropriately with a patient's pupils. Most lensmeters have a marking or dotting device that can be used to mark temporarily the optical center of a spectacle lens. The technique for checking optical centers is as follows:

1. Place the spectacle lens against the lens stop of the lensmeter.
2. Make certain the eyeglasses frame sits squarely on the spectacle table, rim down, temple pieces away from you.
3. Focus the mires and center them with the focused eyepiece target (Figure 1). Use the dotting device to mark the lens while it is held in this

Figure 1 Measuring optical centration of the spectacle lens.

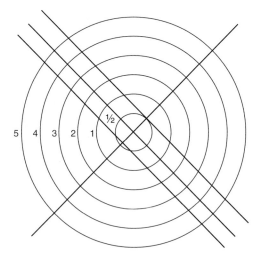

position. The center line (of the 3 lines) is the optical center of the lens. If the lensmeter does not have a dotting device, use a nonpermanent marker to record the approximate center of the lens by noting the point at which the lensmeter light source shines through the eyeglass lens.

CLINICAL PROTOCOL 5-5

Measuring Vertex Distance

1. Ask the seated patient to close both eyes.
2. Gently rest the fixed caliper arm of the distometer on the closed eyelid and carefully place the movable caliper arm against the back surface of the trial lens, phoropter lens, or the patient's eyeglass lens (see Figure 5-16).
3. Record the separation distance between these 2 surfaces from the millimeter scale on the distometer. (The scale allows for an average eyelid thickness.)

▶ *This chapter includes related videos, which can be accessed by scanning the QR codes provided in the text or going to aao.org/PracticalOphthalmologyvideo.*

☝ *This chapter includes related activities, which can be accessed by scanning the QR codes provided in the text or going to aao.org/PracticalOphthalmologyactivity.*

In an ocular alignment and motility examination, the patient is tested for 3 principal properties of the visual system: binocularity (fusion), ocular alignment, and eye movement (motility). Because the subject is complex, this chapter begins with a discussion of commonly used terminology and basic extraocular muscle function before specific examination techniques for assessing binocularity, alignment, and motility are discussed.

Strabismus Terminology

Strabismus is a general term used to describe a misalignment of the eyes in which both eyes are not directed at the object of regard. The Greek word *strabismus* means to squint, to look obliquely or askance; in some countries other than the United States, the terms "strabismus" and "squint" are used interchangeably. Strabismus either can cause or be caused by the absence of binocular vision. *Binocular vision* is the ability of the visual cortex and related pathways to converge the 2-dimensional input from each eye into a single, 3-dimensional visual perception.

Amblyopia is a term used to describe loss of vision due to abnormal visual input in childhood. In physiologic terms, amblyopia represents a failure in the development of cortical visual connections from disuse or an inability to form a clearly focused retinal image during the first few years of life, a critical period in the development of the visual pathways. Strabismus can lead to amblyopia, and amblyopia can lead to strabismus.

A number of terms are used to classify and describe strabismus. Strabismus is called *comitant* when the angle of misalignment is approximately equal in all directions of gaze. Strabismus is called *incomitant* when the angle of misalignment varies with the direction of gaze, such as in the case of a sixth cranial nerve palsy.

Strabismus is further classified as either a heterophoria or a heterotropia. A *phoria* (or *heterophoria*) is a latent tendency toward misalignment that occurs only when binocularity is interrupted, such as when 1 eye is occluded. During binocular viewing, the eyes of a patient with a heterophoria are perfectly aligned. The term "strabismus" usually refers to a *tropia* (or *heterotropia*), a manifest deviation that is present when both

85

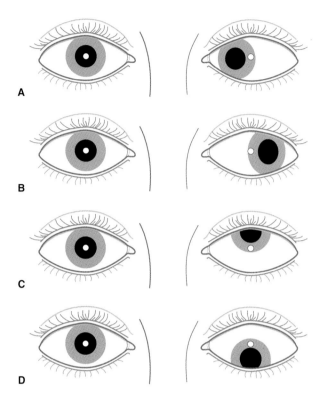

Figure 6-1 Types of heterotropia. **A,** Esotropia. **B,** Exotropia. **C,** Left hypertropia. **D,** Right hypertropia (left hypotropia).

eyes are open (Figure 6-1). A heterotropia that is present only part of the time is called *intermittent,* whereas one that is always present is called *constant.*

Heterotropias and heterophorias are subdivided according to the direction of the deviation. *Esotropia,* a manifest strabismus in which the nonfixating eye is deviated toward the nose, is the most common type of ocular misalignment of childhood. *Exotropia,* in which the nonfixating eye deviates outward toward the temple, is more likely to be intermittent than esotropia. An upward deviation of an eye is called *hypertropia.* By convention, a vertical deviation is referred to as a *right* or *left* hypertropia according to the higher eye, whether or not that eye is the one used for fixation. In reality, if the patient uses the higher eye to fixate, the fellow eye will be hypotropic, but the term *hypotropia* is less commonly used. Table 6-1 lists clinical abbreviations commonly used in the evaluation of strabismus.

Motility Terminology

Eye movements can be monocular (1 eye only) or binocular (both eyes together). Monocular eye movements are called ductions, and 6 terms are used to describe them:

- *adduction* (movement of the eye nasally)
- *abduction* (movement of the eye temporally)
- *elevation* (movement of the eye upward)

Table 6-1   Clinical Abbreviations Used in Evaluation of Strabismus

Alignment of the Eyes	Abbreviation	Usage
Esodeviations	E	Esophoria for distance
	ET	Esotropia for distance
	E(T)	Intermittent esotropia for distance
	E' or ET' or E(T)'	Esodeviations for near
Exodeviations	X	Exophoria for distance
	XT	Exotropia for distance
	X(T)	Intermittent exotropia for distance
	X' or XT' or X(T)'	Exodeviations for near
Hyperdeviations[a]	H	Hyperphoria for distance
	HT	Hypertropia for distance
	H(T)	Intermittent hypertropia for distance
	H' or HT' or H(T)'	Hyperdeviations for near
Extraocular muscles[a]	IO	Inferior oblique
	IR	Inferior rectus
	LR	Lateral rectus
	MR	Medial rectus
	SO	Superior oblique
	SR	Superior rectus
Other abbreviations	Ortho	Orthophoria, no deviation present
	DHD, DVD	Dissociated horizontal deviation, dissociated vertical deviation
	IPD	Interpupillary distance
	NPA	Near point of accommodation
	NPC	Near point of convergence
	OA, UA	Overaction, underaction
	PD	Prism diopters or pupillary distance (meaning is clear from context)

[a]L (left) or R (right) generally precedes these abbreviations.

- *depression* (movement of the eye downward)
- *intorsion*/incyclotorsion (nasal rotation of the superior vertical corneal meridian)
- *extorsion*/excyclotorsion (temporal rotation of the superior vertical corneal meridian)

Binocular eye movements are described as versions and vergences. *Versions* are binocular eye movements in the same direction (eg, to the right, to the left, etc.). One muscle of each eye is primarily responsible for the movement of that eye into a particular field of gaze. Two simultaneously acting muscles (1 from each eye) working to move both eyes in the same direction are called *yoke muscles,* and their movement is said to be *conjugate.* For example, the right medial rectus and the left lateral rectus work together to move the eyes to the left. The 6 positions of gaze in which yoke muscles act together, known as the *cardinal fields of gaze,* are right and up, right, right and down, left and up, left, and left and down (Figure 6-2).

Vergences are normal, disconjugate binocular eye movements in which the eyes move in opposite directions in order to maintain single binocular vision. The primary types of vergences routinely evaluated are *convergence,* the movement of both eyes nasally, and *divergence,* the movement of both eyes temporally.

Figure 6-2 The cardinal positions of gaze and the yoke muscles acting in those positions.

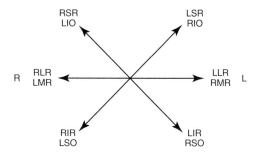

Function of the Extraocular Muscles

There are 7 extraocular muscles: 4 rectus muscles, 2 oblique muscles, and the levator palpebrae superioris muscle. The rectus and oblique muscles move the globe, whereas the levator muscle primarily moves the eyelid and only indirectly affects ocular motility. The relative positions of the extraocular muscles are shown in Figure 6-3.

The medial rectus and the lateral rectus muscles have only horizontal actions. Contraction of the medial rectus muscle results in adduction and contraction of the lateral rectus results in abduction. The superior rectus and the inferior rectus muscles originate nasally relative to their insertions and hence provide more complex motility action. In the primary position of gaze (fixating straight ahead on an object at infinity), the primary action of the superior rectus is elevation; its secondary actions are adduction and intorsion. In primary position, the primary action of the inferior rectus is depression; its secondary actions are adduction and extorsion.

The oblique muscles, as their names indicate, insert into the sclera at oblique angles. The superior oblique muscle passes through the trochlea, a cartilaginous pulley located on the superonasal orbital rim, before inserting in the posterosuperior quadrant of the globe. In primary position, the primary action of the superior oblique muscle is intorsion;

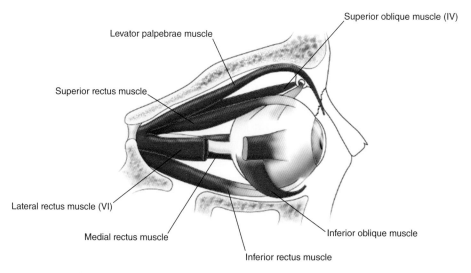

Figure 6-3 The extraocular muscles of the right eye. (Illustration used with permission of The University of Texas Southwestern Medical Center.)

Table 6-2   Actions of Extraocular Muscles from Primary Position

Muscle	Action	Muscle	Action
Superior rectus	Elevation Adduction Intorsion	Inferior rectus	Depression Adduction Extorsion
Superior oblique	Intorsion Depression Abduction	Inferior oblique	Extorsion Elevation Abduction
Medial rectus	Adduction	Lateral rectus	Abduction

secondarily it provides depression (especially in adduction) and abduction. The inferior oblique inserts posterolaterally on the globe near the macula. In primary position, its primary action is extorsion; secondarily it provides elevation (especially in adduction) and abduction. Table 6-2 summarizes the basic actions of the extraocular muscles, and Activity 6-1 demonstrates their use.

ACTIVITY 6-1 Extraocular Muscles
Access all *Practical Ophthalmology* activities at www.aao.org/Practical Ophthalmologyactivity.

Ocular Motility Examination

A thorough history is an essential part of the examination of a patient suspected of having strabismus. As the history is obtained, the examiner has the opportunity to observe the patient in a relaxed, casual manner. Particular attention should be paid to the presence of any unusual head position or movement, and the examiner should note direction of such movement and whether it manifests as a head tilt or a head turn. It is also important to note any tendency of the patient to close 1 or both eyes partially or completely.

The examiner should obtain information about the birth history and subsequent development of the patient, especially if the patient is a child. Areas of particular interest regarding a child include a history of prematurity, known intrauterine infections, genetic syndromes, and developmental delay. The examiner should also obtain information regarding any medications currently being used, or medications used by the mother during pregnancy. It is important to document the age of onset of the strabismus (old photographs can be invaluable in this regard) as well as whether it is constant or intermittent, present at distance or near or both, alternating or unilateral, or worse when the child is tired or ill. Previous treatment by patching, atropine, glasses, prisms, or surgery should be documented. In the case of an older patient, information should be obtained about double vision, the patient's general health, and any history of trauma or medical problems such as diabetes, thyroid disease, or prior surgeries in and around the eyes. In all cases, the examiner should ask about any family history of strabismus or amblyopia.

Overview of Examination

To begin, it is important to make note of visual acuity, as patients with poor vision may not be able to follow fixation targets normally used to test ocular motility and alignment. Tests of binocularity, such as the Titmus fly stereopsis test, are best performed before any test that involves covering one eye, since dissociation of the eyes by monocular occlusion may influence the results of tests of binocularity. Next, versions are tested; this is the evaluation of the ocular movements into the cardinal and midline positions. The ocular alignment is then assessed at distance and near fixations. If a deviation is present, it is measured, preferably with use of prism and cover testing.

Evaluation of Eye Movements

Clinical Protocol 6-1 describes the assessment of ocular motility. The phrase *diagnostic positions of gaze* is applied to the composite of all gaze positions and movements. Common positions of gaze are referred to as follows:

- *primary position*—straight ahead with the head straight
- *cardinal positions*—6 positions in which the prime mover of each eye is 1 muscle (together termed *yoke muscles*): up and right, up and left, right, left, down and right, down and left (Figure 6-2)
- *midline positions*—straight up and down from the primary position

Measuring Strabismus

Strabismus is measured with prisms and quantified in prism diopters. An ophthalmic prism is a wedge of clear plastic or glass with a triangular cross section that has an apex and a base (see Chapter 5). Prism power is measured by the number of centimeters of deflection of a light ray measured 1 meter from the prism and abbreviated as PD (for "prism diopters") or by the superscript delta symbol ($^\Delta$). The notation PD or $^\Delta$ is appended to the numeric measurement of the deviation.

Plastic prisms should be held with the rear surface perpendicular to the direction of the fixation object along the line of sight. This is the frontal plane position, and it closely approximates the angle of minimum deviation. Glass prisms should be held with the rear surface perpendicular to the eye's visual axis or parallel to the iris plane (Prentice position). Prisms are available singly or as bars of small horizontally or vertically oriented prisms that are attached to each other in order of increasing strength.

Tests of Alignment

The most commonly used methods of assessing and quantifying ocular alignment are the red reflex (Brückner) test, corneal light reflex test, and cover tests. Corneal light reflex tests are typically used with patients who have poor fixation or who are unable to cooperate sufficiently for cover testing. Cover tests require that the patient be able to cooperate and fixate with each eye on a target so that accommodation can be controlled and the eyes will make accurate refixation movements during testing. For measuring a deviation, the examiner should choose the best test that the patient can perform, in descending order: (1) prism and cover testing, (2) Krimsky test, and (3) Hirschberg test.

Activity 6-2 is helpful for learning and practicing strabismus evaluation.

 ACTIVITY 6-2 Strabismus Simulator

Red Reflex Test

The red reflex test, also referred to as the *Brückner test,* is the most rapid but the least sensitive test for detecting strabismus. It is performed by using the direct ophthalmoscope, with the bright white light and the lenses set to plano (0 D), to obtain a red reflex simultaneously in both eyes. If strabismus is present, the deviated eye will have a different reflex (lighter, darker, brighter, or dimmer) than that of the fixating eye, depending on the underlying problem (Figure 6-4). This test can also identify differences in the red reflexes when there are opacities in the visual axis (eg, cataracts, retinoblastoma) and moderate to severe anisometropia, and is often used by pediatricians to screen for ocular problems.

Corneal Light Reflex Tests

The corneal light reflex test compares the position of the corneal light reflex in both eyes. In normally aligned eyes, the reflexes should be symmetric on both corneas and in the same position relative to the pupil. Observation of the corneal light reflex constitutes an objective assessment of ocular alignment. For very young and/or uncooperative children, this might be the only feasible way of testing for and measuring strabismus. The most commonly used tests to measure ocular alignment with use of the corneal light reflex are the Hirschberg and Krimsky tests.

Hirschberg test

The Hirschberg test gives an estimation of ocular alignment by directly analyzing the degree of decentration of the corneal light reflex. Figure 6-5 illustrates estimated deviations, and Clinical Protocol 6-2 describes how to measure ocular alignment with the Hirschberg test. This technique is based on the fact that every millimeter of decentration is equal to roughly 7°, or 15$^\Delta$, of deviation off of the visual axis. A light reflex at the pupillary margin (2 mm from the pupillary center) is equal to approximately 15° (30$^\Delta$) of deviation; a reflex in the middle of the iris indicates a deviation of about 30° (60$^\Delta$); and a reflex at the limbus is equivalent to a deviation of 45° (90$^\Delta$).

Krimsky test

The Krimsky test utilizes reflexes from both corneas and is the preferred approach for assessing ocular deviation in a patient with poor vision in the deviating eye. Reflexes from both eyes are produced by an appropriately placed penlight that is centered on the

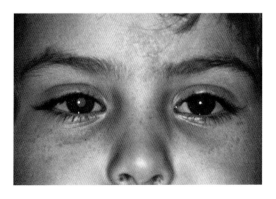

Figure 6-4   The red reflex test. This child has an esodeviation, as evidenced by the lighter, brighter reflex in the nonfixating right eye.

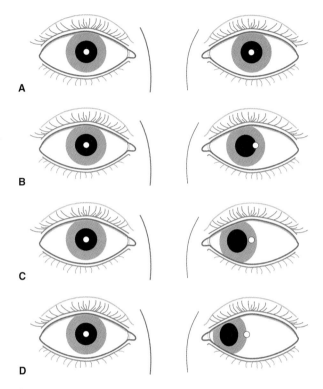

Figure 6-5   Hirschberg test: performing the corneal light reflex test to estimate deviation.
A, Normal alignment. **B,** Pupillary margin, 30ᐃ (15°) esotropia. **C,** Mid-iris, 60ᐃ (30°) esotropia.
D, Limbus, 90ᐃ (45°) esotropia.

patient's fixating eye. Prisms of increasing or decreasing power are placed in front of the fixating eye until the corneal reflection is centered on the deviating eye (Figure 6-6). Clinical Protocol 6-3 summarizes the Krimsky test, and Video 6-1 demonstrates it.

 VIDEO 6-1   Krimsky Test
Courtesy of Steven M. Archer, MD, and Kristina Tarczy-Hornoch, MD, DPhil.
Access all *Practical Ophthalmology* videos at www.aao.org
/PracticalOphthalmologyvideo.

Cover Tests

Cover tests are the most accurate for detection and quantification of strabismus, but they require a high degree of cooperation from the patient and an ability to maintain constant fixation on a target for each eye under monocular conditions. For cover tests to be meaningful, the examiner must closely scrutinize the patient's eye movements when 1 eye is occluded. For a young child, the fixation target can be a toy or a small picture, and several different targets presented in sequence may be needed to keep the child's attention and ensure good fixation. Each eye must be able to move adequately when it fixates. Cover tests are performed at both distance and near, typically 20 feet (6 m) and 14 inches (33 cm), ideally with the patient's refractive correction. In certain situations, it may be useful to measure and compare the deviation both with and without refractive

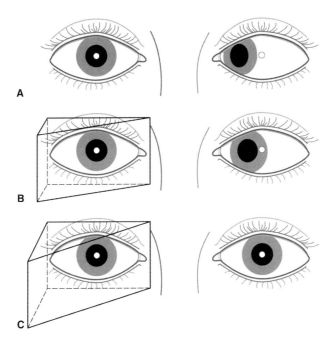

Figure 6-6   Krimsky test: estimating deviation. A decentered corneal light reflex in the left eye **(A)** is gradually centered by placing progressively stronger prisms in front of the fixating right eye **(B, C)**.

correction. A standard occluder should be used, but at times the examiner might need to use their hand or fingers as the occluder.

The cover-uncover test is performed first to establish the presence of a manifest deviation (heterotropia). If no manifest deviation is present, the cross-cover test is then performed to detect a latent deviation (heterophoria).

Cover-uncover test

Clinical Protocol 6-4 describes how to perform the cover-uncover test. This test is usually done with the patient in an upright, seated position, but it can be done with a bedridden patient. The only necessary condition is that the patient be able to maintain fixation with each eye individually on a target. As 1 eye is covered, the examiner observes the opposite, uncovered eye carefully for any movement. If the uncovered eye moves to pick up fixation, a heterotropia is present. Concentrate on the uncovered eye and ignore any movement of the covered eye after the cover is removed. Some patients start with straight eyes prior to the cover-uncover test but develop an overt deviation during or after testing, which indicates that their fusion is easily disrupted. Such a patient has an intermittent heterotropia. For intermittent heterotropias, the corresponding deviation should be denoted with parentheses, for example: X(T) or E(T), as appropriate. Video 6-2 demonstrates the cover-uncover test.

VIDEO 6-2   Cover-Uncover Test
Courtesy of Steven M. Archer, MD, and Kristina Tarczy-Hornoch, MD, DPhil.

Cross-cover test

The cross-cover test is performed by alternately covering each of the patient's eyes without allowing binocular fixation. A deviation that is detected by the cross-cover test that is not detectable by the cover-uncover test is by definition a phoria. When a tropia is present, the cross-cover test demonstrates the total deviation, a combination of the latent (phoria) and manifest (tropia) deviations. The cross-cover test is a dissociative test; therefore, it often results in a deviation considerably larger than the amount initially noted with the cover-uncover test. Video 6-3 demonstrates the cross-cover test; results of the cross-cover test are recorded as in the examples in Table 6-3.

 VIDEO 6-3 Cross-Cover Test (Alternate Cover Test)
Courtesy of Steven M. Archer, MD, and Kristina Tarczy-Hornoch, MD, DPhil.

Prism alternate cover test

The prism alternate cover test is used to quantify the amount of strabismus present. It measures the total deviation, both latent (phoria) and manifest (tropia). It is similar to the cross-cover test in that each eye is alternately covered. A prism is introduced to measure the deviation. Clinical Protocol 6-5 describes the technique for performing the prism alternate cover test, and Video 6-4 demonstrates it.

 VIDEO 6-4 Prism Alternate Cover Test
Courtesy of Steven M. Archer, MD, and Kristina Tarczy-Hornoch, MD, DPhil.

Simultaneous prism-cover test

In some patients, the amount of deviation measured by the prism alternate cover test is considerably larger than the deviation that is usually manifest (ie, the deviation "builds" with the alternate cover test). In these cases, the simultaneous prism-cover test is helpful in determining the actual heterotropia present when both eyes are uncovered. It is performed by covering the fixating eye at the same time that the prism is placed in front of the deviating eye. The test is repeated using successively larger (or smaller) prism powers until the deviated eye no longer shifts when the fixating eye is covered; see Video 6-5 for a demonstration.

 VIDEO 6-5 Simultaneous Prism Alternate Cover Test
Courtesy of Steven M. Archer, MD, and Kristina Tarczy-Hornoch, MD, DPhil.

Table 6-3   Sample Recording Results of Alternate Cover Testing

Example 1		Example 2	
$\overline{cc}$	XT 30$^\Delta$	$\overline{sc}$	RET' 10$^\Delta$ builds to 30$^\Delta$
	X(T)' 20$^\Delta$	$\overline{cc}$	RE(T)' 5$^\Delta$
This example describes a patient wearing corrective lenses (*cc*) who has a constant exotropia of 30 prism diopters at distance and intermittent exotropia of 20 prism diopters at near (near = ').		This example describes a patient who, when not wearing glasses (*sc*), shows a constant right esotropia at near of 10 prism diopters that increases to 30 prism diopters with alternate cover testing. When this patient wears glasses, the right esotropia becomes intermittent and is reduced to 5 prism diopters.	

Other Considerations with Alignment Tests

It is important to document the fixation preference in patients with strabismus, as this can have implications in both obtaining measurements and treatment planning. Clinical Protocol 6-6 outlines how to assess fixation preference in patients with strabismus.

Parents of young children sometimes voice concern about an infant's ocular alignment when no true deviation is present. Often these parents have observed *pseudostrabismus,* which is an artificial appearance of misaligned eyes. Pseudoesotropia usually results from prominent epicanthal folds, a wide nasal bridge, or both. In these cases, the corneal light reflex will be centered when measured by the Hirschberg test and there will be no deviation detectable by the cover-uncover test.

Pseudoexotropia usually results from *positive angle kappa,* which is a disparity between the visual axis and the anatomical axis of the eye (Figure 6-7). The corneal light reflex will appear to be decentered if angle kappa is present, but there is no deviation measured by cover-uncover or cross-cover testing. Nasal decentration simulates an exotropia (positive angle kappa) and temporal decentration simulates an esotropia (negative angle kappa). A mild degree of positive angle kappa is a common finding in many individuals with normal vision.

A patient may present with an anomalous head position that is caused by strabismus. Head tilts and head turns should be recorded, and the examiner should measure and note any strabismus both in primary position (ie, with the head positioned straight) as well as in the anomalous head position.

At times, the examiner will intentionally tilt the patient's head to obtain measurements, most often as part of the evaluation of cyclovertical muscles. This technique is particularly useful to diagnose superior oblique palsies as part of the 3-step test, which involves an assessment of the alignment of the eyes in primary position, in far-right and

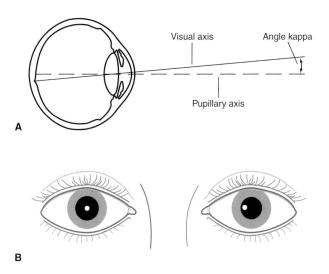

Figure 6-7 Positive angle kappa. **A,** Horizontal section of the right eye. Positive angle kappa is a disparity between the visual and anatomical (pupillary) axes of the eye. In this case, the fovea is slightly temporal to the pupillary axis, and the corneal light reflex is slightly nasal to the center of the cornea. **B,** There is nasal displacement of the corneal light reflex, but no deviation on cover testing.

Figure 6-8   An example of a diagram used to record the ocular motility and alignment. In this case, the patient has an abduction deficit of the left eye with an incomitant esotropia that is worse in left gaze; this is consistent with a partial or recovering left sixth cranial nerve palsy.

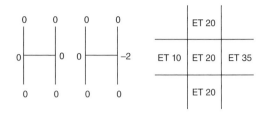

far-left gaze, and with the head tilted to the right and to the left. A detailed description of the technique used to perform the 3-step test can be found in the Basic and Clinical Science Course Section 6, *Pediatric Ophthalmology and Strabismus.*

Many schemes have been devised for recording the findings of alignment testing. One example is illustrated in Figure 6-8. Notation can be made on such a schematic drawing, but the patient's head should be properly aligned before cover test measurements are taken. When measurements are taken with the patient's head in another position, even if it is their habitual position, it should be noted.

The presence of any *nystagmus* (involuntary rhythmic eye movements) should be noted. Latent (occlusion) nystagmus is a conjugate, horizontal jerk nystagmus that occurs under monocular viewing conditions. In this condition, when 1 eye is occluded (as is done for cover testing), nystagmus develops in both eyes, with the fast phase directed toward the uncovered eye.

Accommodative convergence of the visual axes occurs as part of the near reflex. A fairly consistent increment of accommodative convergence (AC) occurs for each diopter of accommodation (A), and the relationship can be expressed as the accommodative convergence/accommodation (AC/A) ratio. The normal AC/A ratio is 3^{Δ} to 5^{Δ} of accommodative convergence for each diopter of accommodation. Abnormalities of this ratio can occur in childhood and are an important cause of strabismus. If the AC/A ratio is abnormally high, the excess convergence tends to produce esotropia during accommodation or focusing on near targets. If the AC/A ratio is abnormally low, the eyes will tend to have an exodeviation when the individual looks at near targets. For a detailed discussion of the clinical implications of this interrelationship, refer to the resources referenced at the end of this chapter.

Tests of Binocularity and Fusion

The ability to use both eyes together is referred to as *fusion* or *single binocular vision.* Single binocular vision results from simultaneous stimulation of corresponding retinal elements that have the same visual direction. For example, an object to a person's left stimulates a spot on the temporal retina of the right eye and a corresponding spot on the nasal retina of the left eye. The brain then perceives the object as a single image in space.

Subjective testing of the patient's fusional ability is an important part of the ocular examination. Such tests evaluate both stereopsis and gross binocular status.

Stereopsis

The term *stereopsis* refers to the simultaneous use of the eyes to perceive details of depth that occur when slightly disparate (noncorresponding) retinal elements are stimulated at the same time. In this way, we order things in space and judge relative nearness of objects. This is distinct from the monocular cues such as overlay of contours and sizes of known objects that allow appreciation of gross depth perception. *Sensory fusion* describes the ability of the brain to blend (fuse) separate images from both eyes into a single image. *Suppression* is active central inhibition of the images that originate from 1 eye; this prevents diplopia in the presence of strabismus. Sensory fusion is necessary to achieve high-grade stereopsis, often referred to as at least 40 seconds of arc (stereoacuity is always quantified in seconds of arc). Patients without demonstrable stereopsis use monocular cues for depth perception, such as differences in sizes of familiar objects. It is possible to fuse without having high-grade stereopsis but not possible to have high-grade stereopsis without sensory fusion.

The tests used to measure stereopsis consist of either polarized images or random-dot stereograms that may be nonpolarized or polarized. Figure 6-9 illustrates the Titmus (fly) test, which is the most common test for near stereopsis. Clinical Protocol 6-7 summarizes the procedure for the Titmus stereoacuity test.

Other Tests of Binocular Status

Several other tests are performed for the evaluation of binocular status. Those most commonly used are the Worth 4-dot test, the Maddox rod test, the Double Maddox rod test, and the 4^Δ base-out test. Because of the subjective nature of the responses to these tests, more than 1 type of test is often performed to confirm or refute the findings. The least dissociative test, or the test that allows the patient to see the same or a very similar image with each eye, will give a response that most closely approximates everyday seeing conditions.

Worth 4-dot test

The Worth 4-dot test, which is performed at both distance and near, provides information about the patient's gross binocular status and identifies the presence of a suppression scotoma. The patient wears a pair of eyeglasses with a red filter over 1 eye and a green

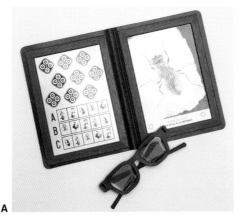
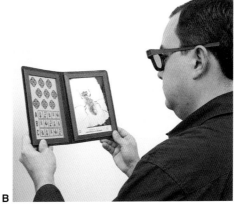

Figure 6-9 The Titmus stereopsis test. **A,** Light-polarizing eyeglasses and targets. **B,** The patient views the target through polarizing filters and reports perception of depth. (Photos by Dan McGarrah.)

filter over the other eye. Traditionally, the red filter is placed in front of the right eye and the green filter in front of the left eye. Red light is visible to the eye behind the red lens, but green light is not visible because the red lens absorbs these wavelengths. Similarly, green light is visible to the eye behind the green lens, but red light is not visible because the green lens absorbs these wavelengths.

The patient looks at a target composed of 4 lighted circles: 1 red, 2 green, and 1 white. Patients with normal ocular alignment and normal sensory status will report seeing a total of 4 lights; this indicates fusion. When the target is presented at distance, the Worth 4-dot test tests central (foveal) fusion. When the patient views the test at near, peripheral fusion is tested. Different responses are obtained and recorded for both distance and near, noting fusion, suppression (right, left, or alternating), or diplopia. See Figure 6-10 for further explanation of this test.

The Worth 4-dot test is clinically useful in the evaluation of *monofixation syndrome*, which describes a sensory state of a central scotoma that is often related to strabismus. In

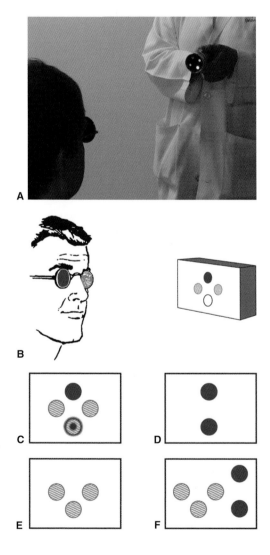

Figure 6-10 The Worth 4-dot test. **A,** The flashlight target, which illuminates the 4 dots, is held by the examiner (as shown). The same flashlight, or a wall-mounted illuminated target with a similar distribution of the 4 lights, can be used for the distance test. The patient wears the same red-green glasses for both tests. (Courtesy of Preston H. Blomquist, MD.). **B,** Looking through a pair of red-green glasses, the patient views a box with 4 lights (1 red, 2 green, 1 white) at 6 m and at 33 cm. The possible responses are as follows: **C,** Patient sees all 4 lights: Peripheral fusion with orthophoria or strabismus with anomalous retinal correspondence. The light in the 6 o'clock position is, depending on ocular dominance, predominantly red or predominantly green. It might also be reported as pink or a mixture of red and green if there is no strong preference for either eye. **D,** Patient sees 2 red lights: Suppression in left eye. **E,** Patient sees 3 green lights: Suppression in right eye. **F,** Patient sees 5 lights: Uncrossed diplopia with esotropia if the red lights appear to the right of the green lights, as in this figure; crossed diplopia with exotropia if the red lights appear to the left. If the red and green are seen in rapid succession, alternating suppression is present. (From Van Noordon GK, Campos EC. *Binocular Vision and Ocular Motility and Management of Strabismus.* 6th ed. Mosby; 2002:221.)

this condition, the Worth 4-dot test can demonstrate the absence of bifoveal fusion with the presence peripheral fusion. The result is fusion with 4 dots at near when the patient is able to view the target from outside of the central scotoma, and 2 or 3 dots at distance when the central scotoma inhibits the patient's view of the target.

Maddox rod test

The Maddox rod test is a binocular test that can be used only with patients who are able to give reliable, subjective responses. It is performed at distance and at near with a muscle light used for fixation. Patients wear their habitual corrective lenses for the test. A striated red Maddox rod is placed before the patient's preferred eye, and the patient is instructed to fixate on the light. The Maddox rod consists of multiple cylindrical lenses stacked together. As a result, when one looks through the rod at a light source, they see a line image that is perpendicular to the orientation of the rod.

Placing the striations horizontally allows the patient to see the red line vertically; placing them vertically allows the patient to see the red line horizontally. The patient is asked if they see a red line while they look at the white fixation light. There are 4 possible responses:

- The line is not seen. (Indicates suppression of the eye that is looking through the Maddox rod).
- The line goes through the light. (Indicates fusion and ocular alignment).
- The horizontal line is above or below the light. (Indicates vertical diplopia and usually the presence of a vertical deviation).
- The vertical line is to the left or to the right of the light. (Indicates horizontal diplopia and usually the presence of a horizontal deviation). The Maddox rod test is a very dissociating test and will often cause a diplopic response from a patient with a horizontal phoria.

The examiner records the patient's responses for both distance and near.

Double Maddox rod test

The double Maddox rod test is used to test for and measure cyclotropias. Maddox rods are oriented vertically and placed in front of each eye, classically with the red Maddox rod over the right eye and the white Maddox rod over the left eye. With the rods aligned vertically, the patient should see 2 horizontal lines. The patient or examiner adjusts the axes of the rods until the patient perceives the lines to be parallel. The amount and direction of angle of rotation required determines the magnitude and direction of the cyclotropia. For example, with the examiner facing the patient, if that patient adjusts either the right eye 10 degrees counterclockwise or the left eye 10 degrees clockwise, it is determined that the patient has 10 degrees of excylotorsion. Note that the amount and direction of cyclotropia is irrespective of which eye the patient adjusts. Of note, careful examination of the fundus during indirect ophthalmoscopy can also identify incyclotorsion or excyclotorsion.

4^Δ base-out test

The 4^Δ base-out test is useful to diagnose a foveal suppression scotoma in patients with a small misalignment or no apparent ocular misalignment, such as those with *monofixation syndrome*. A 4^Δ prism is placed base-out in front of 1 eye while the patient fixes on a target. The typical response in a patient with normal vision is a version movement (both eyes) followed by convergence to reestablish fusion. A patient with a foveal suppression scotoma of the contralateral eye will demonstrate a version without convergence, whereas a patient with a suppression scotoma of the ipsilateral eye will show no movement. Several atypical responses to this test have been described; it should be noted that this test is not valid when acuity is poor in either eye. The 4^Δ base-out test is discussed in greater detail in "Suggested Resources" at the end of this chapter.

Pitfalls and Pointers

- Visual acuity testing for detection of amblyopia is critical in all cases of suspected strabismus.

- A very small angle deviation might not be possible to detect with the corneal light reflex test and might even be difficult to detect with cover tests in very young children.

- The examiner must use ingenuity to keep a very young patient interested and fixating on a target. Such ploys as brightly colored toys, pictures, and storytelling about the objects are useful. A good general rule is "1 toy, 1 look." A well-prepared examiner will always have several interesting toys or pictures on hand.

- When the examiner performs cover tests, they must ensure that the patient is actually fixating on the object of regard with each eye. Inaccurate results are obtained if the patient is unable to fixate reliably on an object due to poor visual acuity or inattention.

Suggested Resources

Adult Strabismus Surgery [Clinical Statement]. American Academy of Ophthalmology; 2017.

Amblyopia [Preferred Practice Pattern]. American Academy of Ophthalmology; 2017. Accessed September 15, 2020. https://www.aao.org/preferred-practice-pattern /amblyopia-ppp-2017

Esotropia and Exotropia [Preferred Practice Pattern]. American Academy of Ophthalmology; 2017. Accessed September 15, 2020. https://www.aao.org/preferred -practice-pattern/esotropia-exotropia-ppp-2017

Orge FH. *Strabismus Simulator* [an online Interactive simulator designed to teach and allow practice of basic strabismus evaluation]. Available on the American Academy of Ophthalmology web site at www.aao.org/interactive-tool/strabismus -simulator. Accessed September 15, 2020.

Pediatric Ophthalmology and Strabismus. Basic and Clinical Science Course, Section 6. American Academy of Ophthalmology; published annually.

von Noorden GK, Campos EC. *Binocular Vision and Ocular Motility: Theory and Management of Strabismus.* 6th ed. CV Mosby Co; 2001.

Wright KW, Strube YNJ, eds. *Pediatric Ophthalmology and Strabismus.* 3rd ed. Oxford University Press; 2012.

CLINICAL PROTOCOL 6-1

Assessing Versions

1. Sit facing the patient. Hold a small fixation target at eye level about 14 inches in front of the patient; the patient should stare in primary position (straight ahead).

2. Ask the patient to follow the target as you move it into the 6 cardinal fields and then up and down along the midline. Elevate the upper eyelid with a finger on your free hand to observe movements in downgaze.

3. Note whether the amplitude of eye movements is normal or abnormal in both eyes. To record the relative underaction or overaction in each gaze position, designate normal as 0 (no overaction or underaction) and use the number 4 to designate maximum underaction or overaction. Thus, underactions are rated using a scale from −1 to −4, and overactions are rated from +1 to +4.

VIDEO 1 Motility Examination
Courtesy of Richard C. Allen, MD, PhD.

CLINICAL PROTOCOL 6-2

Performing the Corneal Light Reflex (Hirschberg) Test

1. Have the patient seated facing you; the patient's head should be straight and their eyes directed in primary gaze.

2. Hold a penlight or muscle light in front of the patient's eyes at a distance of approximately 2 feet; direct the light at the midpoint between both eyes of the patient. Align yourself with the light source. Instruct the patient to look directly at the light.

3. Compare the position of the 2 corneal light reflexes and record the estimated result as prism diopters or degrees of deviation. In parentheses beside the measurement make the notation "(by Hirschberg)."

CLINICAL PROTOCOL 6-3

Performing the Krimsky Test

1. Position the patient, the penlight, and yourself as for the Hirschberg test, above.

2. Choose a prism of a power estimated by the Hirschberg test for the deviation.

3. Place the trial prism in front of the fixating (not the deviated) eye, with the apex of the prism (narrower end) pointing in the direction of the deviation. If a prism bar is available, use it with the flat (back) surface toward the patient, and the apices of the prisms pointed in the direction of the deviation, as with single prisms.

4. Increase or decrease the strength of the trial prism until the light is reflected from each cornea symmetrically.

5. Record the strength of the prism used, and note "(by Krimsky)" beside the measurement. For example, if it was necessary to use a 30^Δ prism to center the corneal reflexes for a patient with an exotropia, record the results as follows:

XT 30^Δ (by Krimsky)

CLINICAL PROTOCOL 6-4

Performing the Cover-Uncover Test

1. Make sure that the patient's usual refractive correction is in place.

2. Have the patient look at a distance fixation target, and position yourself directly opposite the patient, within arm's reach, without obstructing the patient's view.

3. Swiftly cover the fixating eye with an occluder or your hand, and observe the other eye for any movement. Carefully note the direction of movement.

4. Uncover the eye and allow about 3 seconds for both eyes to be uncovered.

5. Swiftly cover the other eye and observe its fellow eye for any movement.

6. Ensure that the patient is maintaining fixation on the same point as established for step 1.

7. Repeat the test for near, using a near fixation point.

CLINICAL PROTOCOL 6-5

Performing the Prism Alternate Cover Test

1. Position yourself directly opposite the patient, within arm's reach, without obstructing the patient's view. With the patient seated upright and looking at a distance fixation point, rapidly shift the occluder from 1 eye to the other several times, without allowing any interval of binocularity. Make sure that each eye fixates on the target after each movement of the cover.

2. Place a prism over 1 eye (usually the patient's dominant eye) while you continue to shift the cover from 1 eye to the other. Remember to orient the prism with the apex toward the direction of deviation. If 1 of the patient's eyes does not move well, as occurs in restrictive or paretic strabismus, it is important to place the prisms over the affected eye. Choose the strength of the initial prism to approximate the deviation estimated by the position of the corneal light reflections.

3. Continue to place prisms of progressively higher power in front of the eye until no movement is noted in either eye (neutralization). To be certain

of neutralization, additional prisms may be introduced until a reversal of movement is noted. The simultaneous use of both horizontally and vertically placed prisms may be necessary to neutralize all deviations. For large deviations, 2 horizontal or 2 vertical prisms should not be stacked on each other because doing so causes significant measurement errors. Instead, prisms should be placed in front of both eyes.

4. Record the results as noted in the examples in Table 6-3; in addition, you may diagram the results in the various diagnostic positions of gaze to further describe the clinical scenario, which is helpful to display comitance or incomitance. Figure 6-8 provides an example of one type of diagram used to record ocular motility and alignment.

5. Repeat the test for near in primary position.

CLINICAL PROTOCOL 6-6

Testing Fixation Preference in Strabismic Patients

1. This test is used to detect a fixation preference (and potentially amblyopia) in a patient with strabismus. This is particularly useful in infants or nonverbal patients who are unable to provide an accurate visual acuity measurement.

2. Position the patient and present an interesting target at near fixation.

3. Determine which eye is fixating on the target (preferred eye).

4. Cover the preferred eye. Observe the shift of the fellow eye (nonpreferred eye) to assume fixation on the target.

5. Uncover the preferred eye. Determine if fixation is maintained by the previously nonpreferred eye or switches back to the preferred eye; note the timing of the fixation switch. Observe the presence or absence of a blink preceding a fixation switch.

6. Record the results as:
   a. alternates fixation (amblyopia unlikely)
   b. prefers OD/OS, holds OS/OD through a blink (amblyopia unlikely)
   c. prefers OD/OS, holds OS/OD to a blink (amblyopia suspected)
   d. prefers OD/OS, holds OS/OD briefly (amblyopia suspected)
   e. prefers OD/OS, will not hold OS/OD (amblyopia likely)

7. Repeat testing, this time with a distance target

CLINICAL PROTOCOL 6-7

Testing for Stereoacuity Using the Titmus Fly Stereopsis Test

1. Check the polarization of the glasses being used to ensure that each eye sees a different image; the left eye should see only the L on the lower left of the Titmus fly test, and the right eye should see only the R.

2. Place the polarizing glasses on the patient. If glasses are usually worn, place the polarizing glasses over them.

3. Hold the fly image, facing the patient, approximately 16 inches (40 cm) away, with the surface of the page parallel to the surface of the glasses.

4. Ask the patient to touch or pinch the wings of the fly. Reassure young children, who might respond with surprise or fright if the image appears too real to them. If the image is perceived as having height, the patient will be observed to attempt to touch the wings as if they were above the page surface.

5. If the fly test is positive, show the patient the 3 rows of animal figures. Ask which figure in each row is coming forward or is above the page.

6. After noting the responses to the animals, direct the patient's attention to the squares with the 4 circles in each. Ask the patient to tell you which circle is coming forward in each square. Alternatively, you may ask the patient to point to the appropriate circle or, particularly with children, to push the button that is popping up.

7. Score the response as the last correctly identified before 2 consecutive circles are missed.

8. Record the stereopsis as seconds of arc, as designated in the instruction booklet that is included with each test. It is advisable to copy the scoring chart for each test and attach it to the back of the test chart for ready reference; you will probably not remember the numbers for each target, and if the test that you are using is not the standard one, the scoring could vary.

9. Be sure that the patient has both eyes open during the test. Some patients are so accustomed to being tested monocularly that they automatically close 1 eye.

10. You might suspect that some patients are using monocular clues to choose the correct responses. If so, turn the book upside down and ask them to describe the images. If they do not describe the images as going behind or sinking into the page, then you have confirmed your suspicion that they were relying on monocular clues instead of stereopsis.

▶ *This chapter includes a related video, which can be accessed by scanning the QR codes provided in the text or going to aao.org/PracticalOphthalmologyvideo.*

The pupil is the window to the inner eye; light passes through it to reach retinal photo-receptors. Because of its potential to reveal serious neurologic or other disease, examination of the pupil is an important element of a thorough ophthalmic evaluation, which requires meticulous attention to detail. Pathologic disorders can alter the size, shape, and location of the pupil, as well as the way the pupil reacts to light and near-focus stimulation. The patient who has a pupillary abnormality generally comes to the attention of the ophthalmologist because of anisocoria (difference in size between both pupils) or reduced pupillary light reaction.

This chapter provides a brief, basic background about pupillary pathway anatomy as well as instructions for the principal tests to evaluate pupillary responses. It also gives a brief overview of the pupillary abnormalities that are most commonly encountered through pupillary evaluation and testing.

Anatomy of Pupillary Pathways

Disorders of the pupil generally arise from dysfunction of the afferent or efferent pupillary pathways. The *afferent* pathway is composed of optic nerve axons that emanate from the retina and optic disc, pass through the chiasm, and exit the optic tract before the lateral geniculate body to synapse in the dorsal midbrain. The *efferent* pathway includes parasympathetic and sympathetic input to the iris muscles.

The size of the pupil is controlled by the opposed actions of the sympathetic and parasympathetic nervous systems that control the tone of 2 smooth muscles, the pupillary sphincter muscle and the pupillary dilator muscle. The pupillary sphincter muscle is supplied by cholinergic fibers of the parasympathetic system via the third cranial (oculomotor) nerve; the pupillary dilator muscle is supplied by adrenergic fibers of the sympathetic system. In general, the pupils tend to be smaller in infants and larger in children and young adults, and become smaller again with advancing age.

Parasympathetic Pathway (Light-Reflex Pathway)

The pupillary parasympathetic pathway subserves the pupillary light reflex (Figure 7-1). The afferent arc begins in the retina and ends in the midbrain tectum. When light stimulates the retinal photoreceptors (rods and cones), electrical impulses are transmitted through the retina by way of retinal ganglion cell axons, which include pupillomotor

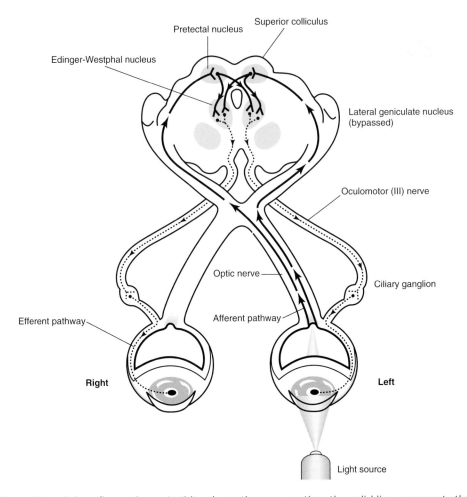

Figure 7-1 Light reflex pathway. In this schematic cross section, the solid line represents the afferent pathway and the dotted line represents the efferent pathway. A light that stimulates the left retina will generate impulses that travel up the left optic nerve and divide at the chiasm. Some impulses continue up the left tract; some cross and travel up the right tract. The impulses arrive at each pretectal nucleus and stimulate cells, which in turn send impulses to the Edinger-Westphal nuclei and down the third cranial nerve to each iris sphincter, causing each pupil to constrict. Because of the double decussation, the first in the chiasm and the second between the pretectal nuclei and the Edinger-Westphal nuclei, the direct pupil response in the left eye equals the consensual response in the right eye. (Reprinted from *Immediate Eye Care: An Illustrated Manual,* Ragge NK, Easty DL, p. 185, © 1990, with permission from Elsevier.)

fibers. The pupillary and visual fibers pass through the optic nerve to the chiasm, where hemidecussation occurs, and then to the optic tract. They bypass the lateral geniculate body, where the visual fibers synapse, to enter the midbrain. The first synapse occurs at the pretectal nuclei, near the superior colliculus. The fibers then decussate a second time in the posterior commissure and synapse at both the ipsilateral and contralateral Edinger-Westphal nuclei, the parasympathetic motor center of the oculomotor nerve.

The efferent fibers from the Edinger-Westphal nuclei then travel superficially in the oculomotor nerve as it leaves the brain stem, and enter the orbit within the inferior division of the oculomotor nerve to synapse at the ciliary ganglion. Postganglionic fibers then travel within the short posterior ciliary nerves, passing through the suprachoroidal space to in-nervate the pupillary sphincter muscle in the iris and the ciliary muscle in the ciliary body. This complex anatomical pattern, with partial crossings at the chiasm and in the posterior commissure, results in the symmetry of the direct and consensual pupillary responses.

Near-Reflex Pathway

The near-reflex pathway subserves pupillary constriction when the eyes fixate on a target at near. The afferent component of the near-reflex pathway is less well defined than the light-reflex pathway. Unlike the light-reflex pathway, which is entirely subcortical, the near-reflex pathway sends fibers to the cerebral cortex bilaterally. Its central fibers are located more ventrally (ie, ventral to the Edinger–Westphal nuclei) in the midbrain than those of the light-reflex pathway. The final common pathway is mediated through the oculomotor nerve with a synapse in the ciliary ganglion.

Sympathetic Pathway

Pain, fear, and certain other psychic stimuli lead to pupillary dilation through the sympa-thetic innervation of the pupillary dilator muscle. The oculosympathetic pathway con-sists of a 3-neuron arc (Figure 7-2). The first-order neurons of the sympathetic pathway originate in the posterior hypothalamus, descend to the intermediolateral gray column of the spinal cord, and synapse at the ciliospinal center of Budge at spinal levels C8 to T2. Preganglionic second-order neurons arise from the intermediolateral column, leave the spinal cord by the ventral spinal roots, and enter the rami communicans. They pass though the area of the apex of the lung and join the paravertebral cervical sympa-thetic chain and ascend through this chain to synapse at the superior cervical ganglion.

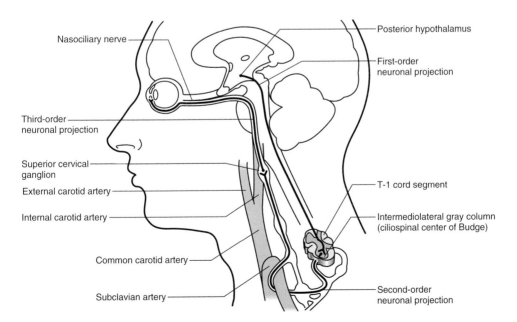

Figure 7-2 Oculosympathetic pathway.

Postganglionic third-order neurons originate in the superior cervical ganglion and enter the cranium with the internal carotid artery. The fibers join the ophthalmic division of the fifth cranial (trigeminal) nerve within the cavernous sinus, reaching the ciliary muscle and pupillary dilator muscle by means of the nasociliary nerve and the long posterior ciliary nerves. Some sympathetic fibers might transiently join the sixth cranial (abducens) nerve within the cavernous sinus.

Examination of the Pupils

A pupillary examination begins with a general observation of the pupils. The pupillary reflexes are then tested by way of the light-reflex test and the swinging flashlight test (to evaluate the direct and consensual pupillary reflexes) and the near-reflex test (to evaluate the near vision response).

General Pupillary Observation

In a room with standardized ambient light, begin a general observation of the pupils by noting the shape of each pupil and the color of the irides. Have the patient fixate a distance target across the room to minimize accommodation and the accompanying miosis. Sit on 1 side of the seated patient and diffusely illuminate both pupils from below the nose with a handheld light (eg, muscle light); use the least amount of light necessary to discern pupil size (Figure 7-3). Carefully measure the pupil diameter in both eyes with a millimeter ruler, the pupil gauge usually printed on the near-vision chart, or an Iowa pupil gauge. Record the size in millimeters in the patient's chart (Figure 7-4).

   If the patient has anisocoria, the pupillary diameters should be measured under both dim and bright illumination. A subtle degree of anisocoria (usually less than 1 mm)

Figure 7-3 Pupils can be seen in dim light by shining a handheld light on the patient's face from below while the patient looks into the darkness. (Reprinted, with permission, from Thompson HS, Kardon RH. Clinical importance of pupillary inequality. *Focal Points: Clinical Modules for Ophthalmologists,* Vol. 10, Module 10. American Academy of Ophthalmology; 1992.)

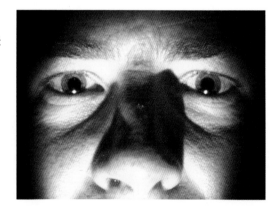

	Size (mm)	Briskness of Light Reaction	RAPD	Near Reaction
Pupil OD	4.5	3+		3+
Pupil OS	4.5	2+	2+	3+

Figure 7-4 Example for recording principal pupillary testing measurements.

can be a normal finding and is called *essential,* or *physiologic,* anisocoria. In physiologic anisocoria, the inequality in pupillary size remains the same under all lighting conditions, and the pupillary light reflexes are equally brisk.

If anisocoria is present, the examiner must document the size in millimeters of the palpebral fissure and note the presence and degree of any ptosis. Ptosis found on the side of a larger, sluggish pupil suggests the possibility of oculomotor nerve paresis. Ptosis found on the side of a smaller pupil requires pharmacologic testing to rule out Horner syndrome, which results from a lesion that affects the sympathetic pathway.

Light-Reflex Test

Shining a light in 1 eye normally causes both pupils to constrict equally, a result of the hemidecussation of pupillomotor fibers in both the chiasm and the midbrain tectum. The pupillary reaction in the illuminated eye is called the *direct reflex,* and the reaction in the nonilluminated eye is called the *consensual reflex.* Clinical Protocol 7-1 describes the basic test used to evaluate these light reflexes as they occur in both eyes simultaneously.

Swinging Flashlight Test

The swinging flashlight test is done after the light-reflex test to compare the direct and consensual responses in each eye individually (Clinical Protocol 7-2). This test is used to detect the presence of a *relative afferent pupillary defect* (RAPD), also called a Marcus Gunn pupil, a critical neuro-ophthalmic sign. During the swinging flashlight test, the examiner briskly alternates illumination from 1 eye to the other several times, and notes the pupillary response. A normal response is for the pupils to become initially constricted and to remain so as the light is swung from eye to eye. However, if 1 pupil consistently dilates and then constricts as the light is alternated, a relative afferent pupillary defect is present in the eye that is directly illuminated when dilation occurs.

It is worth noting that a term, *hippus,* is used to describe a situation, common in younger individuals, in which normal, small-amplitude oscillation of the pupils is observed despite consistent illumination. If the swinging flashlight test is performed too rapidly, an RAPD might be falsely presumed or diagnosed.

An RAPD can be detected even when 1 pupil is bound down by adhesions, paralyzed, or pharmacologically dilated, as long as the contralateral pupil is not. Swinging the light to the eye with optic nerve disease might show no pupillary change in that eye if the pupil is immobile. In such a situation, the degree of consensual response in the normal eye reflects optic nerve activity in the affected eye, and swinging the light to the intact eye should result in further pupillary constriction.

Near-Reflex Test

When a person looks at a near target, 3 reactions normally occur:

- accommodation (contraction of the ciliary muscle, which results in increased lens thickness and curvature)
- convergence (contraction of the medial rectus muscles)
- miosis (contraction of the pupillary sphincter muscle)

Table 7-1   Pupillary Findings in Common Clinical Situations

Clinical Entity	General Features	Neuro-anatomical Site of Lesion	Response to Light and Near Stimulation
Essential (physiologic) anisocoria	Round, regular	Benign, normal finding	Both brisk
Traumatized iris	Irregular, notched pupil border on slit-lamp examination	Pupillary iris sphincter muscle	Both variable; depend on extent of damage
Relative afferent pupillary defect (Marcus Gunn pupil)	Round, regular; positive swinging flashlight test	Optic nerve or extensive retinal damage	Affected pupil shows better consensual than direct light reaction
Midbrain pupils	Mid-dilated (5–7 mm) bilaterally	Dorsal midbrain	Poor to light, better to near
Tonic pupil (Adie syndrome)	Acutely dilated, eventually can become miotic; sector pupil palsy, vermiform movement	Ciliary ganglion	Absent to light, better to near, tonic redilation
Pharmacologically dilated pupil	Very large, round, usually unilateral	Iris sphincter	Fixed at 8–9 mm
Oculomotor palsy (nonvascular)	Mid-dilated (5–7 mm), mild to severe ptosis, unilateral	Third cranial nerve; suspect aneurysm	+/–fixed
Horner syndrome	Small, round, mild ptosis, unilateral	Sympathetic pathway	Both brisk
Argyll Robertson pupil	Small, irregular, bilateral	Midbrain	Poor to light, better to near

(continues next page)

This combination of actions is called the *near synkinesis*. The term *synkinesis* indicates concurrent or simultaneous movements or contractions. The pupillary near reflex should be normal if the light reflex is normal, but the opposite is not true (see "Light–Near Dissociation" later in this chapter). Therefore, if the light reflex is normal, the near reflex need not be tested. Clinical Protocol 7-3 describes the near-reflex test.

Abnormal Pupils

Pupillary evaluation can reveal a variety of ophthalmic and neurologic abnormalities, including iris muscle damage, lesions of the sympathetic or parasympathetic pathways, optic nerve

Table 7-1 (continued)

Aniscoria?	Response to Mydriatics	Response to Miotics	Response to Other Pharmacologic Agents
No change	Dilates	Constricts	Normal
Greater in light	Dilates	Variable constriction; depends on extent of damage	NA
No change	Dilates	Constricts	Normal
No change	Dilates	Constricts	NA
Greater in light	Dilates	Constricts	Pilocarpine 0.1% constricts
Greater in light	Already maximally dilated	No constriction	Pilocarpine 0.5%–2% will not constrict
Greater in light	Dilates	Constricts	Pilocarpine 0.5%–2% will constrict
Greater in darkness	Dilates	Constricts	Cocaine 4%–10%: poor or no dilation; hydroxy-amphetamine 1%: poor or no dilation if third-order neuron damage, dilates otherwise
No change	Poor	Constricts	NA

or retinal pathology, and dorsal midbrain lesions. This section discusses the primary findings commonly encountered when the pupils are examined as well as the implications of those findings. Table 7-1 summarizes the characteristics of pupils in a variety of clinical situations.

Iris Abnormalities

Trauma, surgery, inflammation, or ischemia can damage the iris and alter its appearance. The pupil can be somewhat dilated, sluggishly reactive, and irregular because of traumatic sphincter rupture. There might be notches in the pupillary margin. Additional sequelae of trauma include iritis and reactive miosis. Inflammation can result in anterior and posterior synechiae, which affect the appearance and reactivity of the pupil. Various disorders can cause iris neovascularization with closure of the chamber angle. Developmental anomalies and genetic disorders can be associated with such iris abnormalities as coloboma (congenital absence of part of an ocular tissue), aniridia (absence of the iris), and polycoria (more than 1 pupillary opening in the iris). Iris abnormalities are best observed at the slit lamp.

Relative Afferent Pupillary Defect

A relative afferent pupillary defect, or Marcus Gunn pupil, is detected with the swinging flashlight test, described earlier. An RAPD indicates unilateral or asymmetric damage to the anterior visual pathways (eg, optic nerve disease or extensive retinal damage). Thus, the absence of such a defect means that there is either symmetric damage to the afferent visual system or no damage. It is also not present in patients with cataract or other media opacities, refractive errors, functional visual loss, or cortical lesions. The RAPD is often proportional to the amount of visual loss. It is graded from 1+ to 4+, with 4+ designating an amaurotic pupil, an extreme example in which the eye shows no direct light reaction as a result of profound optic nerve damage. Alternatively, an RAPD can be quantified with use of neutral-density filters placed over the good eye until the defect can no longer be detected.

Light–Near Dissociation

Light–near dissociation occurs when the pupillary near reflex is significantly better than the light reflex. Light–near dissociation can result from damage to bilateral structures that constitute the afferent limb of the pupillary light reaction (eg, bilateral optic atrophy) or from damage to the fibers that mediate the pupillary light reflex in the dorsal aspect of the midbrain. Mesencephalic fibers for the near reflex are located more ventrally than fibers for the light reflex. Thus, the near-reflex fibers are sometimes spared from the effect of compressive or superficial inflammatory lesions that involve the dorsal midbrain.

Light–near dissociation is evident in dorsal midbrain (Parinaud) syndrome, which arises most commonly from a pineal-region tumor that compresses the dorsal midbrain, but it also can be caused by multiple sclerosis, stroke, or hydrocephalus. The patient has mid-dilated pupils with light–near dissociation, upgaze palsy, eyelid retraction, and convergence-retraction nystagmus. The light–near dissociation arises from compression of the superficially located fibers needed for the light reflex; the more ventral near fibers are spared.

Another syndrome that shows light–near dissociation is Argyll Robertson pupil, a rare but classic sign of neurosyphilis (particularly tabes dorsalis). Unlike dorsal midbrain compression, both pupils are miotic. Other causes of light–near dissociation include Adie tonic pupil (discussed in more detail later in this chapter), severe afferent damage, and Wernicke encephalopathy. Certain disorders, such as diabetes mellitus (probably the most common cause of light–near dissociation) and amyloidosis, cause light–near dissociation because of their associated peripheral autonomic neuropathies.

Horner Syndrome

Horner syndrome results from damage to ocular sympathetic fibers at any level along the sympathetic pathway (central, preganglionic, or postganglionic neurons). Features of this syndrome include:

- mild ptosis (often less than 2 mm, due to paresis of the Müller muscle)
- miosis (due to paralysis of the pupillary dilator muscle)

- ipsilateral decrease in facial sweating (anhidrosis or hypohidrosis)
- apparent enophthalmos
- heterochromia iridis (usually in congenital cases)

Other signs include lower eyelid reverse ptosis (the margin of the lower eyelid is higher than normal) and transient decrease in intraocular pressure. The associated anisocoria is more apparent in dim illumination. A dilation lag is noted when there is a shift from bright to dim illumination.

Testing

Pharmacologic testing to confirm the diagnosis of Horner syndrome consists of the instillation of an eyedrop of 4%–10% cocaine solution in each eye. It works by blocking the reuptake of norepinephrine from sympathetic nerve endings, which allows the norepinephrine to remain in contact with its effector muscle for a longer period. Cocaine will dilate an eye with intact sympathetic innervation. If the sympathetic pathway on 1 side is interrupted at any level, norepinephrine is not released from the nerve endings, in which case the cocaine will have no effect and the pupil on that side will remain relatively miotic.

Cocaine testing is considered the gold standard for pharmacologic confirmation of Horner syndrome, but cocaine can be difficult to obtain. Apraclonidine has also been used to confirm the diagnosis of Horner syndrome. Apraclonidine has weak α_1-adrenergic agonist action, which, in most normal eyes, produces no significant effect on the pupil. However, in sympathetically denervated eyes, the iris dilator muscle develops adrenergic supersensitivity, and apraclonidine will cause pupil dilation. Following instillation of 0.5% or 1% apraclonidine in each eye, reversal of anisocoria after 30–45 minutes is diagnostic of Horner syndrome. Note that the pupils only are observed during apraclonidine testing for Horner syndrome, as the ptosis will reduce with or without the condition due to normal stimulation of the Müller muscle.

Once the diagnosis of Horner syndrome is confirmed with the cocaine test, hydroxyamphetamine can be used to differentiate central and preganglionic lesions from postganglionic lesions. The hydroxyamphetamine test cannot be performed on the same day as the cocaine test because cocaine interferes with the action of hydroxyamphetamine. One eyedrop of hydroxyamphetamine (Paredrine 1%) is instilled in each eye. Because hydroxyamphetamine stimulates the release of norepinephrine from sympathetic postganglionic nerve terminals, it will fail to dilate the pupil in patients who have postganglionic lesions but will dilate the pupils in those with central or preganglionic lesions.

Differentiation of lesions is clinically useful because central and preganglionic lesions are more likely to be harbingers of serious disease than are postganglionic lesions. For example, central lesions arise from central nervous system vascular events and tumors. Preganglionic lesions can be caused by apical lung tumors (Pancoast tumors), chest surgery, and thoracic artery aneurysm. The causes of postganglionic lesions include cluster headaches, dissection of the internal carotid artery, and neck trauma.

Do not perform applanation tonometry, test corneal sensation, or otherwise irritate or touch the corneas before pharmacologic testing; any resulting epithelial defect can lead to unequal absorption of the diagnostic eyedrops and perhaps a false-negative or a false-positive test result.

The Fixed and Dilated Pupil

The differential diagnosis of a fixed, dilated pupil is important to master. This sign can be seen in the following conditions:

- Adie tonic pupil
- oculomotor nerve palsy
- pharmacologic blockade
- traumatic iris sphincter rupture
- angle-closure glaucoma

Adie tonic pupil

Adie tonic pupil is typically seen as unilateral mydriasis, often accompanied by ipsilateral loss of accommodation, in an otherwise healthy young woman. Acutely the pupil is large, but it diminishes in size over months to years and can become miotic eventually. The pupil shows sluggish, sectoral, or no reaction to light and a better response to an accommodative target. Redilation after the near response is tonic (slow). When present, slow, worm-like (vermiform) contractions of the iris help in making the diagnosis. The precise cause of the disorder is unknown. Postganglionic parasympathetic denervation is present, and the lesion is thought to localize to the ciliary ganglion or short posterior ciliary nerves. Holmes-Adie syndrome includes other features, notably diminished deep tendon reflexes and orthostatic hypotension. The condition can be diagnosed by its hypersensitivity to weak miotic eyedrops (*denervation supersensitivity*); an Adie tonic pupil constricts in response to 0.1% pilocarpine eyedrops, which affect a normal pupil only minimally.

Oculomotor nerve palsy

Compression of the third cranial (oculomotor) nerve results in the typical features of oculomotor nerve palsy: severe ptosis; deficits in elevation, depression and adduction; and a dilated, poorly reactive pupil on the affected side. Because the parasympathetic fibers are located in the peripheral (superficial) portion of the oculomotor nerve as it exits the brain stem, they are typically affected by a compressive lesion (eg, tumor, aneurysm) and spared by a vasculopathic lesion (eg, diabetes mellitus). When acute third cranial nerve palsy is accompanied by pupillary mydriasis, an aneurysm at the junction of the internal carotid and posterior communicating arteries must be vigorously and urgently investigated with appropriate neuroimaging. Other causes of oculomotor palsy include brain tumor, basal meningitis, and uncal herniation. Vasculopathic (diabetic, hypertensive) oculomotor nerve palsy usually spares the pupil.

Pharmacologic blockade

Pharmacologic blockade is one of the most frequent causes of a dilated and fixed pupil in an otherwise healthy patient. It results from purposeful or inadvertent instillation of atropinelike drugs into the eyes. A scopolamine patch used to prevent nausea caused by motion sickness or from anesthesia during surgery is a common cause of accidental pupillary dilation. Pharmacological blockade can be differentiated from a dilated pupil that accompanies third cranial nerve palsy or Adie tonic pupil by the absence of ptosis and motility abnormalities and by failure of the pupil to constrict upon instillation of pilocarpine 1% eyedrops into the eye. These eyedrops would cause constriction of a mydriatic pupil that accompanies an oculomotor palsy.

Other causes

Another cause of pupillary mydriasis is traumatic iris sphincter rupture. Careful slit-lamp examination will reveal irregular pupillary borders at the sites of sphincter rupture. Acute angle-closure glaucoma classically presents with a mid-dilated and poorly reactive pupil; look for a red eye with corneal edema and increased intraocular pressure.

Pitfalls and Pointers

- Unilateral blindness, or a unilateral relative afferent pupillary defect, does not cause anisocoria. Whereas the pupil on the defective side might react only sluggishly or not at all to direct light stimulation, it will constrict consensually when the normal contralateral eye is stimulated (due to the double decussation of pupillomotor fibers).

- A relative afferent pupillary defect indicates that the afferent visual pathway is defective on 1 side in comparison with the contralateral pathway (the adjective "relative" emphasizes this). There is no such thing as a bilateral relative afferent pupillary defect.

- When you perform the swinging flashlight test, be careful to spend equal time illuminating each pupil to avoid differential bleaching of photoreceptors and possible artifactitious relative afferent pupillary defect. Marked anisocoria or prolonged occlusion can also cause differential photoreceptor bleaching that can confound pupillary testing.

- Recognize that pupil-involving oculomotor nerve palsy is often a harbinger of cerebral aneurysm. Perform the workup expeditiously, and obtain a neurosurgical consultation immediately; delay in diagnosis can have life-threatening consequences.

- When you perform pharmacologic pupillary testing, instill eyedrops in both eyes for comparison.

- Media opacities such as cataract or even dense vitreous hemorrhage almost never cause a relative afferent pupillary defect.

Suggested Resources

Burde RM, Savino PJ, Trobe JD. *Clinical Decisions in Neuro-Ophthalmology*. 3rd ed. Mosby-Year Book; 2002.

Falardeau, J and Kardon R. *Anisocoria*. Focal Points: Clinical modules for Ophthalmologists. American Academy of Ophthalmology; March 2013.

Neuro-Ophthalmology. Basic and Clinical Science Course, Section 5. American Academy of Ophthalmology; published annually.

CLINICAL PROTOCOL 7-1

Perfoming the Light-Reflex Test

1. Under dim room illumination, ask the patient to maintain fixation on a distance target, such as a large letter on the Snellen acuity chart.

2. Shine a bright handheld light directly into the right eye by approaching it from the side or from below. Do not stand in front of the patient or allow the patient to look directly at the light, which would stimulate the near reflex and preclude accurate light-reflex testing.

3. Record the direct pupillary response to light in the right eye in terms of the briskness of the response, graded from 0, which indicates no response, to 4+, which indicates a brisk response (see "Briskness of Light Reaction" in Figure 7-4).

4. Repeat steps 1–3 for the left eye.

5. Repeat steps 1 and 2 in the right eye; observe the consensual reflex by noting the response to the light of the nonilluminated (left) pupil. The rapidity of the response and change in pupil size should normally be equivalent to that seen in the direct light reaction and is graded on the same numeric scale.

6. Repeat steps 1, 2, and 5 in the left eye.

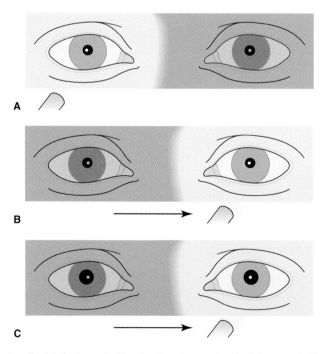

Figure 1 Swinging flashlight test. **A,** Illuminating the patient's right eye. **B,** Illuminating the patient's left eye. **C,** Dilation, which indicates a relative afferent pupillary defect.

Video 1 demonstrates the light reflex test and pupil evaluation.

 VIDEO 1   Evaluation of Pupils
Courtesy of Lindreth G. DuBois, MEd, MMSc, CO, COMT.
Access all *Practical Ophthalmology* videos at www.aao.org
/PracticalOphthalmologyvideo.

CLINICAL PROTOCOL 7-2

Performing the Swinging Flashlight Test

1. Under dim room illumination with the patient fixating a distance target, illuminate the patient's right eye directly with a bright handheld light, in a manner identical to that used to test the light reflex (Figure 1A). Note the pupillary constriction in both eyes.

2. Move the light beam immediately and swiftly over the bridge of the patient's nose to the left eye, and note the pupillary response in that eye. Take care to illuminate each pupil from the same angle. Normally, the pupil will either constrict slightly or remain at its previous size (Figure 1B). If, instead, the pupil dilates when the light illuminates it (ie, the direct light reflex is weaker than the consensual reflex), a relative afferent pupillary defect is present, which usually indicates a disorder of the optic nerve or severe retinal pathology (Figure 1C).

3. Quickly swing the light back to the right eye and evaluate the response. A normal response is again a mild constriction or no change in size at all. Net pupillary constriction or dilation is an abnormal response.

4. Repeat steps 1–3 rhythmically, spending equal intervals illuminating each pupil, until it is clear whether pupillary responses are normal or whether 1 pupil consistently dilates.

5. Record a relative afferent pupillary defect (RAPD) as 1+ to 4+; 1+ indicates a mild afferent defect and 4+ indicates an amaurotic pupil, a severe defect in which the affected eye shows no direct light response (see RAPD in Figure 7-4).

CLINICAL PROTOCOL 7-3

Performing the Near-Reflex Test

1. Under normal room illumination, ask the patient to fixate a distance target.

2. While seated next to the patient, move a detailed target toward the patient's line of vision at near. (The patient's thumb is sometimes an excellent near target, as use of it provides proprioceptive as well as visual near clues to ensure adequate near efforts.) A flashlight should not be used for this purpose.

3. Instruct the patient to shift fixation to the near target. If the patient's thumb is being used as a target, the examiner holds the patient's thumb and moves it, and asks the patient to view it intently.

4. Observe the pupillary reflex when the patient shifts fixation to the near target. Normal pupils constrict upon viewing the near target.

5. Repeat steps 1–4 several times.

6. Record the near reaction in terms of the briskness of the response, graded from 0, for no response, to 4+, for brisk response (see "Near Reaction" in Figure 7-4).

Visual Field Examination

▶ *This chapter includes a related video, which can be accessed by scanning the QR code provided in the text or going to aao.org/PracticalOphthalmologyvideo.*

The field of vision is that portion of a subject's surroundings that is visible at any one time. The visual field properly includes central fixation or foveal vision, conventionally measured by visual acuity tests, and extrafoveal (or peripheral) vision. Visual acuity, or foveal vision, and the peripheral visual field are tested in different ways and provide information on different aspects of visual function. Visual acuity testing measures the eye's greatest resolution, the ability to identify forms. Visual field testing measures peripheral sensitivity, the ability to detect light or motion at different locations.

The visual field of each eye can be tested separately by 1 or more tests. The visual fields are routinely screened with the confrontation fields test. If macular disease is suspected to be causing a central visual field defect, a device called an *Amsler grid* is used to test the central area of each eye's visual field. If a visual field defect is detected by screening, or if symptoms suggest a high likelihood of peripheral field loss, further evaluation is conducted by manual or automated procedures known as perimetry. Perimetry is used to document the presence and severity of a visual field defect and to monitor progression of previously known visual field loss.

The Visual Field

The visual field is an inverted and reversed map of corresponding retinal points. The normal visual field extends about 50° superiorly, 60° nasally, 70° inferiorly, and 90° temporally from fixation. The visual field can be divided into central, intermediate, and peripheral zones. The central zone includes an area from the fixation point to a circle 30° away (a 5 mm radius from the fovea). The central zone contains the temporal physiologic blind spot; this corresponds to the optic nerve head, which is centered about 15° nasally from the fovea. The intermediate zone extends from 30° to 50° and the peripheral zone is the area beyond 50°.

A *scotoma*, one type of *visual field defect*, is a place in the visual field where an object cannot be seen and that is surrounded by normal visual field. A *relative scotoma* is an area in the visual field where test objects of low luminance cannot be seen, but larger or brighter ones can. An *absolute scotoma* is an area where no test object can be seen (eg, the physiologic blind spot). Other types of visual field defects include arcuate defects and hemianopias.

Perimetry is the measurement of the visual field with either moving objects (kinetic perimetry) or stationary test stimuli (static perimetry). In kinetic perimetry, points along the edge of the visual field are determined by finding the weakest light stimulus that evokes a visual sensation (visual threshold). The line that joins points having the same threshold is called an *isopter*. In static perimetry, the use of static targets that change in brightness gives a threshold map of different points.

The normal field of vision varies with the size, color, brightness, and movement of the test stimulus, or target; with the background illumination; and with a patient's alertness and familiarity with the test. Unlike all other portions of the ophthalmic examination, visual fields are conventionally recorded on charts that represent the field *as the patient sees it* (ie, the temporal field of the right eye is to the right), and the field for the right eye is always placed to the right when the visual field maps of both eyes are compared.

The visual field is a 3-dimensional concept that is presented in 2 dimensions (Figure 8-1A). Different types of perimetry give maps with different appearances. A visual field performed by kinetic perimetry (eg, with the Goldmann perimeter) is plotted on polar graph paper (Figure 8-1B) with radial meridians (measured counterclockwise from 0° at the right-hand horizontal) and circles of eccentricity (concentric rings every 10° out from fixation). With such a map obtained by kinetic perimetry, the examiner looks down onto the "hill of vision," with its contours represented by isopters. Most maps produced by automated static perimetry present an array of sensitivity values; these values can also be pictured by the program in gray tones—the gray scale. (Figure 8-1C). Darker shading indicates less visual sensitivity.

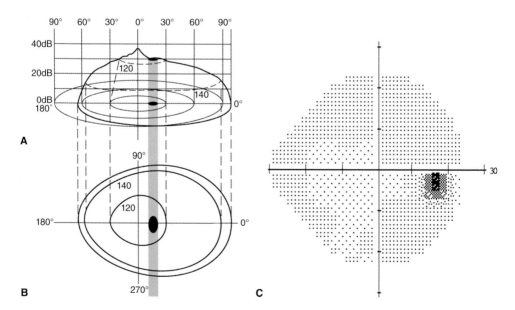

Figure 8-1   The normal visual field and the maps produced by different types of perimetry. **A,** Three-dimensional model of the right eye's "island of vision surrounded by a sea of blindness." The horizontal plane indicates degrees (circles) of eccentricity and meridians. The vertical axis is plotted in decibels of visual sensitivity. **B,** Topography of the visual field represented by plotting isopters on polar coordinates with kinetic perimetry. **C,** Grayscale rendering computed by automated perimetry. (Part C courtesy of Preston H. Blomquist, MD.)

Screening Tests

Visual field screening is routinely done at a patient's initial eye examination. The confrontation fields test can screen for moderate to severe visual field defects, but confrontation testing is often unreliable for detecting mild visual field loss, as in early glaucoma. The Amsler grid, used when the patient has symptoms of central distortion or loss, helps evaluate macular function. Both screening tests are discussed in the following sections.

Confrontation Fields Testing

Confrontation testing of a patient's visual fields is done in a face-to-face position at a distance of about 1 meter (3 feet). By convention, the right eye is tested first, although if there is a marked difference in visual acuity it is advisable to begin with the better eye. The eye not being tested must be completely occluded, by using a handheld or press-on occluder, by putting a folded facial tissue under an elastic eye occluder, or by asking the patient to cover the eye with the palm of the hand. When the patient's left eye is covered, the examiner's right eye should be closed, and vice versa, to permit comparison. The examiner presents fingers midway between themselves and the patient, and tests all 4 quadrants (Figure 8-2).

To assess the patient's visual field, the patient's responses are compared to the examiner's normal visual field. To outline the visual field determined by the confrontation screening method, the examiner's hand is slowly brought inward from different directions, testing each of the patient's meridians. Clinical Protocol 8-1 provides instructions for performing the confrontation fields test.

Amsler Grid Test

The Amsler grid is used to test the central 10° of each eye's visual field. It helps test for suspected macular disease that produces a central scotoma as well as for metamorphopsia (distortion). The Amsler grid is a white or red pattern of lines with a central spot; it is printed on a black background (Figure 8-3A). When viewed at a distance of 30 cm (about 12 inches) with near correction, the lines are 1° apart. A patient with no abnormalities perceives the lines as straight and complete. Patients with abnormalities report distorted

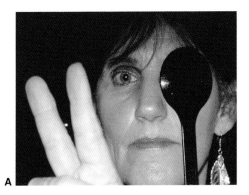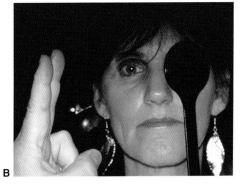

Figure 8-2   The confrontation fields test. **A,** Correct presentation of fingers, side by side frontally. **B,** Incorrect presentation, so that 1 finger hides the other. (Reprinted, with permission, from Walsh TJ, ed. *Visual Fields: Examination and Interpretation.* 3rd ed. Ophthalmology Monograph 3. Oxford University Press; 2011.)

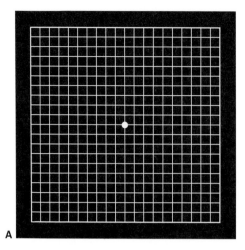
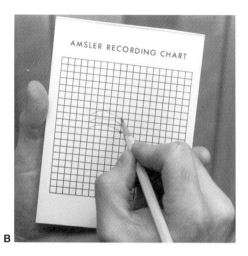

A   B

Figure 8-3   The Amsler grid. **A,** The test pattern has white or red lines on a black background. **B,** The patient draws the central field defect on the preprinted pad that has black lines on a white background.

or missing lines, which they can record themselves on a preprinted black-on-white version of the grid (Figure 8-3B). Clinical Protocol 8-2 gives instructions for Amsler grid testing.

Special Situations

Confrontation testing to screen for visual field defects might not be possible in infants, obtunded patients, and patients with optic nerve disease. Alternative screening methods for such patients are described in the following sections.

Reflex eye movement test for infants
Test the visual field of infants and toddlers by making use of their involuntary fixational reflexes. First, get the child's attention in a frontal gaze. While the child is watching your face, silently bring an interesting toy or other object from the periphery to elicit fixational head and eye movements.

Blink reflex test
Quickly flicking your hand toward a sighted patient's open eye normally elicits a blink reflex. This test can help identify a dense hemianopia or quadrantanopia if a patient does not respond as expected.

Manual Perimetry

A perimeter is an instrument that measures the visual field by the patient's subjective responses. It is used to quantify or confirm a visual field defect discovered or suspected through screening; to detect subtle field defects not detected by confrontation testing, such as those associated with early glaucomatous damage; and to monitor changes in a previously known condition.

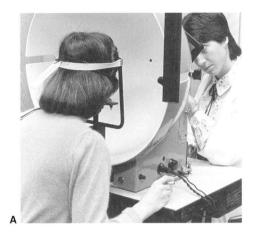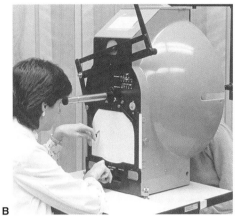

A
B

Figure 8-4 Goldmann perimetry. **A,** From the patient's side. **B,** From the examiner's side.

The Goldmann perimeter is used to perform kinetic perimetry; it tests the entire visual field, with use of different target sizes and intensities, and plots the visual field in degrees of arc. The Goldmann perimeter is a hemispheric dome with a white background that is illuminated to a level near the lower limit of photopic vision. A movable pantographic device permits a light target to be projected within the dome, continuously or intermittently, at various sizes and brightness levels. The examiner directly observes the patient's visual fixation from behind the dome through a telescope, and the patient responds to stimuli with a buzzer (Figure 8-4).

Six different target sizes are available, each 4 times the size of the previous target: 0 (0.0625 mm^2), I (0.25 mm^2), II (1 mm^2), III (4 mm^2), IV (16 mm^2), and V (64 mm^2). Target brightness (intensity) is measured in decibels (dB). Gray filters allow the brightness of the target to be reduced in 5-dB steps from intensity level 4 to 1 and in 1-dB steps from e to a. Perimetry almost always begins with target size I and intensity 4e (this isopter line would be labeled "I4e" on the diagram). Larger targets (II to V) are chosen if this isopter is revealed to be constricted. The choice of targets is usually limited to 2 or 3 of the following: I2, I4, II4, IV4, and V4.

Automated Perimetry

Automated static perimetry can often detect smaller or shallower defects than kinetic perimetry. Because the testing is tedious and time consuming, most modern static perimeters are computerized, and new automated instrumentation continues to be developed. The Humphrey Visual Field Analyzer is the most commonly used computerized system, and comes with an elaborate software package with which to perform various statistical evaluations. Automation has the capability to compare results statistically with those of individuals with normal vision who belong to the same age group as well as with previous tests for the same patient. Also, automated perimetry does not require operators as highly skilled as are needed for manual perimetry, and it eliminates certain operator errors. Some patients, such as young children and individuals who need vigorous encouragement to maintain fixation, might not be good candidates for automated perimetry.

Test Targets and Strategies

The standard target size for automated perimetry is equivalent to a Goldmann size III (4 mm²) white target. The number of points tested determines test time. Since automated static perimetry is fatiguing for the patient, the number of test points should be limited as much as possible. The most commonly used tests explore 50–120 test points. Different software programs test different areas of the visual field, depending on the specific disorder known or suspected. Program selection depends on whether the visual field examination is done for diagnostic testing of a suspected defect or for follow-up of a progressive condition. For example, a glaucoma test includes extra points to detect such common glaucomatous visual field defects as a nasal step or an arcuate defect, whereas neurologic visual field testing emphasizes points along the vertical meridian and within the central field, where many neurologic visual field defects are found.

For most patients with glaucoma or a neuro-ophthalmologic condition, a 30° or a 24° field is appropriate. The Central 30-2 test is an example of a program that evaluates the central 30° with 76 points. It is commonly used for monitoring glaucoma patients and for detecting neurologic visual field defects. The Central 24-2 test (54 points) provides a 24° field from fixation with an extension of the nasal field to 30°, with use of a 6° grid. The 2 in the designation "24-2 test" indicates a grid that straddles the horizontal and vertical meridians. The 24-2 test is generally preferred for testing most patients (instead of a 30-1 or 24-1 test, which align the grid onto the vertical and horizontal meridians).

Deficits less than 6° in diameter or located in the far periphery may be missed by the 30-2 and 24-2 tests. For patients with central visual field loss or very advanced glaucomatous disease, the Central 10-2 test may be appropriate for sequential testing, because it tests the central 10° field with a 2° grid. For patients with peripheral visual field defects, Goldmann perimetry may be useful.

Interpretation of a Computerized Printout

Printed test results show basic patient information such as age and pupillary diameter. The raw data from automated static perimetry are shown as reliability measures and as the numeric plot, which are the actual sensitivity values at each tested point (Figure 8-5). The printout also presents statistical calculations that show how the patient's data varies from the expected (normal) data. The examiner must look at the reliability measures, the numeric plot, the probability maps, and the global indices.

The reliability measures are the proportion of fixation losses, false-positive errors, and false-negative errors. Fixation loss is the proportion of times that the patient responded inappropriately, because of wandering fixation, to a stimulus at the presumed blind spot. The false-positive error rate is the proportion of times that the patient responded when no stimulus was presented. The false-negative error rate is the proportion of times that the patient did not respond when a suprathreshold stimulus (ie, a luminance that had been seen earlier in the test) was presented. The printout flags these parameters with "xx" when low reliability is suspected. The examination may be unreliable if 1 or more of the following occur:

- fixation losses are greater than 25%, especially if accompanied by the lack of a well-demarcated blind spot
- false-positive responses are greater than 15%

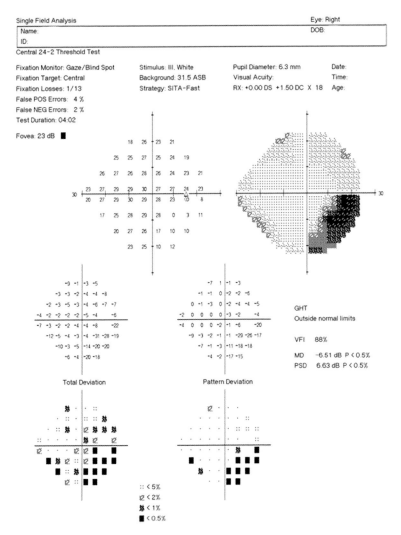

Figure 8-5 Computerized printout record of automated static perimetry. (Courtesy of Preston H. Blomquist, MD.)

- false-negative responses are greater than 33%
- duration of the test is long (it usually runs under 5 minutes for experienced test takers)

The numeric plot gives the measured threshold values at each test point. Recall that a higher number means a dimmer light, and thus a more sensitive visual area. The grayscale plot provides a graphic representation of the raw data. The darker the area on the grayscale plot, the greater the loss of sensitivity for a given target size. Because data between test points are extrapolated, the grayscale plot might not be accurate; however, the grayscale plot can be useful to show patients when educating them about the results of their testing. The total deviation plot indicates the difference between the measured visual sensitivity and that of age-matched normal values at each location. The total deviation probability map indicates the significance of any abnormality. One should remember, however, that statistical significance does not always mean *clinical* significance.

The pattern deviation plot is derived by subtracting the overall generalized depression of a measured field from the total deviation plot to highlight superimposed patterns of localized visual field loss, which are frequently more diagnostic. A probability analysis, based on the adjusted deviation values, is again displayed.

The global indices are MD (mean deviation from age-corrected normal) and PSD (pattern standard deviation). MD is the average decibel value of the entire total deviation plot and is flagged if there is substantially depressed sensitivity, whether generalized or localized. PSD is a measure of the variability across the total deviation plot. For each global index, the statistical significance, which is the probability of finding the obtained value in a healthy person, is given.

The Glaucoma Hemifield Test (GHT) is reported after performance of a Central 24-2 or a Central 30-2 visual field test. It is derived by comparing corresponding zones in the superior and inferior portions of the visual field. The 5 possible results of the GHT are: "Within normal limits," "Outside normal limits," "Borderline," "General reduction of sensitivity," and "Abnormally high sensitivity."

Automated visual field results are not self-explanatory. The examiner must distinguish artifact from disease to account for an abnormal test.

Common Visual Field Defects

An abnormal visual field test result should be described in the medical record according to which eye is involved and the shape of the field abnormality, its location, and its symmetry. These attributes as well as certain typical perimetric patterns help to localize a lesion along the visual pathway. Table 8-1 lists some common descriptions of visual field defects, some of which are discussed in the next paragraphs.

Figure 8-6 shows a variety of commonly seen shapes of visual field defects together with a diagram of their anatomical origins. One of the most common shapes is a scotoma, a localized defect surrounded by detectable visual field. Some examples of common scotomas associated with glaucoma are shown in Figure 8-7. These scotomas often extend from the blind spot or appear to make the visual field smaller (peripheral constriction).

An arcuate scotoma is a monocular isolated paracentral defect, so called because it yields an arclike shape when plotted. This crescentic form is caused by the normal course

Table 8-1   Terms Used to Describe Visual Field Defects

Type of Defect	Terms
Monocular field defects	Localized defects: wedge-shaped temporal field defect, arcuate nasal field defect, central scotoma, enlarged blind spot, cecocentral scotoma, annular scotoma Generalized defects: generalized depression, peripheral constriction
Binocular field defects	Homonymous hemianopias: with macular splitting, with macular sparing, with unilateral sparing of temporal crescent Bitemporal hemianopias Binasal hemianopias Quadrantanopias

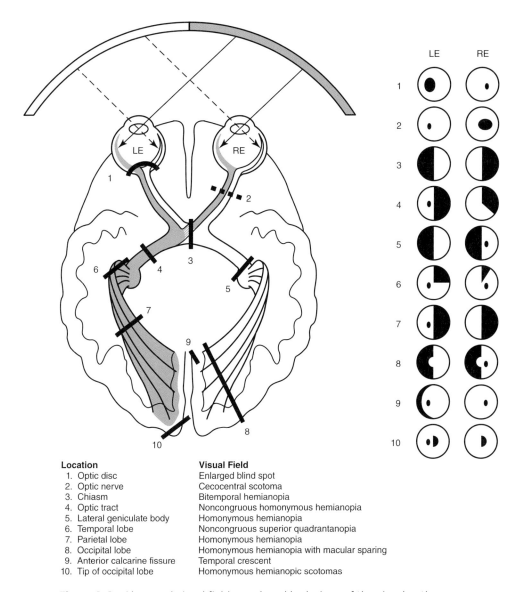

Location	Visual Field
1. Optic disc	Enlarged blind spot
2. Optic nerve	Cecocentral scotoma
3. Chiasm	Bitemporal hemianopia
4. Optic tract	Noncongruous homonymous hemianopia
5. Lateral geniculate body	Homonymous hemianopia
6. Temporal lobe	Noncongruous superior quadrantanopia
7. Parietal lobe	Homonymous hemianopia
8. Occipital lobe	Homonymous hemianopia with macular sparing
9. Anterior calcarine fissure	Temporal crescent
10. Tip of occipital lobe	Homonymous hemianopic scotomas

Figure 8-6   Abnormal visual fields produced by lesions of the visual pathways.

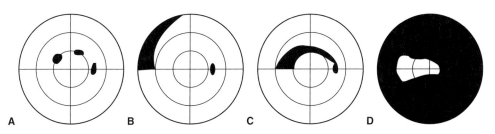

Figure 8-7   Visual field defects produced by glaucomatous optic neuropathy (right eye). **A,** Paracentral scotomata. **B,** Superior nasal step. **C,** Arcuate scotoma. **D,** Advanced peripheral constriction.

of the retinal ganglion cell nerve fibers. Defects in the arcuate zone can connect with the blind spot (Seidel scotoma), appear as 1 or more scattered paracentral scotomas, or end at the horizontal raphe (nasal step). A nasal step is a scotoma that, when plotted, abuts onto the horizontal meridian and appears as a steplike loss of vision at the outer limit of the nasal field. An altitudinal defect is one that causes loss of the upper or lower visual field. There can also be generalized depression in which visual sensitivity is diffusely reduced.

A binocular visual field defect in each eye's hemifield is called a *hemianopia*. Incomplete hemianopias are referred to as *quadrantanopias* and *sectoral defects*. A chiasmal or retrochiasmal lesion produces visual field defects that respect the vertical meridian and remain in 1 hemifield of each eye (see Figure 8-6). Retinal and optic nerve lesions produce visual field defects that can cross the vertical meridian (see Figure 8-7).

A hemianopia can be homonymous (ie, impairing visual function on the same side of each eye), bitemporal, or binasal. Quadrantanopias and altitudinal defects are described as being superior or inferior.

Retrochiasmal field defects that are similar between the 2 eyes are called congruous, and defects that are asymmetric or differently sized for each eye are incongruous. Because corresponding fibers from the 2 retinas lie close together as they near the visual cortex, lesions of the posterior radiations tend to be congruous, while anterior retrochiasmal lesions are more frequently incongruous.

Localizing Visual Field Defects

The physician needs to know the typical patterns obtained in perimetry to determine the probable location of a lesion. A decision-making approach based on knowledge of neuroanatomy helps the examiner make an accurate medical interpretation (Figure 8-8).

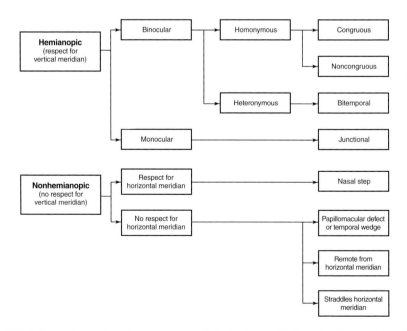

Figure 8-8   Interpretation tree for visual field defects. (From Trobe JD, Glaser JS. *The Visual Fields Manual: A Practical Guide to Testing and Interpretation.* Triad; 1983.)

Progression

Visual fields often must be tested on several occasions to get a reliable picture of the patient's status. Chronic diseases such as glaucoma can produce progressive visual field loss that might be detected before optic nerve or other changes are visible (Figure 8-9).

Pitfalls and Pointers

Remember the "rules of the road" when interpreting visual field defects:

- Unilateral optic nerve disease causes unilateral visual field defects.
- Nasal retinal nerve fibers cross in the chiasm to go to the contralateral optic tract; temporal retinal nerve fibers remain uncrossed.
- Lesions that involve the chiasm and retrochiasmal pathways cause visual field defects that respect the vertical meridian.
- Retrochiasmal lesions produce a contralateral homonymous hemianopia.
- The more posterior the lesion occurs in the postchiasmal pathway, the more likely the defects are congruous.

Suggested Resources

Glaucoma. Basic and Clinical Science Course, Section 10. American Academy of Ophthalmology; published annually.

Heijl A, Patella VM. *Effective Perimetry.* 4th ed. Carl Zeiss Meditec; 2012.

Walsh TJ, ed. *Visual Fields: Examination and Interpretation*. Ophthalmology Monograph 3. 3rd ed. Oxford University Press; 2011.

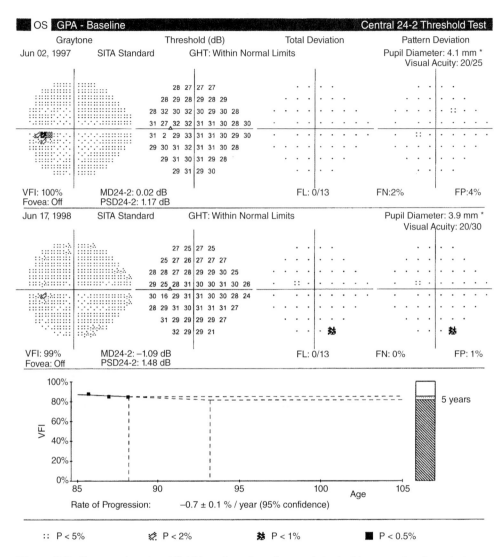

Figure 8-9 Progressive visual field loss from baseline as detected by repeat automated perimetry in a patient with chronic glaucoma. (Courtesy of Misha F. Syed, MD, MEHP.)

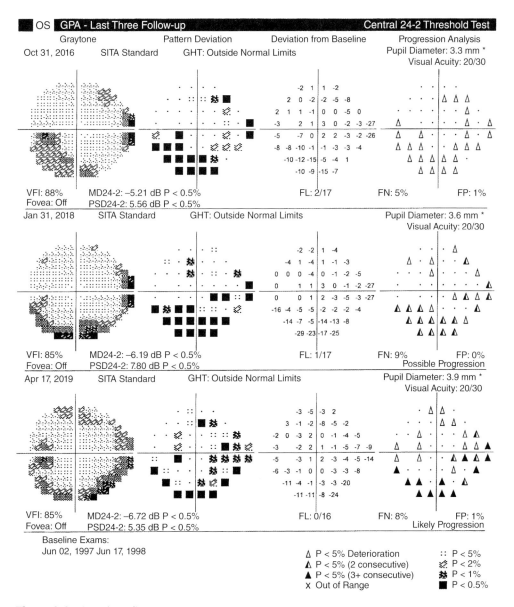

OS GPA - Last Three Follow-up   Central 24-2 Threshold Test

Graytone	Pattern Deviation	Deviation from Baseline	Progression Analysis

Oct 31, 2016   SITA Standard   GHT: Outside Normal Limits   Pupil Diameter: 3.3 mm *
                                                                  Visual Acuity: 20/30

VFI: 88%   MD24-2: −5.21 dB P < 0.5%   FL: 2/17   FN: 5%   FP: 1%
Fovea: Off   PSD24-2: 5.56 dB P < 0.5%

Jan 31, 2018   SITA Standard   GHT: Outside Normal Limits   Pupil Diameter: 3.6 mm *
                                                                  Visual Acuity: 20/30

VFI: 85%   MD24-2: −6.19 dB P < 0.5%   FL: 1/17   FN: 9%   FP: 0%
Fovea: Off   PSD24-2: 7.80 dB P < 0.5%   Possible Progression

Apr 17, 2019   SITA Standard   GHT: Outside Normal Limits   Pupil Diameter: 3.9 mm *
                                                                  Visual Acuity: 20/30

VFI: 85%   MD24-2: −6.72 dB P < 0.5%   FL: 0/16   FN: 8%   FP: 1%
Fovea: Off   PSD24-2: 5.35 dB P < 0.5%   Likely Progression

Baseline Exams:
Jun 02, 1997 Jun 17, 1998

△ P < 5% Deterioration   :: P < 5%
▲ P < 5% (2 consecutive)   ⚇ P < 2%
▲ P < 5% (3+ consecutive)   ⚉ P < 1%
X Out of Range   ■ P < 0.5%

Figure 8-9 (continued)

CLINICAL PROTOCOL 8-1

Performing the Confrontation Fields Test

Test Setup

1. Seat the patient and occlude the eye not being tested.
2. Face the patient at a distance of about 1 m (40 inches), and close your eye that is directly opposite the patient's occluded eye.
3. Ask the patient to fixate on your nose or on your open eye.

Check for Scotoma

1. *Finger counting.* Hold your hands midway between yourself and the patient in opposite quadrants about 30° from central fixation (60 cm [24 inches] from your mutual axis); your hands should be stationary. Quickly present, then retract, a finger or fingers on 1 hand in 1 quadrant of the monocular field, and ask the patient to state the number of fingers presented. To avoid confusion, limit the number of fingers shown to 1, 2, and 5, and hold the fingers side by side in the frontal plane. Repeat this in all 4 quadrants, testing at least 2 times per quadrant.

   a. Test patients who cannot count fingers by waving your hand and asking if the patient perceives the motion. With patients who can perceive only light, test for the ability to determine the direction of light projection by pointing a muscle light or penlight toward the pupil while the patient's other is eye completely shielded. Repeat this in all 4 quadrants.

   b. Test young children with a finger-mimicking procedure. First, teach the child to hold up the same number of fingers as you do, then conduct the test as usual. Test rapidly, because a child will soon glance directly at your hand (although this involuntary movement can also indicate a normal response).

2. *Simultaneous finger counting.* Present fingers simultaneously in opposite quadrants, and ask the patient to state the total number of fingers presented. Use the following combinations: 1 and 1, 1 and 2, and 2 and 2. This test can reveal a more subtle field defect than finger counting in each quadrant separately. Sometimes a patient with a relative scotoma can detect fingers presented to the defective hemifield but has problems with simultaneous targets.

3. *Simultaneous comparison.* Hold both palms toward the patient, close to the line of sight, in opposite superior, then inferior, quadrants. Ask the patient to state whether 1 hand appears darker or less distinct. This test is very subjective and relies on equal illumination but can reveal a subtle defect in a hemifield.

   a. A similar test can be done by asking the patient to compare the relative hue or intensity of 2 identically colored objects, such as the red caps of 2 eyedropper bottles. Hold the targets in separate quadrants. If there is a hemianopia, the patient might describe 1 cap as red and the other as faded or colorless. This test can also be done

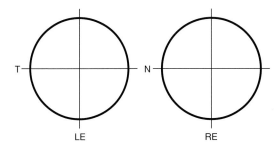

Figure 1 Sample chart for plotting the visual field as the patient sees it.

with 1 colored item by bringing it across from a defective to a normal area, to determine whether the patient perceives a sudden change in intensity.

b. Check a central scotoma by comparing central and eccentric locations with use of hands or other identical objects.

Diagram the Confrontation Field

If an abnormality is detected, sketch a 360° visual field chart, labeled for the right and left eye and the temporal and nasal field, and plot the visual field as the patient sees it (Figure 1). If the patient can count fingers in all 4 quadrants, correctly counts fingers simultaneously, and notes no difference on simultaneous comparison, the examiner may record the results as "full to 3-stage confrontation."

CP Video 8-1 demonstrates performance of confrontation visual fields testing.

VIDEO 1 Confrontation Visual Fields
Courtesy of Lindreth G. DuBois, MEd, MMSc, CO, COMT
Access all *Practical Ophthalmology* videos at aao.org
/PracticalOphthalmologyvideo.

CLINICAL PROTOCOL 8-2

Performing the Amsler Grid Test

Test Setup

With the patient wearing appropriate reading spectacles or trial lenses for near correction, ask the patient to hold the testing grid perpendicular to the line of sight, approximately 30 cm (about 12 inches) from the eye. Occlude the eye not being tested.

Check for Scotoma

1. Ask the patient to fixate steadily at the central spot of the grid.

2. Ask the patient whether any of the squares or straight lines appear distorted or missing.

Diagram the Test Result

Have the patient draw the area of visual distortion or loss on the preprinted Amsler grid notepad (see Figure 8-3B). Be sure to note the date, patient's name, and tested eye. Test both eyes and record all results, whether abnormal or not.

9

External Examination

▶ *This chapter includes related videos, which can be accessed by scanning the QR codes provided in the text or going to aao.org/PracticalOphthalmologyvideo.*

The external ocular examination consists of a 3-part stepwise sequence that focuses the examiner's senses on the patient: inspection (looking), palpation (feeling), and auscultation (listening). These methods are accompanied by specific clinical measurements as necessary. A fixed sequence of examination steps helps ensure that the examiner has covered all anatomical details and physiologic functions of the external eye. With experience, screening a patient's external features will occur almost automatically. The patient's history and appearance should lead the examiner to the appropriate testing techniques, so the many available examination tasks described in this chapter need not be applied in their entirety to every patient.

A thoughtful and thorough external examination can yield considerable information that directs the course of the rest of the examination. This chapter details the application of the 3 principal steps in the external ophthalmic examination and provides instruction in a variety of measurement and evaluation techniques that are commonly used in this part of a comprehensive ophthalmic examination.

Situating the Patient

The patient usually sits in the examining chair for the examination. Young children often do well sitting on their parent's lap. An uncooperative infant or toddler can be laid flat on a bed or padded table and immobilized by having the parent hold the child's upstretched arms firmly against the sides of the child's head while leaning against the child's legs and body. Very young infants can be swaddled (Figure 9-1).

General Observation

Before the detailed external ocular examination begins, the examiner usually conducts a brief visual survey of the entire patient, being attentive for signs of medical, dermatologic, and neurologic disease. This general physical observation may occur during casual pre-examination conversation or history taking. By observing the patient's specific actions and appearance, especially the facial features around the eyes, the examiner can often find clues to the patient's attitude, overall well-being, and general physical or ocular problem. Sometimes an examiner can recognize a disease pattern by an initial intuition. Other times, the history will direct the examiner's attention to a specific abnormality.

Figure 9-1 How to bundle a baby for an eye examination. **A,** Fold a sheet into an equilateral triangle and lay the supine infant on it, with the infant's head just above the top edge. **B,** Fold 1 side over the infant to pin 1 arm against the body; tuck the edge of the sheet under the child's body and tuck the bottom flap of the sheet up over the baby's feet. **C,** Hold the other arm against the baby's side while you pull the other edge over the baby's body and tuck the edge underneath the child.

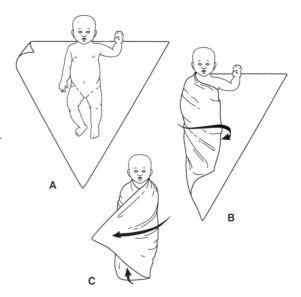

Observing the patient in a lighted room before the stepwise ocular inspection gives many clues to anatomical deformities and illness. During this observation, note the patient's demeanor, mental status, complexion, and apparent nutritional health, along with any abnormal movements, disabilities, or stigmata. Some conditions with obvious features are quickly recognizable, such as albinism and Down syndrome. The extremities, especially the hands, can give clues to systemic diseases, such as rheumatoid arthritis. Focusing on the face and ocular adnexa can reveal skin conditions, such as rosacea and other disorders that can affect the eyes.

During the external examination, the examiner looks for any disturbance in the following sequence:

- head and face: bones, muscles, nerves and blood vessels; skin; lymph nodes; mouth, nose, and paranasal sinuses
- orbit
- eyelids
- lacrimal system
- globe

Inspection

The inspection is a visual survey of the external eye and, like the general observation, often begins while the physician is talking to the patient. The basic equipment for the external examination should be readily available to the examiner (Table 9-1). Clinical measurements that are taken during the external examination are assessed for symmetry and compared with expected values. Each visible or palpable mass is measured in the longest dimension and its perpendicular.

Table 9-1   Equipment for Examining the External Eye

Equipment	Use
Illuminators:	
Room light or natural sunlight	Gross observation of skin abnormalities and other diseases; globe evaluation
Finnoff transilluminator ("muscle light")	Evaluation of masses or lesions of the eyelid and globe; transscleral illumination; estimation of anterior chamber depth
Penlight or pocket flashlight	Diffuse illumination at bedside; evaluation of masses or lesions of the eyelid and globe; near PD measurement
Handheld illuminator with slit aperture	Assessment of axial and peripheral anterior chamber
Blue or UV light source	Tear outflow testing with fluorescein
Direct ophthalmoscope	Transpupillary retroillumination; magnified examination of skin or eye lesions
Retinoscope	Detection of refractive changes caused by abnormal corneal topography and lens opacities
Magnifiers:	
Condensing lens	Assessment of eyelid lesions
Loupes (2×–3×)	Assessment of eyelid and eye lesions
Slit-lamp biomicroscope	Assessment of skin and external ocular lesions
Measuring devices:	
Millimeter ruler	Measurement of lesion dimensions, eyelid positions, intercanthal and interpupillary distances, globe displacement, and corneal diameter
Exophthalmometer	Measurement of exophthalmos and intercanthal distance
Calipers or gauge	Measurement of corneal diameter
Ophthalmodynamometer	Measurement of ophthalmic arterial pressure
Listening devices:	
Stethoscope	Auscultation of orbit, neck, and chest
Blood pressure cuff	Measurement of brachial arterial pressure
Retractors:	
Cotton-tipped applicators	Raising and lowering eyelids; eyelid eversion
Metallic retractors	Eyelid double eversion; opening eyelid of a young child
Pharmaceuticals and supplies:	
Fluorescein solution or strips	Tear film testing and ocular surface status
Schirmer strips	Tear film testing
pH indicator paper	Tear pH testing
Anesthetic eyedrops	Tear film testing and easing pain

Table 9-1   Equipment for Examining the External Eye (continued)

Equipment	Use
Anesthetic gel	Lacrimal probing
Wire swab	Nasal examination
Tongue depressor	Mouth and throat examination
Lacrimal set:	
Punctal dilator	Punctal dilation
Lacrimal probes	Lacrimal probing
Lacrimal cannula with 3 mL syringe	Lacrimal irrigation
Nasal speculum	Nasal examination
Protective devices:	
Examination gloves	Examiner and patient protection
Safety spectacles	Examiner protection

Head and Face

Obtain different perspectives of the patient's head and face, beginning at a talking distance and then proceeding to closer inspection and magnified views. A sketch or photograph of the patient's face can be made to document any abnormalities. Measuring the occipitofrontal circumference of the head with a tape measure, along with other growth measurements, such as height and weight, helps to assess children with developmental delay.

Inspect the face for symmetry and craniofacial bone development, and look for evidence of old trauma, clefting syndromes, and hemifacial atrophy. After this, evaluate the mobility of the facial muscles. Any suspected motor or sensory abnormality is tested by special techniques (Clinical Protocol 9-1). If corneal sensation testing is indicated, that may be performed at this time.

Inspect the facial skin for dermal and vascular changes. Observe the skin's color, texture, tone, and moisture. A magnifying lens such as the +20 D condensing lens used in indirect ophthalmoscopy, the direct ophthalmoscope, 2×–3× binocular loupes, and low magnification with the slit-lamp biomicroscope can help assess individual skin lesions. Common skin abnormalities are classified by the most distinctive characteristic (Table 9-2). The distinguishing attributes of skin abnormalities that should be noted are size, elevation, color, margination, depth of involvement, distribution, surface changes, and degree of tissue destruction or ulceration.

Lymph nodes are normally not visible or palpable. Gross enlargement of any node should be noted. The examiner may palpate for preauricular and cervical lymph nodes before inspecting other external features, particularly when infection, granulomatous disease, or malignancy is being considered.

Examine the inside of the mouth and nose with a penlight to look for changes in the oral and nasal mucous membranes. Note whether the parotid or other salivary glands are enlarged or tender.

Sinus examination is feasible if the light source is very bright and the room is completely dark. To examine each frontal sinus, point the transilluminator upward through the

Table 9-2   Common Abnormalities and Characteristics of the Skin

Abnormality	Characteristics
Erythema	Dilated blood vessels
Macule	Focal area of dilated blood vessels, without palpable elevation
Papule	Focal area of dilated blood vessels, with elevated accumulation of inflammatory and other cells
Nodule	Solid inflammatory lesion that extends into deep dermis
Vesicle	Small blister filled with clear fluid
Bulla	Large blister filled with clear fluid
Pustule	Blister or abscess filled with pus
Cyst	Encapsulated lesion filled with liquid or viscous fluid
Papilloma	Hypertrophied epidermis and vessels with normal surface
Verruca	Papillomatous growth covered by keratotic epidermis
Hyperkeratosis	Accumulation of keratinizing epidermal cells
Scaling	Dried squamous cells
Crusting	Dried blood, pus, or sebum
Eczema	Crusts on an erythematous base
Erosion	Ruptured vesicle or bulla
Ulcer	Loss of epidermis and papillary layer of dermis
Fissure	Linear ulcer
Eschar	Hemorrhagic ulceration

supraorbital ridge while covering the orbit with your hand. To examine each maxillary sinus, point the transilluminator downward, behind the infraorbital rim, and look into the patient's open mouth and through the palate to see the glow of light from clear, air-filled sinuses.

Orbit

The anatomical relationship between the 2 orbits should be noted. Common measurements to be taken for this purpose are the intercanthal distances and the interpupillary distance.

A millimeter ruler is used to measure the intercanthal distances (ie, the distance between the 2 medial canthi and the distance between the 2 lateral canthi). The normal distance between the medial canthi (about 30 mm) is nearly one-half the interpupillary distance. The distance between the lateral canthi is routinely measured during exophthalmometry (discussed later in this chapter).

The interpupillary distance (IPD, or PD) is the distance between the centers of both pupils. The PD is routinely obtained during spectacle lens fitting with a corneal reflection pupillometer, an optical instrument that measures the distance between the 2 corneal reflections (assuming orthophoria). In the clinic, it is convenient to use a millimeter ruler to measure the distance between either the temporal pupillary border or limbus of 1 eye and the nasal pupillary border or limbus of the other eye as the patient stares at a distance target (Figure 9-2). Clinical Protocol 9-2 describes the binocular technique. The average distance PD is about 61 mm, with differences related to sex and ethnicity; the corresponding near PD is about 4 mm less.

Check the position of both globes, first by looking directly at the patient. Look for apparent exophthalmos or enophthalmos with the following technique:

1. Ask the patient to tilt the head forward.
2. Look over the patient's forehead and eyebrows from above, sighting along the plane of the face. You may need to stand up.
3. Elevate both upper eyelids as the patient maintains primary position.
4. Note the position of the front of each globe in relationship to the other. Record any disparity between the 2 eyeballs of more than 2 mm.

Measurement of the axial (anteroposterior) position of the globes by exophthalmometry is important in documenting and following orbital disease. An exophthalmometer measures the distance from the lateral orbital margin to the corneal apex (Figure 9-3). An average value is 17 mm. Measurements are larger in tall people, in those with large skulls or small orbits, and in some patients with axial myopia. Although absolute values help in following an individual patient, the most important initial measurement is the

Figure 9-2 Measuring the interpupillary distance (IPD) by recording the distance between the 2 corneal light reflections. IPD can also be measured between the nasal limbus of 1 eye and the temporal limbus of the other eye.

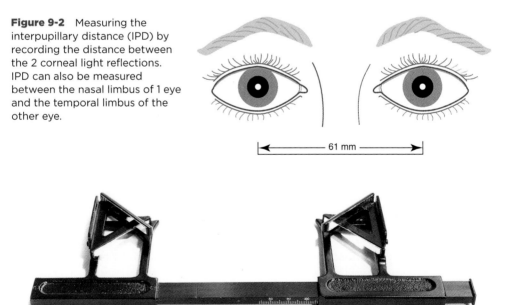

61 mm

Figure 9-3 Exophthalmometer. (Reprinted by permission from Vaughan DG, Asbury T. *General Ophthalmology.* 10th ed. McGraw-Hill/Appleton & Lange, 1983. Reproduced with permission of the McGraw-Hill Companies.)

difference between the 2 eyes. *A difference of more than 2 mm is considered abnormal.* The examiner must make sure that the orbital rims are stable and symmetric, because trauma and facial deformities can affect the measurements. Clinical Protocol 9-3 includes instructions for performing exophthalmometry.

Orbital masses might not only produce proptosis but also displace the globe vertically or horizontally, or even cause retraction of the globe (enophthalmos). The examiner should measure displacement of the globe in any direction. Instructions for doing so are in Clinical Protocol 9-4. Pulsation of the globe should also be noted. Frequently, the patient has to be examined in various seated and supine positions to make ocular pulsations apparent.

Eyelids

Evaluate the symmetry and relative position of the eyebrows. Check to see whether there is any compensatory lifting or wrinkling on 1 side compared with the other. Note the position of the eyelashes relative to the globe, the number or density of the eyelashes, their color, and any regions of missing eyelashes. Note the position, movement, and symmetry of the eyelids, including the presence of any scars from previous surgery or injury.

Specific abnormalities of the eyelids and eyelashes are described, drawn, or photographed for the medical record. Shining a transilluminator through the eyelid can help differentiate a solid from a cystic eyelid mass. Table 9-3 lists common eyelid abnormalities.

With the eyelids open, the upper eyelid usually hides the top 1.5 mm of the cornea. The eyelid creases of the upper and lower eyelids divide the eyelid skin into adherent tarsal portions and loosely attached preseptal portions. The lower eyelid crease is more evident in the young. The nasojugal and malar folds of the lower eyelid become more prominent with aging. Table 9-4 lists many normal adult values relative to eyelid structure and function.

To assess eyelid closure, ask the patient to blink and then to close both eyes gently. Normal eyelid movements are necessary for the lacrimal pump to draw tears into the puncta, canaliculi, and lacrimal sac. Any gap that allows exposure of the ocular surface (ie, lagophthalmos) is noted and measured.

Eyelid position relative to the cornea is estimated by observation of the position of the upper and lower eyelid margins relative to the superior and inferior corneal limbus, respectively. Judging the margin–limbus distances is useful for screening. For any patient with blepharoptosis, the examiner must measure interpalpebral fissure height, upper eyelid margin–corneal reflex distance, upper eyelid crease position, and levator function. Clinical Protocol 9-5 outlines these steps. Figure 9-4 illustrates a method of noting the results of these measurements in the medical record. The degree of blepharoptosis is graded as shown in Table 9-5.

Upper eyelid retraction is assessed with the patient's gaze in the primary position; where the upper eyelid margin crosses the globe in relation to the superior limbus should be noted. Eyelid retraction is classified as listed in Table 9-6. Patients with eyelid retraction might also exhibit eyelid lag (von Graefe sign), which is a delayed or fluttering eyelid movement on downward pursuit.

To detect lower eyelid retraction, first have the patient fixate on a target, such as your finger. While you look at the suspect eye, have the patient follow your finger as you

Table 9-3   Common Abnormalities of the Eyelids, Eyelashes, and Eyebrows

Abnormality	Description
Abnormal eyelid position or function:	
Lagophthalmos	Insufficiency or weakness of eyelid closure
Blepharospasm	Involuntary contraction of the orbicularis oculi muscle
Blepharoptosis	Abnormal drooping of the eyelid (owing to congenital, mechanical, myogenic, aponeurotic, or neurogenic causes)
Protective ptosis	Drooping of the upper eyelid (owing to ocular surface discomfort or inflammation)
Pseudoptosis	An eyelid that appears to sag (owing to contralateral eyelid retraction, a small or displaced globe, or an overhanging brow)
Brow ptosis	Drooping of the eyebrow
Ectropion	Outward turning of the eyelid margin (owing to involutional, cicatricial, or paralytic causes)
Entropion	Inward turning of the eyelid margin (owing to involutional, cicatricial, or spastic causes)
Eyelid lag	Delayed movement of the upper eyelid during downward pursuit of the eye
Abnormal eyelashes or eyebrows:	
Trichiasis	Misdirection of 1 or more eyelashes
Madarosis	Patchy or diffuse loss of eyelashes
Poliosis	Whitening of eyelashes
Distichiasis	Extra row of eyelashes
Synophrys	Confluent eyebrows that meet in the midline
Abnormal eyelid fold:	
Dermatochalasis	Redundant eyelid skin
Blepharochalasis	Chronic lymphedema with wrinkled eyelid skin
Epicanthus	Vertical fold at the medial canthus
Epiblepharon	Horizontal fold near the lower eyelid margin

Table 9-4   Normal Adult Values of Eyelid Structure and Function

Eyelid Structure and Function	Value
Blinking rate	15–16 blinks per minute
Palpebral fissure length	25–30 mm
Palpebral fissure height	8–12 mm
Distance from upper eyelid margin to corneal light reflex	3–5 mm
Distance from upper eyelid margin to upper eyelid crease	8–11 mm
Levator excursion	10–15 mm

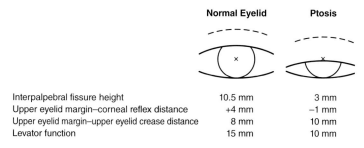

Figure 9-4   Method of recording ptosis measurements.

	Normal Eyelid	Ptosis
Interpalpebral fissure height	10.5 mm	3 mm
Upper eyelid margin–corneal reflex distance	+4 mm	−1 mm
Upper eyelid margin–upper eyelid crease distance	8 mm	10 mm
Levator function	15 mm	10 mm

Table 9-5   Method of Grading Degree of Upper Eyelid Blepharoptosis

Severity	Interpalpebral Fissure Height	Margin–Reflex Distance
Mild	7 mm	+1.5 mm
Moderate	6 mm	+0.5 mm
Severe	5 mm	−0.5 mm

Table 9-6   Method of Grading Degree of Upper Eyelid Retraction

Severity	Upper Eyelid Margin Position
Mild	Eyelid margin intersects the upper limbus
Moderate	Up to 4 mm of sclera of the superior globe is visible
Severe	More than 4 mm of sclera shows

move it downward until the lower eyelid margin of the patient's other eye rests at the lower limbus. Observe whether any sclera shows between the eyelid margin and limbus of the involved eye; this is an indication of eyelid retraction.

Lacrimal System

Observe the lacrimal gland by raising the patient's upper eyelid and instructing the patient to look downward and medially, thereby prolapsing the palpebral lobe. The orbital lobe is sometimes palpable at the superotemporal orbital rim. Observe and note any lacrimal gland masses (see also "Lacrimal System" under "Palpation" later in this chapter).

Observe the lacrimal puncta for apposition to the globe and patency. Look for punctal eversion, stenosis, occlusion, and functional obstruction by redundant conjunctiva. Inspect the area of the lacrimal sac for swelling and erythema. Note whether there is an overflow of tears.

Globe

To examine the entire ocular surface and sclera, hold the eyelids open and ask the patient to look up, down, right, and left. Twirling a cotton applicator at the upper and lower eyelid creases helps to raise and lower the eyelids and avoids direct touching of the eyelids or globe with the fingers. This technique is illustrated in Figure 9-5.

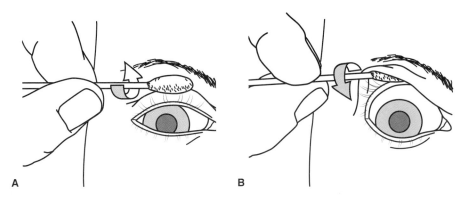

A   B

Figure 9-5 No-touch technique for raising the upper eyelid. **A,** Apply a cotton-tipped applicator to the skin of the upper eyelid at the eyelid crease as the patient looks down. **B,** Twirl the applicator stick between the thumb and forefinger to bunch up the excess eyelid skin and elevate the upper eyelid margin, then elevate the eyelid skin by raising the applicator stick toward the superior orbital rim.

The volume of the tear meniscus should be assessed by inspection. Indicator paper can be used after a chemical injury to check the tear pH.

Inspect the bulbar conjunctiva. Note the type and extent of any conjunctival discharge and classify it as watery, serous, mucoid, mucopurulent, or purulent.

The palpebral conjunctiva is first examined inferiorly. Ask the patient to look up while you gently pull the lower eyelid downward. Evaluate the tarsal conjunctiva, normally about 3–4 mm wide at its central portion, and as much of the remaining lower palpebral conjunctiva as possible. To expose the upper tarsal conjunctiva, evert the upper eyelid as the patient looks down. Clinical Protocol 9-6 presents several techniques for eyelid eversion. The central upper tarsus is normally 9–10 mm wide, and the overlying tarsal conjunctiva generally is the best place to evaluate conjunctival papillae and follicles. Exposure of the retrotarsal conjunctiva and upper fornix might require the use of an eyelid retractor (double eversion of the eyelid).

Examine the anterior globe in sufficient ambient lighting. Subtle color changes of the conjunctiva and sclera (eg, icterus, age-related hyaline plaques at the insertion of horizontal rectus muscles) are better seen with the naked eye in natural sunlight than with slit-lamp illumination. One or more intrascleral nerve loops are often present, usually 4 mm from the superior limbus.

Measurements of the corneal diameter, when needed, are usually obtained with a millimeter ruler, although calipers and gauges give a more accurate reading. The observer must sight exactly perpendicular to the ruler to avoid parallax error. The horizontal corneal diameter is about 10 mm in the newborn and reaches the adult length of 11–12 mm by age 2–3. The vertical diameter is more difficult to assess because the exact location of the superior and inferior limbus is harder to define. The corneal diameter is measured in patients suspected to have a developmental disorder of the globe.

Better ways than gross inspection are available to evaluate corneal topography, but a quick look from the patient's side, aligning your view along the iris plane, helps to discern severe ectasia, as in keratoconus. Another way to detect a corneal deformity is to

Table 9-7   Method of Grading the Anterior Chamber Angle

Angle Grade	Diffuse Light Yields	Slit Light Shows	Interpretation
IV	Full illumination of nasal iris	AC depth = corneal thickness	Angle closure very unlikely
III	⅔ illumination of nasal iris	AC depth = ½ corneal thickness	Angle closure unlikely
II	⅓ Illumination of nasal iris	AC depth = ¼ corneal thickness	Angle closure possible
I	< ⅓ Illumination of nasal iris	AC depth < ¼ corneal thickness	Angle closure likely

inspect the contour of the lower eyelid border as the patient looks down. For example, Munson sign is the angular curvature of the lower eyelid that is produced by keratoconus. The retinoscope and direct ophthalmoscope can also be used to detect refractive changes caused by abnormal corneal topography.

The depth of the anterior chamber can be checked during the external examination. Diffuse penlight and slit-beam techniques for doing so are described in Clinical Protocol 9-7. In the diffuse penlight technique, the angle of the anterior chamber is classified by the extent of illumination of the nasal iris when the penlight is held near the temporal limbus (Table 9-7). Gonioscopy is performed whenever an anterior chamber angle abnormality is suspected (see Chapter 11).

Suspected lesions inside the eye can be assessed with a transilluminator or bright penlight. Clinical Protocol 9-8 describes specific techniques of transscleral illumination and transpupillary retroillumination.

Palpation

Feeling for abnormalities involves tactile, proprioceptive, and temperature senses. The considerate examiner avoids sudden, unexpected touches on or around the eyes, particularly in patients with poor vision and in sighted people who have their eyes closed. Explaining the examination's goals helps to reassure patients during palpation.

A screening examination is done routinely as follows:

1. Use the middle fingers to check for preauricular lymph nodes.
2. Use the index fingers and thumbs to open the eyelids wide apart.
3. Ask the patient to gaze in different directions to expose most of the ocular surface as you inspect the globe.
4. Judge and record any mass according to its size, shape, composition, tenderness, and movability.

A more detailed examination is done when necessary, such as in suspected trauma or with a congenital anomaly. Cranial nerve function might also need to be assessed (see Clinical Protocol 9-1).

Head and Face

Note frontal bossing and other anomalous bony changes. Tenderness over the maxillary or frontal sinus can be a sign of paranasal sinusitis.

Palpation of the temporal artery in elderly patients might reveal tenderness with hardening and tortuosity during acute episodes of giant-cell arteritis. Palpation of the neck vessels is done to check for carotid arterial pulses and for a jugular venous hum (Figure 9-6).

Certain types of infections produce enlarged lymph nodes. Palpation for an enlarged preauricular (superficial parotid) lymph node is done by placing the fingers below the patient's temple, just in front of the tragus. This node is normally neither tender nor palpable. Palpate the submandibular lymph nodes, which are located under the angle of the jaw. Superficial cervical lymph glands—the jugular, post-sternocleidomastoid, and supraclavicular nodes—are palpated in patients with suspected lymphadenopathy. The locations of these lymph nodes are shown in Figure 9-7.

Orbit

Clinical Protocol 9-9 describes the methods of palpating the orbital margins and contents of patients with head trauma who might have fractures. A step-off can indicate a facial fracture. Simultaneous palpation of both sides makes it easier to identify abnormalities. In all cases of suspected orbital trauma, the examiner must first be certain of the integrity of the globe before any manipulations are done. If a ruptured globe is suspected, do not palpate directly. Instead, hold the eyelids of an injured eye open by directing the upper eyelid onto the brow and the lower eyelid onto the cheek without pressing on the globe. Note discrepancies from the normal anatomy in the medical record.

Eyelids

Gentle palpation of the closed eyelids is done by sliding the examining finger over the eyelid skin. This maneuver can be facilitated by stretching the skin and having the patient rotate the globe so that the examiner does not press on the cornea. A mass can sometimes be felt even when it is difficult to see. The examiner should note the presence of an eyelid

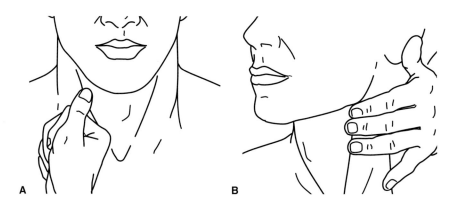

Figure 9-6 Palpation of the carotid pulse. **A,** Placement of the examiner's thumb from the front. **B,** Placement of the examiner's fingers from behind.

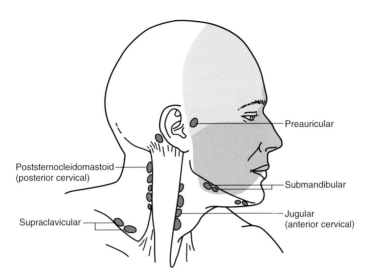

Figure 9-7 Lymph nodes inspected or palpated during the external ophthalmic examination. Shaded areas show the lymphatic drainage of the ocular adnexa to the preauricular and submandibular nodes.

mass and whether the eyelid margin or conjunctiva is involved. The dimensions of an eyelid lesion should be measured with a millimeter ruler. Generally, the longest diameter and its perpendicular are recorded, along with the lesion's consistency and movability.

To test for the presence of a Bell phenomenon (activated superior rectus function when efforts are made to close the eyelids against resistance), ask the patient to shut the eyelids and to keep them closed while you gently pry the eyelids open and peek at the position of the globes. Determining which part of the globe lies behind the interpalpebral fissure is important if there is incomplete eyelid closure (so as to know whether corneal exposure is occurring).

Lacrimal System

Any mass of the lacrimal gland or lacrimal sac is evaluated for size and tenderness. A patient with epiphora should undergo compression of the sac to learn if material can be expressed from the puncta. Clinical Protocol 9-10 describes lacrimal sac compression and the dye disappearance test, which are the principal diagnostic tests for a patient with excess tears.

Globe

Applying fingertip pressure onto the eyeball through the eyelid can help determine whether congested vessels can be blanched (which suggests conjunctival vascular dilation) or not (such as with ciliary flush or episcleritis) and whether a nodule is movable (which suggests a conjunctival phlyctenule or episcleral nodule) or not (such as with nodular scleritis). The location of any focal tenderness should be noted.

Schirmer testing, used for patients with dry eye, is described in Clinical Protocol 9-11. The examiner uses sterile filter paper strips (30 mm long, plus a 5 mm wick) to assess the amount of tear fluid. The Schirmer test *without* anesthetic measures both basal tears (from the accessory lacrimal glands) and reflex tears (from the main lacrimal gland). The test *with* anesthetic measures predominantly basal tear secretion. The examiner usually selects only 1 of these 2 tests. Each test measures the relative degree of aqueous tear production, because the amount of conjunctival mucus and meibomian gland lipids collected by the test strips is negligible. A measurement (*with* anesthetic) of >10 mm/5 min is regarded as indicating normal tear production. A measurement of 5–10 mm/5 min is equivocal and could be normal or abnormal, because tear production varies by age and other factors. A value of <5 mm/5 min suggests a dry eye state. Measurements *without* anesthetic tend to be about 5 mm/5 min greater because the strips cause some irritation.

Auscultation

Auscultation for an orbital bruit is performed by placing the bell of the stethoscope over the closed eyelids as the patient briefly holds their breath. A small pediatric bell works well. The noise of eyeball movement can be eliminated by instructing the patient to open the eyelids of the opposite eye and fixate on a straight-ahead target. The stethoscope bell can also be placed over the frontal sinus and on the temple to listen around the orbit.

Faint rumbling sounds heard over the globe can be normal. An orbital bruit can signify the presence of a carotid-cavernous fistula or an arteriovenous malformation. The bruit is usually accentuated during systole and decreases with compression of the ipsilateral carotid artery or both jugular veins.

The neck can be examined for a carotid bruit by listening over the carotid bifurcation, just below the jaw angle. Chest auscultation is necessary to ensure that a cardiac murmur is not being transmitted to the neck. Some ophthalmologists include blood pressure measurement in their initial eye examination.

Pitfalls and Pointers

- Be professional and nonjudgmental during the external examination. Be aware that the patient is probably "examining the examiner" and is sensitive to offhand remarks and nonverbal signs that could be misinterpreted. Conversing with the patient helps to distract the patient from your observation and palpation tasks.

- Wash your hands between patients. Washing your hands with warm water in the room just before starting the examination shows the patient that you follow recommended precautions and often alleviates some anxiety. Warm, dry, clean, and manicured hands are appreciated by everyone.

- Ensure that all examining equipment is properly cleaned by clinic protocol (tonometry tips, goniolenses, etc.). If your slit lamp has a steel or plastic chin rest, clean it after use with each patient.

- Don't rush to examine the obvious lesion and ignore the rest of the external examination. Sit back, get an overview, and proceed carefully and thoroughly through the stepwise procedure. Recall that the reason the patient is in your office may be quite different from what you first suspect or is advertised by a consult note.

- Don't forget to compare the abnormal eye with the fellow eye. Back-and-forth comparisons between both sides of the face can reveal a subtle asymmetry.

- Compare your findings with previous records. Looking at old photographs, including driver's licenses, can reveal an unrecognized but long-standing ptosis or asymmetry. If necessary, have the patient bring in old photographs from home. The examiner should also have photographs taken whenever possible to document trauma, presurgical appearance, and any lesion that might be growing. When photographs are not possible, careful drawings included within the medical record can greatly aid future caregivers in the assessment of the evolution of pathology.

- Be careful when measuring the eyelid fissure height. The position of the eyelids will change depending upon eye position, facial muscle activity, alertness, and external stimuli such as phenylephrine eyedrops. Check the palpebral fissure in primary position, with the eyes gazing at a distance target. Don't forget to observe the brow for ptosis, compensatory elevation, and wrinkling.

- Be gentle. Pressure on the globe can elicit the oculocardiac reflex and produce bradycardia in susceptible individuals. Be sure to warn the patient about what to expect during procedures such as eyelid eversion.

Suggested Resource

Orbit, Eyelids, and Lacrimal System. Basic and Clinical Science Course, Section 7. American Academy of Ophthalmology; published annually.

CLINICAL PROTOCOL 9-1

Performing a Neurosensory Examination of the Head and Face

Assessing Facial Nerve Function

1. Ask the patient to squeeze their eyes closed forcefully and note whether the orbicularis oculi muscles completely bring the eyelids together.

2. Compare the relative strength of both orbicularis oculi muscles by using your fingertips to pry the eyelids open. The needed force should be the same for both sides.

3. Ask the patient to smile and show their teeth. Note the symmetry of the facial expression.

4. When there is weakness of 1 side of the lower face, check for a supranuclear lesion by asking the patient to raise both eyebrows and to wrinkle the forehead. A central facial palsy spares the forehead and orbicularis oculi muscles; a peripheral lesion often does not.

Eliciting Blink Reflexes

1. Without mentioning it to the patient, note the frequency and completeness of normal blinks. Expect to see a complete blink every 4 seconds.

2. If involuntary blinks are absent, swat your hand toward the patient to assess whether a blinking movement can be elicited.

3. Gently tap on the patient's glabella if a central nervous system disorder is suspected. A normal response produces only a few blinking movements; repetitive blinks (as in parkinsonism) are abnormal.

Assessing Facial Sensation

1. Using your fingertip, tissue paper, or cotton wisp, lightly touch 1 side of the patient's face and then the contralateral, corresponding side. Ask the patient to compare the affected side with the normal side. Repeat for all 3 trigeminal nerve dermatomes and for the distribution of each principal sensory nerve (Figure 1).

2. Map the area of reduced sensation (eg, the zone of hypesthesia that results from an infraorbital nerve damaged by an orbital floor fracture).

3. Perform simultaneous testing of both sides of the face if abnormal cortical function is suspected.

Testing Corneal Sensation

1. Without touching the eyelashes or stimulating the visual startle reflex, touch the cornea with a clean cotton wisp, facial tissue wick, fragment of dental floss, or puff of air from a small syringe. A brief touch should

Figure 1 Assessing facial sensation.

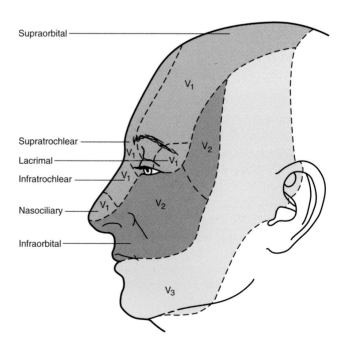

produce a reflex blink with a faint subjective sensation. The response may be graded on a scale of 0 to 4+.

2. Use an esthesiometer, an instrument that has a nylon filament of adjustable length, to quantify the degree of sensation for patients in whom recovery or further loss is anticipated.

CLINICAL PROTOCOL 9-2

Measuring Binocular Interpupillary Distance

1. Ask the patient to fixate a distance target.
2. Facing the patient at an arm's-length distance, position yourself just below the patient's gaze. Align your eyes with the patient's eyes as the patient maintains distance fixation over your head.
3. Rest the millimeter ruler lightly across the bridge of the patient's nose.
4. Close your right eye and use your left eye to line up the zero point of the ruler with the temporal limbus of the patient's right eye (Figure 1).
5. Keep the ruler steady. Close your left eye and open your right eye.
6. Read the measurement that aligns with the nasal limbus of the patient's left eye (Figure 2).
7. Repeat the above sequence to confirm a reproducible reading.
8. Near PD is measured in a similar way by having the patient stare at your nose instead of the distance target.

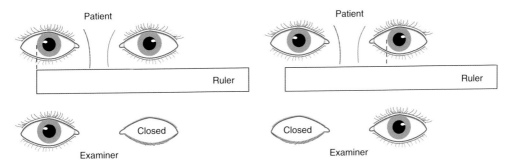

Figure 1 Aligning with the patient's right eye.   **Figure 2** Aligning with the patient's left eye.

CLINICAL PROTOCOL 9-3

Performing Exophthalmometry

1. Position yourself directly in front of the patient. Your left eye measures the patient's right eye, and your right eye measures the patient's left eye.
2. Hold the exophthalmometer so that the angled mirrors are oriented upward, above the fixation foot plates.

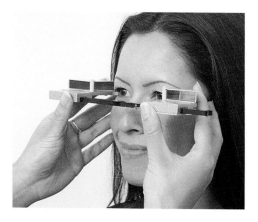

Figure 1 Position of the foot plates.

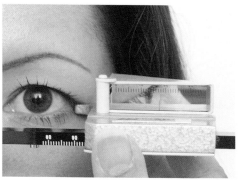

Figure 2 The mirror image of the corneal curvature is visible on the ruler.

3. If a patient's previous intercanthal reading is known, set the last recorded distance between the patient's lateral canthi on the scale. If this is the patient's first reading, place the instrument so that the foot plates rest on both lateral orbital rims at the level of the outer canthi (Figure 1).

4. With your left eye, sight along the right-hand mirror of the instrument at the reflection of the patient's right eye.

5. Instruct the patient to occlude their left eye with a hand or occluder and to look toward your eye to achieve straight-ahead alignment.

6. Using your open left eye, align the instrument's 2 vertical markers (usually a long vertical line in the center of the proptosis scale and a corresponding mark or line on the instrument's base).

7. Read the distance from the lateral orbital rim to the corneal apex by noting where the mirror image of the patient's anterior-most corneal curvature falls along the mirror's millimeter ruler (Figure 2). Note that you see the anterior corneal surface from the side; the reading is the anterior extent of the corneal apex on the gauge.

8. Obtain a similar measurement for the patient's left eye by using your right eye to align the appropriate vertical markers on the opposite mirror of the instrument.

9. Record the readings for each eye and the distance between the lateral canthi as shown in Figure 3.

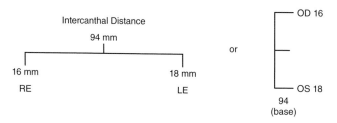

Figure 3 Recording exophthalmometry results.

CLINICAL PROTOCOL 9-4

Measuring Globe Displacement

Horizontal Displacement

1. Imagine a vertical straight line down the middle of the patient's face that aligns the center of the glabella and the philtrum of the upper lip.

2. Hold a millimeter ruler horizontally across the bridge of the patient's nose, perpendicular to the imaginary vertical line (Figure 1).

3. Measure the distance from the center of the nasal bridge to the medial limbus of the right eye as the patient stares at a distance target. Occlude the contralateral eye if strabismus is present.

4. Repeat the measurement for the left eye. The difference between the 2 measurements is the amount of horizontal displacement.

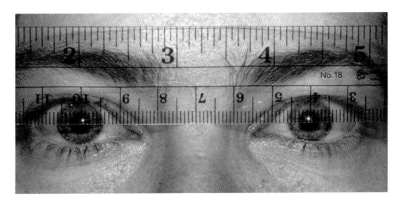

Figure 1 Horizontal displacement measurement. (Reprinted from *Clinical Tests: Ophthalmology,* by Huber and Reacher, 1989.)

Vertical Displacement

1. Hold a straightedge horizontally along the patient's nasal bridge to visually align the lateral canthi.

2. Hold a millimeter ruler vertically, perpendicular to the horizontal straightedge, to pass through the center of the pupil of the patient's right eye.

3. Measure the distance from the edge of the horizontal straightedge to the pupillary center (or corneal light reflex).

4. Repeat the measurement for the left eye. The difference between the 2 measurements is the amount of vertical displacement.

CLINICAL PROTOCOL 9-5

Measuring Eyelid Position

Interpalpebral Fissure Height

1. Ask the patient to fixate a penlight in primary gaze position.
2. Hold a millimeter ruler vertically, close to the patient's open eye, to measure the distance between the center of the upper and lower eyelid margins (Figure 1).
3. Record the interpalpebral fissure height in millimeters for each eye.
4. To recheck the measurements, obtain and add together the following 2 measurements:
   a. The distance between the upper eyelid margin and the corneal light reflex (normally about 4 mm).
   b. The distance between the lower eyelid margin and the corneal light reflex (normally about 6 mm).

Video 1 demonstrates taking eyelid measurements.

 VIDEO 1 Eyelid Measurements
Courtesy of Richard C. Allen, MD, PhD.
Access all *Practical Ophthalmology* videos at aao.org /PracticalOphthalmologyvideo.

Upper Eyelid Margin–Corneal Reflex Distance

1. Hold a penlight directly in front of the patient, so that the patient observes it in primary gaze and a corneal light reflex is present.
2. Use a millimeter ruler to measure the distance between the center of the upper eyelid margin and the corneal light reflex (Figure 2).
3. Record the margin–reflex distance for each eye. Use a negative number if the light reflex is obstructed by the eyelid.

Upper Eyelid Crease Position

1. Use a penlight or other near target to bring the patient's gaze into the primary position.
2. Measure the distance between the upper eyelid margin and the upper eyelid crease (Figure 3).
3. Record the upper eyelid crease position for each eye. Note if the upper eyelid crease is absent and cannot be accurately measured.

Levator Function

1. Either hold a thumb on the brow or place the palm of your hand against the patient's forehead. This maneuver prevents the frontalis muscle from assisting with upper eyelid elevation, thereby isolating the action of the levator muscle.

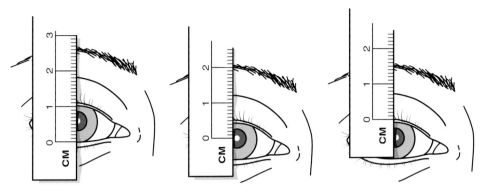

Figure 1 Measuring the interpalpebral fissure height.

Figure 2 Measuring the upper eyelid margin–corneal reflex distance.

Figure 3 Measuring the upper eyelid crease position.

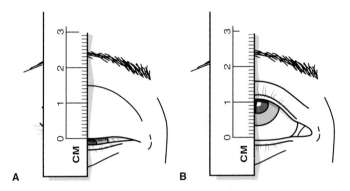

Figure 4 Measuring levator function. **A,** Aligning with patient's upper eyelid margin. **B,** Aligning the new location of the upper eyelid margin.

2. Ask the patient to look down, and align the zero point of the millimeter ruler with the patient's upper eyelid margin; take care not to touch the patient's eyelids or eyelashes (Figure 4A).

3. Do not move the ruler. Ask the patient to look up as far as possible. Keeping the ruler steady, measure the new location of the upper eyelid margin (Figure 4B). The difference between the 2 measurements (ie, the total amount of upper eyelid excursion) gives the levator function.

4. Record the levator function in millimeters for each eye.

CLINICAL PROTOCOL 9-6

Everting the Eyelid

Examining the Lower Conjunctiva and Fornix

1. With the patient looking down, press the skin below the lower eyelid with your thumb or forefinger against the maxillary bone and tug down (Figure 1A).

Figure 1 Examining the lower conjunctiva and fornix. **A,** Lower eyelid position. **B,** The patient is asked to look up.

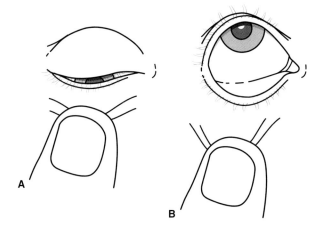

2. Ask the patient to look up, which allows the lower fornix to prolapse and exposes most of the lower palpebral conjunctiva (Figure 1B).

Examining the Upper Conjunctiva

Steps for the 2-hand method:

1. Using your thumb and forefinger to grasp some eyelashes, pull the upper eyelid margin away from the globe (Figure 2A).
2. Place an applicator stick horizontally at the upper eyelid crease, along the upper border of the tarsus, to act as a fulcrum (Figure 2B). Hold the applicator stick in the hand that is temporal to the eye being examined.
3. Pull the upper eyelid margin outward and upward to fold the upper eyelid over the applicator stick (Figure 2C). Withdraw the applicator stick and hold the eyelid margin in place against the skin overlying the superior orbital rim with the thumb in order to view the upper tarsal conjunctiva (Figure 2D). Eversion of the upper eyelid is easier if the patient is looking down.

Steps for the 1-hand method:

1. With the patient looking upward, use your hand that is temporal to the eye being examined and place your thumb against the lower eyelid to hold it in place (Figure 3A).
2. Place the tip of the index finger against the upper eyelid to hold the upper eyelid upward; instruct the patient to look down and to hold that gaze (Figure 3B).
3. Pinch the upper and lower eyelids together, an action that should permit the upper eyelid to hang over the lower eyelid margin (Figure 3C).
4. Lay the side of your index fingertip across the upper eyelid, just above the upper border of the tarsus, and push on the upper tarsal border.

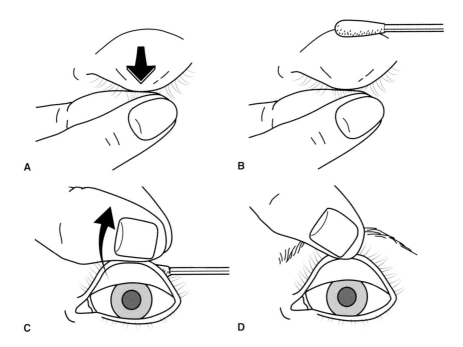

Figure 2 Examining the upper conjunctiva, 2-hand method. **A,** Upper eyelid position.
B, Applicator stick acting as a fulcrum. **C,** Upper eyelid folding over the applicator stick.
D, Eyelid held in place with the thumb.

5. Pinch the upper eyelid outward between your index finger and thumb (Figure 3D).
6. With finger and wrist rotation, flip the upper eyelid over to expose the upper palpebral conjunctiva. The index finger maintains a steady downward pressure on the upper eyelid crease as the finger is pulled away. The thumb provides the upward rotary action that turns the eyelid over. The thumb holds the upper eyelid margin in place against the superior orbital margin (Figure 3E).

Exposing the Upper Fornix
Steps for the 1-hand method:

1. Evert the upper eyelid by the 2-hand or 1-hand method.
2. Firmly hold the upper eyelid margin against the superior orbital margin with your thumb.
3. With your free hand, use your forefinger to press the lower eyelid upward over part of the cornea and backward against the globe. This action should compress the orbital contents sufficiently to cause most of the upper fornix to protrude.

Steps for the retractor method:

1. With the patient looking down, use your thumb and forefinger to grasp some eyelashes of the upper eyelid and pull the eyelid margin away from the globe.

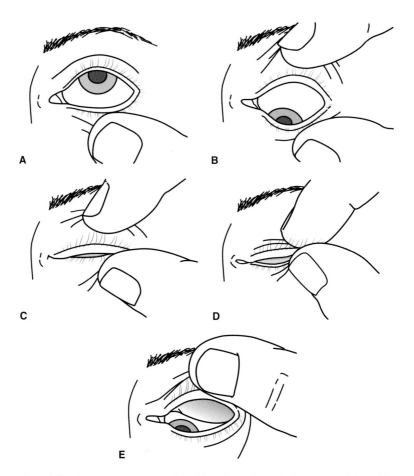

Figure 3 Examining the upper conjunctiva, 1-hand method. **A,** Lower eyelid position. **B,** Examiner's fingers holding the eyelids apart. **C,** Bringing the eyelids back together. **D,** Pinching the upper eyelid outward. **E,** Everting the upper eyelid.

2. With your free hand, place the edge of an eyelid retractor at the upper border of the tarsus of the upper eyelid, with the retractor handle facing down (Figure 4A).

3. Rotate the handle of the retractor upward and hold the retractor in place to view the upper tarsal conjunctiva (Figure 4B).

4. Continue to rotate the retractor and allow its curved end to press the cul-de-sac outward. This action everts the eyelid and exposes the upper fornix by suspending the upper eyelid on the retractor (Figure 4C). Pressing on the globe from below accentuates the protrusion of the upper fornix.

Tip: Instillation of an eyedrop of proparacaine into each eye prior to eyelid manipulation for forniceal examination can aid patient comfort.

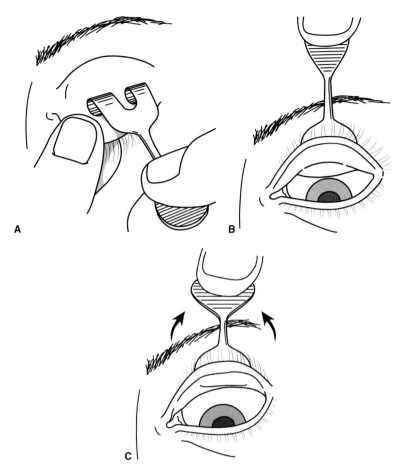

Figure 4 Exposing the upper fornix, retractor method. **A,** Placing the eyelid retractor.
B, Rotating the handle upward. **C,** Continued rotation presses the cul-de-sac outward.

Video 1 demonstrates eyelid eversion.

VIDEO 1 Eyelid Eversion
Courtesy of Richard C. Allen, MD, PhD.

CLINICAL PROTOCOL 9-7

Estimating Anterior Chamber Depth

Penlight With Diffuse Beam

1. While facing the patient, hold a penlight near the temporal limbus, and shine the light across the front of the right eye toward the nose. Keep the beam parallel to the plane of the normal iris.

2. Observe the medial aspect of the iris. Normally, the iris is completely illuminated (Figure 1A). An eye with a shallow anterior chamber will have two-thirds of the nasal portion of the iris in shadow (Figure 1B).

3. Grade the angle as open (grade IV or III), intermediate (grade II), or narrow (grade I).

4. Repeat the test for the left eye.

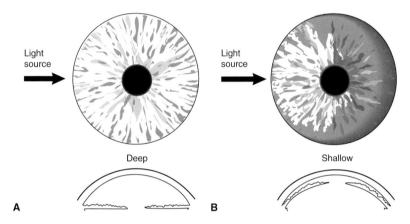

Figure 1 Estimating anterior chamber depth. **A,** Normal iris with complete illumination. **B,** Iris with shadow, indicating shallow anterior chamber.

Slit Lamp With Slit Beam (van Herick method)

1. Direct the thin slit beam perpendicular to the peripheral cornea.

2. View the anterior chamber angle at a 60° angle from the beam.

3. Grade the peripheral angle width by comparing the distance between the corneal endothelium and the iris with the corneal thickness. In an open angle, the peripheral chamber depth equals the corneal thickness. When the peripheral depth is one-fourth or less of the normal corneal thickness, gonioscopy should be done to evaluate the angle.

Video 1 demonstrates slit-lamp assessment of angles.

  VIDEO 1 Slit-Lamp Assessment of Angles
Courtesy of Lindreth G. DuBois, MEd, MMSc, CO, COMT.

CLINICAL PROTOCOL 9-8

Illuminating the Inner Eye for External Viewing

Illumination Through the Sclera

1. In a darkened room, place the tip of the transilluminator against the eyelid. The light could also be held directly against the patient's anesthetized globe if the bulb is not hot.

2. Identify the red reflex, which is normally seen exiting through the dilated pupil and glowing through most of the sclera.

3. If a corneal opacity that obscures a clear view of the inner eye is present, note the shape of the pupil.

4. With transscleral illumination, look for a mass in the eye wall. Move the light source over the surface of the globe while examining the light reflected through the pupil and sclera. The pupil will be dark when the transilluminator is placed over a solid lesion. A solid lesion inside the eye wall will also obscure the faint scleral glow when the light is held against the adjacent or opposite sclera.

Illumination Through the Pupil

1. Shine a coaxial bright light, such as the direct ophthalmoscope, into the patient's eye from a distance of about 50 cm.

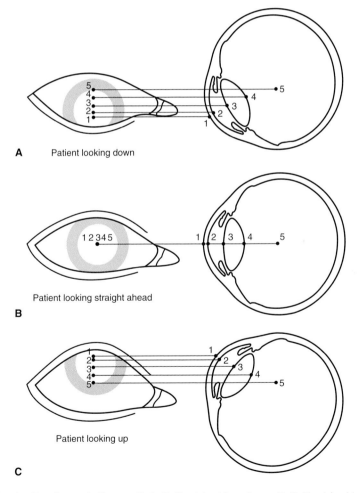

Figure 1 Illumination through the pupil. **A,** Patient looking down. **B,** Patient looking straight ahead. **C,** Patient looking up.

2. Look for any obscuration of the reflected light. Opacities near the pupillary axis appear as dark shadows at the pupillary plane against the normal red reflex.

3. Localize an opacity by asking the patient to look slowly up and down or by shifting the direction of the light; opacities visible against the red reflex will shift with eye movements according to their position relative to the pupillary plane (Figure 1). Determine in which direction the opacity appears to move, in relationship to the pupillary axis:

    a. *No movement.* An opacity in the pupil, such as an anterior lens opacity, will remain stationary.

    b. *Same direction.* An opacity anterior to the pupil (eg, in the cornea) shifts in the same direction as the patient's direction of gaze.

    c. *Opposite direction.* An opacity posterior to the pupil (eg, in the posterior lens or vitreous) shifts in the opposite direction.

CLINICAL PROTOCOL 9-9

Palpating the Orbit

Orbital Rim

1. Palpate the anterior portion of the orbit by placing a finger between the orbital margin and the globe. Standing behind the patient can make it easier to methodically trace, with the pad of the finger, the margin around the orbital rim.

2. Begin laterally. The lateral orbital margin is generally about 5 mm from the lateral canthus.

3. Slowly move upward (clockwise on the patient's right orbit and counterclockwise on the left orbit). Locate the supraorbital notch (foramen) by gently moving your fingertips along the orbital rim, at the junction of the medial one-third and lateral two-thirds of the superior orbital margin.

4. Move your fingertips medial to the supraorbital notch. Feel for the trochlea, normally palpable 4 mm posterior to the orbital margin. The upper border of the medial canthal ligament can be felt just below this point.

5. Move your fingertips along the inferior orbital margin, which should form a smooth, continuous contour. A vertical line that extends from the supraorbital notch intersects the palpable infraorbital foramen 4 mm below the inferior orbital margin.

6. Move your finger along the outer orbital rim and feel the marginal tubercle of the zygomatic bone. Approximately 6 mm above this point is the junction of the frontal and zygomatic bones, which is palpable at the supraorbital margin. The frontozygomatic suture is about 10 mm from the lateral canthus.

Orbital Contents

1. After completing the circumference of the orbital rim, gently touch the patient's closed eyelids.

a. Any thrill or pulsation movement should be noted.

b. If a sinus fracture is suspected, move the fingers around the globe to detect any crepitus within the confines of the orbital margin.

c. Press gently into the periocular tissues to feel for the anterior extension of a retrobulbar or anterior orbital mass.

2. Judge the resiliency of the retrobulbar tissues by cautiously pushing the globe posteriorly through the patient's closed eyelids. Normally the eye can be displaced into the orbital fat about 5 mm. By comparing the 2 orbits, the degree and ease of globe retropulsion are assessed.

3. Ask the patient to perform a Valsalva maneuver. Judge whether any pressure is transmitted to the orbits by keeping your fingertips pressed onto both globes through the patient's closed eyelids during the maneuver.

CLINICAL PROTOCOL 9-10

Measuring Lacrimal Outflow in the Tearing Patient

Lacrimal Sac Compression

1. Apply pressure by gently pushing your index finger or a cotton-tipped applicator stick over the lacrimal fossa, inside the inferomedial orbital rim (not on the side of the nasal bone).

2. Note any mucus or mucopurulent material that can be expressed back through the canaliculi and puncta. Reflux confirms a completely obstructed nasolacrimal duct (Figure 1). If no reflux is found, then proceed with the dye disappearance test.

Dye Disappearance Test

1. Instill fluorescein into both eyes with a moistened fluorescein strip or an eyedrop of fluorescein solution.

2. Observe the tear film, preferably with a cobalt-blue light, to ensure that fluorescein is visible in the preocular tear film of both eyes.

3. Wait 5 minutes. The patient may blink normally but should avoid wiping the eyes.

4. Use a cobalt-blue light to examine the tear meniscus.

a. The tear film should be clear, which indicates complete disappearance of the fluorescein dye.

b. If the tears are still tinged yellow, the lacrimal outflow system has a functional or anatomical blockage (Figure 2).

c. Record any asymmetric clearance by indicating which side retains the dye longer.

5. For patients with delayed clearance of fluorescein, determine the level of occlusion by lacrimal probing and irrigation.

Figure 1 Lacrimal sac compression. (Courtesy of Francis C. Sutula, MD. Reprinted from *Orbit, Eyelids, and Lacrimal System,* Basic and Clinical Science Course, Section 7; 1996.)

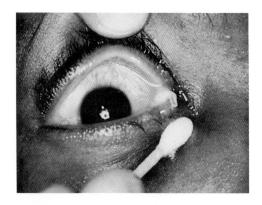

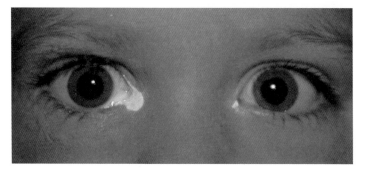

Figure 2 Dye disappearance test. (Reprinted from *Orbit, Eyelids, and Lacrimal System,* Basic and Clinical Science Course, Section 7; 1996.)

CLINICAL PROTOCOL 9-11

Conducting Tear Production Tests for the Dry Eye

Schirmer I Test ("Schirmer Without Anesthetic")

1. Seat the patient in a dimmed room with the back of the head stabilized against the headrest of the examining chair.

2. Remove any excess moisture from the patient's eyelid margin and cul-de-sac with a facial tissue or cotton-tipped applicator. Do not instill any eyedrops into the eye before the test.

3. Fold a packaged, sterile filter paper strip at the indentation mark. To avoid contaminating the sterile strips, bend the round wick end of the test strips at the notch 120° before opening the pouch.

4. Open the pouch and remove a strip. Use the strip with the angled end for the right eye. Grasp the strip by the non–wick end to avoid contaminating the wick end with your fingertips.

5. Ask the patient to look up. Draw the lower eyelid gently downward, and make sure that the eyelid margin has been adequately dried with a

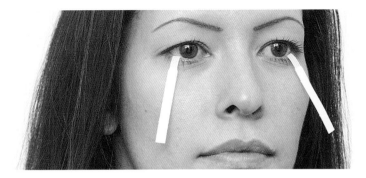

Figure 1   Schirmer test. (Photo by Dan McGarrah.)

cotton-tipped applicator. By convention, the strip with 1 corner cut off is used for the right eye.

6. Hook the rounded, bent end of the test strip over the lower eyelid margin of each eye and release the lower eyelid to hold the strip in place. The strip is typically placed at the junction of the inner two-thirds and the outer one-third of the eyelid margin. It should not touch the cornea. The notch should point toward the lateral canthus. Check to make sure that the short end of the strip is inserted all the way to the notch.

7. Ask the patient to gaze slightly above the midline with the eyelids open (Figure 1). The patient may continue normal blinking. Patients are permitted to keep their eyes closed during the test, but squeezing should be discouraged.

8. At this point, try to avoid any interruptions to the patient and note the time. After 5 minutes have elapsed, remove both strips.

9. Measure the distance between the indentation mark and the farthest extent of wetting. Standardized strips are packaged in an envelope with a millimeter scale. Do not include the bent wick end in the final measurement.

10. Record the result in the chart as follows: Schirmer I testing (without anesthetic): right eye: X mm/5 min; left eye: Y mm/5 min. If complete wetting occurs before 5 minutes, this time may be noted.

Basic Secretion Test ("Schirmer with Anesthetic")

1. Instill 1 drop of proparacaine 1% eyedrops into both eyes.

2. Wait 1 minute while the patient keeps both eyes closed.

3. Gently blot the cul-de-sac dry with a tissue or cotton swab.

4. Proceed with steps 1–10 of the Schirmer I test.

10 Slit-Lamp Biomicroscopy

The slit-lamp biomicroscope (commonly called the *slit lamp*) is an instrument that permits magnified examination of the eye with various kinds of illumination. A unique feature of the slit lamp is that its slit-shaped beam of light allows the examination in cross-section of living ocular tissues that are transparent or translucent. The slit lamp enhances the external examination by allowing a binocular, stereoscopic view; a wide range of magnification (6× to 40×); and illumination of variable shapes and intensities.

This chapter discusses the uses of the slit lamp in general and its parts and their functions in detail, including the principles of slit-lamp illumination. Various diagnostic and measurement techniques conducted with a slit lamp also are covered. Specific applications of slit-lamp techniques to the anterior segment examination are discussed in Chapter 11; detailed instructions for performing Goldmann applanation tonometry with the slit lamp appear in Chapter 12; instructions for indirect slit-lamp biomicroscopy of the posterior segment are included in Chapter 13.

Uses of the Slit Lamp

The slit lamp allows for detailed examination of all tissues of the eye and adnexa. It is routinely used for examination of the anterior segment and anterior vitreous. Most of the anterior segment tissues (except the anterior chamber angle and the posterior surface of the iris) are directly visible with the slit lamp alone, without special lenses. Optical constraints of the instrument and the eye prevent visualization of the angle of the anterior chamber and those structures that are posterior to the anterior vitreous unless various hand-held lenses are used (as discussed later in this chapter and in Chapters 11 and 13).

In addition to being a tool for examination, the slit lamp is often used for tonometry, linear measurement of tissues or lesions, ophthalmic photography, and laser therapy. It can also be used to aid in contact lens fitting and minor surgical procedures, such as removal of foreign bodies in the conjunctiva or cornea.

Parts of the Slit Lamp

A typical slit lamp is illustrated in Figure 10-1. The Haag-Streit 900 model is shown because it is the most commonly encountered; several other slit lamps, whose differences from the Haag-Streit instrument are usually relatively minor or are easily mastered, are also available.

The slit-lamp biomicroscope consists of 3 principal portions: the viewing, or observational, arm, which contains the eyepiece and magnifying elements; the illumination arm, which contains the light source and its controls; and the patient-positioning frame. These portions are connected to a base, which has a joystick that the examiner uses to

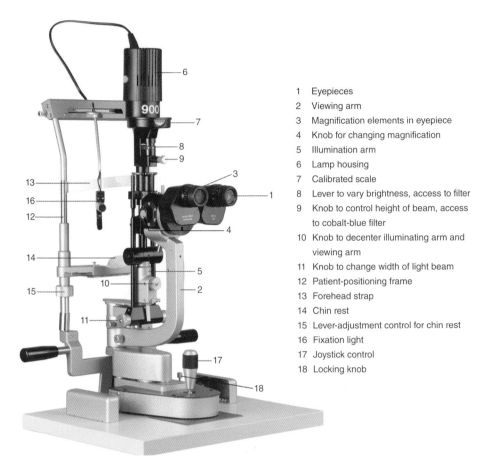

1 Eyepieces
2 Viewing arm
3 Magnification elements in eyepiece
4 Knob for changing magnification
5 Illumination arm
6 Lamp housing
7 Calibrated scale
8 Lever to vary brightness, access to filter
9 Knob to control height of beam, access to cobalt-blue filter
10 Knob to decenter illuminating arm and viewing arm
11 Knob to change width of light beam
12 Patient-positioning frame
13 Forehead strap
14 Chin rest
15 Lever-adjustment control for chin rest
16 Fixation light
17 Joystick control
18 Locking knob

Figure 10-1 Parts of the slit lamp (Haag-Streit 900). The numbers correspond to descriptions given in the text. (Courtesy of Haag-Streit USA, Inc.)

move the viewing and illumination arms about. The entire unit is wired to a transformer power source on a supporting platform. The specific parts of the instrument are detailed below; numbers in parentheses correspond to the numbers in Figure 10-1.

The Viewing Arm

The examiner looks through a pair of eyepieces (1), also known as *oculars,* mounted on top of the viewing arm (2), which typically provide 3.5× magnification. A knurled focusing ring around each ocular can be twisted to suit the examiner's refractive error, and the two oculars can be pushed together or spread apart, much like the eyepieces of field binoculars, to accommodate the examiner's interpupillary distance. The oculars are attached to a housing that contains the instrument's magnification elements (3). Depending on the model, magnification can be adjusted with a lever below the housing (10× or 16×) or a knob just behind the oculars (4) (5 increments, from 6.3× to 40×).

The Illumination Arm

For most illumination techniques, the illumination arm (5) and the viewing arm are kept parfocal, that is, the image of the source of illumination and the image being viewed by the examiner are both in focus at the same location at any given time. The illumination arm can also be swung on its pivoting base 180°, which allows the examiner to direct the light beam anywhere between the nasal and the temporal aspect of the eye being examined. Atop the illumination arm is a lamp housing (6) that contains the light bulb that is the instrument's light source.

At the base of the lamp housing a window exposes a disk that shows a calibrated scale (7) that indicates the length of the beam being used; this scale is also used to measure lesions. Below the scale is a lever for varying the brightness of the light beam; it also allows access to various filters, including the cobalt-blue and red-free filters (8). Just below this is a projecting knurled knob (9) that, when twisted, varies the length (height) of the light beam (12 mm full height) and activates the cobalt-blue filter when twisted all the way to the left. The rod to which this knob is connected can be pushed side to side to turn the light beam from vertical to horizontal. On the principal lower frame of the illumination arm, a knob facing the examiner (10) can be loosened to decenter the illuminating arm nasally or temporally (that is, make it not parfocal with the illuminating arm); this feature is useful for indirect lateral illumination and the sclerotic scatter lighting technique. Accessible by either hand, knurled dual knobs for changing the width of the light beam (11) are located at the bottom of each side of the metal shafts that support the lamp housing and are attached to the lower frame of the illumination arm. With this control, the beam width can be varied from a narrow slit to 8 mm.

The Patient-Positioning Frame

The patient-positioning frame (12) consists of 2 upright metal rods to which are attached the forehead strap (13), for the patient to rest the forehead against during examination, and the patient chin rest (14). Just below the chin rest is a knob for adjusting its height (15). A fixation light (16) is attached to a swing arm that projects from a crosspiece above the two upright rods; the crosspiece and rods form the patient positioning frame. The examiner positions this light in front of the eye not being examined in order to direct the patient's gaze during biomicroscopy. Alternatively, the patent may simply be asked to look at the examiner's ear.

The Base

The slit lamp's joystick control (17) is located on the base of the instrument, within easy reach of the examiner when they are looking through the oculars. The joystick is used to shift the viewing and illumination arms forward, backward, and laterally. On some instruments, the joystick is twisted and rotated to lower and elevate the light beam. A locking knob (18) in the base, near the common support of the viewing and illumination arms, can be loosened to allow mobility of focus. The knob is tightened to prevent the slit lamp from shifting when it is not in use. Under the instrument's supporting platform is a knob for turning the slit lamp's power transformer on and off (not shown); it usually has 3 settings for degrees of brightness. The transformer should be turned off in between uses to avoid burnout of the illumination bulb. The entire slit lamp is typically mounted on a table whose height can be adjusted by pressing a lever located underneath it (not shown).

An applanation tonometer for measuring intraocular pressure can be attached to the slit lamp. This is not shown in Figure 10-1 but is discussed in Chapter 12.

Preparing and Positioning the Patient

The first step in positioning the patient is to adjust the table with the slit lamp mounted on it for the height of the patient. The slit lamp's viewing and illumination portions should be well back from the chin rest and forehead strap before the examiner attempts to position the patient; otherwise, the patient's nose, or even eye, can be bumped by the slit-lamp apparatus.

The patient's head is then positioned and steadied for slit-lamp examination by means of the chin rest and forehead strap. The chin rest consists of a concave plastic cup, which can be cleaned with an alcohol wipe. The chin rest should be cleaned in front of the patient so they know that the chin rest is clean; in some cases, the chin rest is attached to a stack of disposable tissue papers, which can be torn away to expose fresh tissue for each patient. The forehead strap, where makeup and dirt could be expected to accumulate, should also be cleaned with an alcohol wipe. Cleaning of the positioning frame between patients helps prevent the transmission of infectious diseases such as viral conjunctivitis.

With the patient's forehead and chin firmly in place, the height of the chin rest can be raised or lowered by means of a knob below the chin rest (15). The patient's lateral canthus should be brought level with the black demarcation line that is just below the level of the forehead strap on the supporting rod of the patient-positioning frame.

The patient's chin should be well seated in the chin rest and the forehead pressed firmly against the forehead strap. Some patients tend to drift backward and might need to be reminded or helped to keep the forehead against the strap.

It can be difficult to position the slit lamp and its headrest close to obese patients, because their upper bodies tend to push objects away. Such patients can be accommodated by the slip lamp being kept further away and the patient leaning forward.

For patients who are tall or have long legs, the table on which the instrument is mounted can apply uncomfortable pressure to the thighs or knees. In such cases, the footrest on the patient's chair should be folded up to allow the patient's legs to dangle more. When lowering the slit lamp, one should always be mindful that there is enough space above the patient's knees so as not to crush them. When moving the illumination arm, one should also be mindful of the patient's nose. Children often have difficulty reaching the chin rest and forehead strap and can do so more easily if they kneel on the seat of the examination chair.

Adjust the settings on the slit lamp so that the patient is not initially subjected to uncomfortably bright light when the instrument is turned on. This can be accomplished by dimming the light source or using a very narrow beam of light at first. It is always considerate for the examiner to ask if the patient is comfortable before they begin the examination. Patients often want the chin rest or table height raised or lowered slightly. The stool on which the examiner sits should be adjusted to a comfortable height so that the examiner's back is straight, and the slit lamp's oculars should be adjusted for the examiner's interpupillary distance.

Principles of Slit-Lamp Illumination

The slit lamp illuminates the tissues of the eye in several different ways, any or all of which can be useful, depending on the clinical situation. The beginning ophthalmology resident should strive to master all of these techniques of illumination early on, in order to be able to use the slit lamp to its full advantage.

The slit lamp offers 6 main illuminating options, each with its own special properties and particular uses:

- diffuse illumination
- direct (focal) illumination
- specular reflection
- retroillumination
- indirect lateral illumination
- sclerotic scatter

All of these illumination techniques are described in detail in the following sections.

Diffuse Illumination

Diffuse illumination is most commonly used to briefly scan the adnexa and ocular surface, such as the eyelids, eyelashes, conjunctiva, and sclera. Diffuse illumination with white light should be performed with a full-height, broad beam that is directed onto the surface of the eye or adnexa at an angle of 30°–50° from either the temporal or nasal side (Figure 10-2). The brightness level needs to be lowered so that the broad beam is not uncomfortably bright for the patient. Low magnification should be used.

The cobalt-blue filter produces blue light in which fluorescein dye fluoresces with a yellow-green color. Diffuse illumination with blue light is used for evaluation of fluorescein staining of ocular surface tissues or the tear film (Figure 10-3) and to discern the fluorescein pattern during Goldmann applanation tonometry (see Chapter 12).

The red-free filter produces light-green light, which facilitates the evaluation of rose bengal staining (Figure 10-4).

Direct Focal Illumination

Direct focal illumination is the most common illumination technique used. There are 3 types: the parallelepiped, the optical section, and the conical beam.

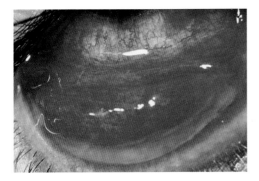

Figure 10-2 Diffuse illumination with white light. The beam has been widened to its fullest extent here to evaluate membranous (adenoviral) conjunctivitis.

Figure 10-3 Diffuse illumination with the cobalt-blue filter (to enhance the fluorescence of fluorescein dye) is used here to demonstrate the dendritic corneal ulceration of herpes simplex epithelial keratitis. The fluorescein dye is staining the corneal stroma. In contrast, intact corneal epithelium prevents uptake of fluorescein dye into the cornea. (Reproduced, with permission, from Coleman AL, *Eye Care Skills on CD-ROM,* American Academy of Ophthalmology, 2001.)

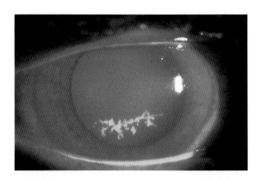

Figure 10-4 Diffuse illumination with the red-free (green) filter is here used to enhance visibility of rose bengal red dye, which has stained keratin in intraepithelial (squamous) neoplasia.

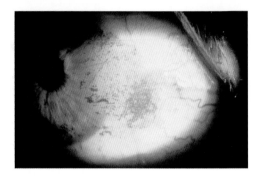

Directing a full-height, medium-width beam (1–3 mm) obliquely onto the cornea will allow a quadrilateral block of light (*parallelepiped,* or corneal prism) to illuminate it (Figure 10-5). The anterior surface of the parallelepiped represents the anterior surface of the cornea, the posterior surface represents the posterior surface of the cornea, and the other 2 faces of the parallelepiped (perpendicular to the surface faces) show the cornea in cross-section. The same kind of illumination may be used to examine the crystalline lens.

After direct focal examination with the medium beam, the parallelepiped is narrowed to the thinnest possible beam, which allows only the cross-sectional illumination of the cornea. This thin beam (0.1 mm–0.4 mm), called an *optical section,* is especially useful for evaluating the depth of lesions (Figure 10-6), thinning of the cornea, and the depth of the anterior chamber. The corneal epithelium appears as a thin, optically empty (black) line at the surface of the optical section, while the rest of the cornea and the lens are reflective of light and so have a silvery appearance.

The *conical beam* is achieved by narrowing the vertical height of the parallelepiped to less than 1 mm to produce a small circular or square spot of light and focusing the beam between the cornea and the anterior lens. The anterior chamber is normally optically clear (black). By setting the slit lamp for the brightest intensity and making the room as dark as possible, the small beam can be used to grade cell and flare in the anterior chamber (see Chapter 11).

Specular Reflection

Specular reflection, or reflected illumination, is used mainly for examination of the corneal endothelium, although it can be used to examine the tear film as well. It depends on the creation of a zone of specular reflection, an area of very bright illumination produced by the reflection of light directly to the examiner's eyes. Zones of specular reflection

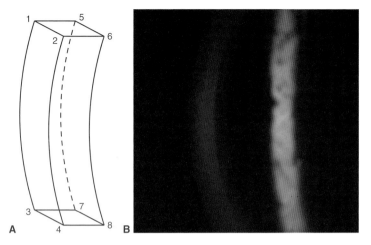

Figure 10-5 Corneal parallelepiped. **A,** The corneal parallelepiped (medium-width beam) achieved with direct focal illumination; face 1-2-3-4 represents the surface of the corneal epithelium; face 5-6-7-8 is the corneal endothelium; and faces 2-6-4-8 and 1-5-3-7 represent cross-sections of the cornea. **B,** Clinical photograph of the corneal parallelepiped of a normal eye. (Part B courtesy of Amanda Ortega, OCT-C.)

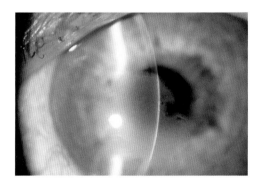

Figure 10-6 The optical section provides a purely cross-sectional view. Here it is used to visualize superficial (intraepithelial) keratin in corneal intraepithelial (squamous) neoplasia.

exist, for example, on the surface of a sunlit lake. Most of the surface of the lake appears relatively dark because the sunlight is reflected somewhere other than straight to the observer; but very bright patches are seen on the lake in locations from which sunlight is reflected directly to the observer—these are the zones of specular reflection. When such an area of reflection is established on the corneal endothelium, it is possible for the examiner to see individual endothelial cells and their cellular outlines. This is because minute irregularities in the tissue cause some of the light in the zone of reflection not to be reflected to the examiner, and the irregularities then stand out as dark areas in an otherwise bright zone.

To achieve specular reflection, the examiner directs a medium to narrow beam of light (it must be thicker than an optical section) toward the eye from the temporal side. The angle of illumination should be wide (50°–60°) relative to the examiner's axis of observation. A bright zone of specular reflection will be evident on the temporal, midperipheral corneal epithelium. Placing the surface of the slit beam on this zone of epithelial reflection will yield a zone of specular reflection on both the epithelial (anterior) and endothelial (posterior) faces of the parallelepiped (Figure 10-7). By using high

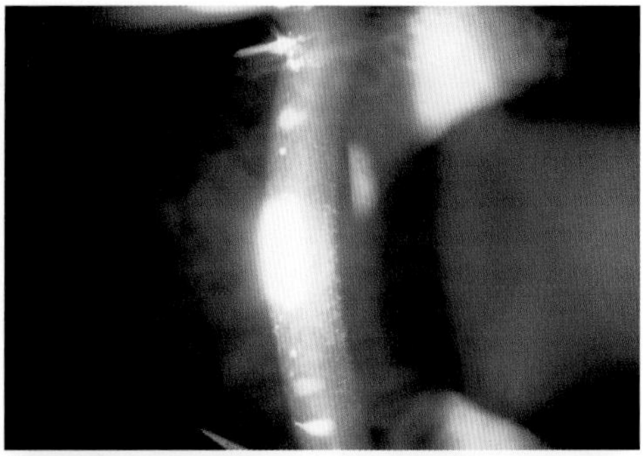

Figure 10-7 Specular reflection can make visible deep corneal guttae (orange peel-like, dark indentations of the endothelium caused by focal excrescences of Descemet membrane) in early Fuchs corneal dystrophy.

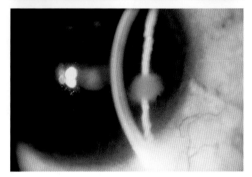

Figure 10-8 Superficial calcium (in Bowman layer) is made evident by transillumination of the cornea by light reflected from the iris; the corneal parallelepiped is to the left of the ovoid calcium deposit, which is highlighted by the (out of focus) light from the iris.

magnification (16× or above) and focusing carefully with the joystick, the examiner can bring the endothelial cells, in the form of a mosaic pattern, into view. The technique requires some practice, so beginners should not be discouraged if they are unable to see the cells the first several times they make the attempt.

Retroillumination

Retroillumination uses light reflected off of deeper structures, such as the iris or retina, to illuminate more anterior structures. A medium-width beam of light is projected onto a part of the eye that lies deeper than the area to be studied, so that the latter can be seen by reflected light while the examiner focuses on the tissues to be examined. For example, to examine the cornea, the light is projected onto the iris while the examiner's view is focused on the cornea (Figure 10-8). Similarly, the iris may be examined by directing light onto the surface of the lens or the retina. This technique allows visualization of abnormalities of the posterior cornea, iris transillumination defects, and cortical or posterior subcapsular cataract (Figure 10-9). It is best to assess for iris transillumination defects through an undilated pupil and for lens opacities with a dilated pupil.

Transillumination from the retina is achieved by shortening the slit beam to the height of the pupil and aligning the illumination beam to be nearly parallel with the patient's visual axis. Generally, the illuminating arm and viewing arm are set to be parfocal. By turning the knob near the lower aspect of the illuminating arm (see label 10 in Figure 10-1), one can focus on the nasal iris, for example, while the light beam is at the temporal area of the pupil. The diffuse red glow from the fundus will serve to highlight pathology of the more anterior structures.

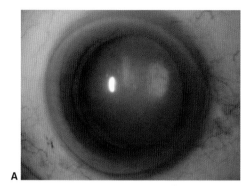

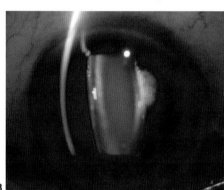

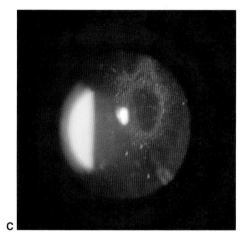

Figure 10-9 Posterior subcapsular cataract. **A,** Diffuse illumination. **B,** Direct (focal) illumination. **C,** Retroillumination. (Courtesy of Fasika A. Woreta, MD.)

Indirect Lateral Illumination

For indirect lateral illumination, the light is directed just adjacent to the lesion to be examined, thus reducing scatter from direct illumination (Figure 10-10). This type of illumination is most useful for translucent lesions such as some corneal opacities and iris nodules.

Sclerotic Scatter

Sclerotic scatter is especially useful for detecting subtle corneal opacities. Like transillumination, sclerotic scatter requires making the illumination arm not parfocal with the

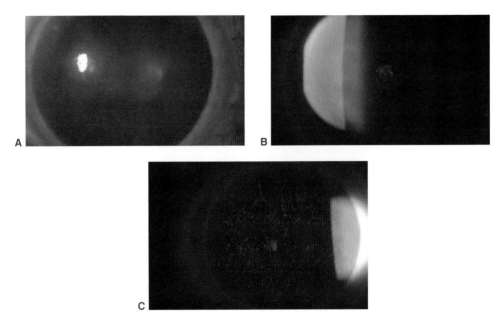

Figure 10-10   Diffuse illumination, indirect lateral illumination, and retroillumination. **A,** Diffuse illumination is used to examine an eye with lattice corneal dystrophy. **B,** Indirect lateral illumination of the same eye makes visible the lattice lines. By looking to the side of the projected light beam, the refractile lines can be seen. **C,** Retroillumination of the same eye shows the delicate branching lattice lines. (Images by William Anderson, CRA, FOPS.)

viewing arm. A medium-width beam is directed onto the limbus, by rotation of the illuminating arm temporally, while the examiner views the center of the cornea. When sclerotic scatter (total internal reflection of light) is achieved, the opposite limbus glows, thus highlighting any corneal opacities (Figure 10-11).

Special Techniques

Certain accessory instruments and attachments to the slit lamp allow examinations that cannot be performed with the slit lamp alone. Instructions in the use of the slit lamp for measurement of structures and abnormalities are detailed in this section. Use of the slit lamp for gonioscopy, fundus examination, tonometry, photography, and laser therapy are mentioned only briefly here, either because these topics are covered in more detail elsewhere in this book or because further discussion is beyond the scope of this book.

The Slit Lamp as a Measuring Device

The dimensions of ocular structures and lesions can be measured, and then noted in the record in millimeters or tenths of a millimeter, by matching the length of the slit-lamp beam to the horizontal and vertical extents of the subject of interest. Most slit lamps have a knob that, when turned, changes the height of the beam; the knob is associated with a millimeter scale (this is usually above the knob; see labels 9 and 7 in Figure 10-1). A reasonably accurate linear measurement can be made by varying the height of the beam until it corresponds to the height of a lesion. This is easily accomplished for vertical

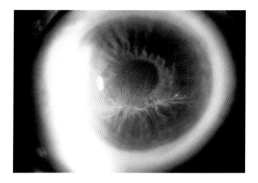

Figure 10-11 Sclerotic scatter produces a diffuse glow of the limbus and a backlighting of any corneal opacities, as with cornea verticillata (whorl-like changes) secondary to epithelial deposition of the oral drug amiodarone, shown here.

measurements because the beam of the slit lamp is routinely oriented vertically. Horizontal measurements can be made by rotating the uppermost, cylindrical portion of the part of the slit lamp that contains the illuminating bulb (in the case of the Haag-Streit 900 instrument), in order to produce a horizontal beam. (Other slit-lamp models might have slightly different mechanisms for obtaining horizontal beams.) Clinical Protocol 10-1 provides instructions for this method of lesion measurement.

Gonioscopy

Gonioscopy is examination of the angle of the anterior chamber (where the peripheral cornea meets the peripheral iris) by means of a refracting or reflecting contact lens (gonioprism, or goniolens) that is placed against the patient's anesthetized cornea. The goniolens allows light from the slit lamp to enter and exit the angle; this would otherwise not be possible due to total internal reflection. Some goniolenses also permit visualization of the posterior vitreous and the retina (including the peripheral vitreous, retina to the ora serrata, the macula, and the optic nerve head). Instructions for performing gonioscopy are found in Chapter 11.

Fundus Examination with the Slit Lamp

Examination of the posterior segment (vitreous and retina) is possible with the slit lamp and accessory lenses. High-plus condensing fundus lenses are handheld lenses used for fundus examination by indirect slit-lamp biomicroscopy. The +90 D and +78 D lenses are used most often today. In the past, a Hruby lens, a high-minus (−55 D) plano-concave lens, was often attached to the slit lamp. When swung into position in front of the patient's eye, the Hruby lens allows for light from the slit lamp to be focused into the posterior segment of the eye, which permits examination of the fundus. This lens is no longer commonly used. Further details of and instructions for indirect slit-lamp biomicroscopy will be discussed in Chapter 13.

Goldmann Tonometry

A Goldmann applanation tonometer attached to the slit lamp is used to measure intraocular pressure. The procedure requires the use of fluorescein dye and the slit lamp's cobalt-blue filter. Clinical Protocol 12-1 provides instructions.

Slit-Lamp Photography

Digital slit-lamp cameras can be mounted onto existing slit lamps to permit clinical photography. Mounting hardware that allows the use of a cell phone camera to obtain slit-lamp images through one eyepiece is also available.

Pitfalls and Pointers

- Remember to set the oculars to your refractive error, or to plano if you use the slit lamp while wearing your glasses; otherwise it can be difficult to obtain a clearly focused view.

- Difficulties occur if the patient is not made reasonably comfortable just prior to, and during, the slit-lamp examination. Proper positioning of the patient is important before the examination is started. Whenever possible, the intensity of light exposure should be kept at levels that are comfortable for the patient.

- It is important to look at the eyelids, other adnexa, and the conjunctiva with relatively dim, diffuse illumination before focusing on the cornea with a parallelepiped or an optical section.

- To take advantage of the full value of the slit lamp, the examiner must become skilled in using all the methods of illumination and understand when each is best employed.

CLINICAL PROTOCOL 10-1

Measuring Lesions Linearly with the Slit-Lamp Beam

1. Set the brightness knob under the slit-lamp table to the first (lowest-intensity) setting.
2. Set the brightness lever on the illuminating arm to full brightness.
3. With 1 of the knurled knobs at the bottom of the illuminating arm (on the Haag-Streit 900), adjust the slit-lamp beam to be slightly thicker than an optical section.
4. Place the illuminating arm directly in front of the viewing arm so that the slit-lamp beam is parallel to the patient's visual axis.
5. Focus the vertically oriented slit-lamp beam onto the lesion to be measured.
6. Twist the protruding, knurled knob (just below the brightness lever on the Haag-Streit 900) to vary the height of the beam until it equals the height of the lesion.
7. Read the scale (at the base of the bulb housing) that indicates the height of the beam in tenths of a millimeter.
8. Rotate the bulb housing 90° to orient the beam horizontally, and repeat steps 6 and 7 to measure the horizontal dimension of the lesion; the bulb housing may be rotated less than 90° to perform diagonal measurements.
9. Record the measurements in the patient's record.

11 Anterior Segment Examination

Whereas the external examination provides an overview of gross abnormalities of the adnexa and certain anterior ocular structures, the anterior segment examination consists of a more detailed study of the tissues of the anterior segment, from the cornea to anterior vitreous, by use of the slit-lamp biomicroscope.

The examination of the anterior segment should always be thorough and systematic. More detailed examination of the lacrimal glands, periorbital skin, and anterior chamber angle may be performed when indicated by history, symptoms, or initial examination.

The components of the slit-lamp biomicroscope and basic principles of its illumination capabilities are detailed in Chapter 10. This chapter describes the basic components of the anterior segment slit-lamp examination and highlights normal examination findings as well as common or important abnormalities. In a limited way where appropriate, this chapter reinforces how the various types of slit-lamp illumination and procedures are best applied for examining individual anatomical components.

Overview of the Anterior Segment Examination

The slit-lamp examination of the anterior segment should proceed from a gross anatomical view to a more detailed view. This means that for each anatomical region, examination should begin with relatively low magnification and either diffuse lighting with a broad beam or direct focal illumination, as appropriate. By beginning at lower magnification, the examiner is less likely to overlook gross abnormalities. When the initial biomicroscopic examination suggests the possibility of an abnormality that requires further investigation, the more specialized slit-lamp illumination techniques and higher magnification can be applied.

The components of the anterior segment examination, listed below, follow an anatomically logical order:

* lacrimal gland and periorbital skin
* eyelids and eyelashes
* conjunctiva
* episclera and sclera
* tear film
* cornea
* anterior chamber
* iris
* crystalline lens
* retrolental space and anterior vitreous

The following text describes the anterior segment examination in terms of structures and findings that are evaluated and provides instructions in various specialized biomicroscopic and other techniques that might be required for complete evaluation.

Lacrimal Gland and Periorbital Skin

Biomicroscopic evaluation of the lacrimal gland and the periorbital skin is necessary only if the patient's history or a previous evaluation have suggested the presence of an abnormality that needs investigation.

The lacrimal gland is the main contributor to the aqueous layer of the tear film and consists of an orbital lobe and a palpebral lobe. The palpebral lobe is the most anterior portion and is the only portion visible on slit-lamp examination. It can be seen by lifting upward on the temporal aspect of the upper eyelid with a thumb while the patient's ipsilateral eye is directed inferonasally. The normal palpebral lobe of the gland is slightly pink. Enlargement may be due to inflammation, lymphoid lesions or lymphoma, or epithelial tumors (Figure 11-1). The size of the gland varies from person to person, so each lacrimal gland should be examined for symmetry.

To examine the periorbital skin, employ low magnification and diffuse illumination with white light and a broad beam. Various manifestations of dermatitis may be investigated, including erythema (redness of the skin); eczema (Figure 11-2), which occurs with atopic dermatitis; urticaria (hives, epidermal edema, or angioedema); and vesicular or bullous dermatitis (as occur with herpes simplex, varicella zoster, or pemphigus vulgaris).

Slit-lamp examination can be used to examine both benign lesions (seborrheic keratosis, squamous papilloma) and malignant tumors (squamous cell, basal cell, sebaceous cell carcinoma, or melanoma spread from the cheek). Infectious lesions of the periorbital area include preseptal cellulitis, zoster, and molloscum contagiosum. Pigmentary changes of the skin not caused by tumors include vitiligo (patchy loss of cutaneous pigment), hyperpigmentation secondary to chronic inflammation or trauma, and Addison disease.

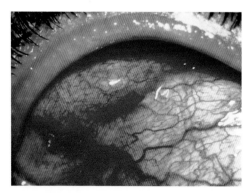

Figure 11-1 Enlarged, inflamed palpebral lobe of the right lacrimal gland.

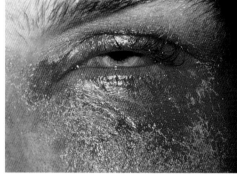

Figure 11-2 Eczematoid (allergic contact) blepharoconjunctivitis caused by topical ophthalmic medication (atropine).

Eyelid and Eyelashes

The eyelid consists of 2 regions, or lamellae: anterior and posterior (Figure 11-3). The lamellae are approximately demarcated by a subtle marking called the *gray line* that runs horizontally along the margin of the eyelid, posterior to the eyelash follicles and anterior to the meibomian gland orifices. The gray line represents the most superficial portion of the orbicularis oculi muscle (the muscle of Riolan). An incision through (or, more precisely, just behind), the gray line separates the eyelid into its 2 lamellae. The anterior (skin–muscle) lamella contains the eyelashes and their follicles, the sebaceous glands of Zeis (which empty into the eyelash follicles), and the sweat glands of Moll. The posterior (tarsoconjunctival) lamella contains the sebaceous meibomian glands that lie within the fibrous tarsal plate and open onto the posterior surface of the margin of the eyelid.

Most lesions of the eyelid are benign; blepharitis is the most common finding of the eyelid. Low magnification, broad beam, and white light are used for slit-lamp examination of lesions of the eyelid.

Benign Lesions of the Eyelid

A *hordeolum*, also known as a stye, is an acute infection of a sebaceous (Zeis or meibomian) gland of the eyelid, most commonly caused by the bacteria *Staphylococcus aureus*. An external hordeolum is acute inflammation of a Zeis gland in the anterior lamella of the eyelid (Figure 11-4). An internal hordeolum is acute inflammation in a meibomian gland of the posterior lamella of the eyelid (Figure 11-5). Examination of an internal hordeolum requires eversion of the eyelid (see Chapter 9).

A *chalazion* is a subacute or chronic lipogranuloma within the eyelid from an obstructed sebaceous gland (Figure 11-6). Hordeola that do not resolve within a few days show gradually diminishing amounts of inflammation over days to weeks and can evolve into chalazia. Chalazia can be superficial or deep, depending on the location of the glands

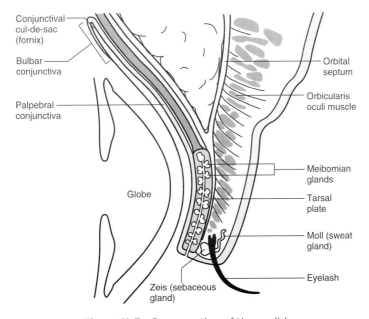

Figure 11-3 Cross-section of the eyelid.

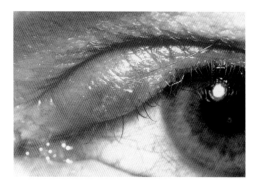

Figure 11-4 External hordeolum (stye).

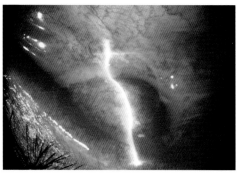

Figure 11-5 Internal hordeolum (acute chalazion).

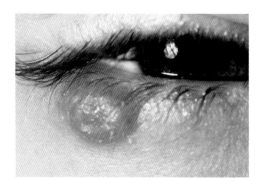

Figure 11-6 Chalazion.

that are blocked. Zeis glands are located more superficially, and the tarsal meibomian glands are deeper. Chalazia that protrude anteriorly (toward the skin of the eyelid) produce a domelike elevation of the skin. Chalazia that develop more posteriorly manifest a yellowish mass of lipid and granulomatous inflammation (visible through the palpebral conjunctiva). Very large posterior chalazia can also cause elevation of the skin of the eyelid.

Folliculitis is an acute abscess of an eyelash follicle, rather than a sebaceous gland. Folliculitis is nearly always caused by staphylococcal infection. Other common benign lesions of the eyelid include seborrheic keratosis, molluscum contagiosum, squamous cell papilloma, epidermal inclusion cysts, and hidrocystomas.

Blepharitis

Blepharitis (inflammation of the eyelid) is classified as anterior, if it affects the eyelid skin, bases of the eyelashes, and eyelash follicles, or posterior, if it affects the posterior glands.

Anterior blepharitis can present with erythema and edema of the eyelid margin, madarosis (eyelash loss), and telangiectasias in the eyelid. It can be bacterial in origin, seborrheic, or caused by mites.

Staphylococcal blepharitis is a common condition typified by the presence of "collarettes"—thin, honey-colored flakes that surround and lie among the eyelashes (Figure 11-7). In *seborrheic blepharitis*, greasy dandrufflike flakes ("scurf") or scales are found on the eyelashes (Figure 11-8). *Demodectic blepharitis* is caused by infestation of the eyelash follicles with a mite, *Demodex folliculorum*, and is especially common in elderly patients (Figure 11-9). This form of blepharitis is typified by the presence of waxy-appearing, cylindrical cuffs or "sleeves" around the bases of eyelashes (Figure 11-10). Figure 11-11 diagrammatically depicts the difference in appearance between collarettes, seborrheic scurf, and cylindrical cuffs.

Posterior blepharitis arises from disorders of the meibomian glands. Meibomian dysfunction implies hypersecretion of the glands, often along with abnormally thick secretions. The dysfunction is indicated by fullness, excessive secretion, or inspissation of the glands as well as by irregularity of their orifices (Figure 11-12). It can occur as an isolated problem, but it is especially common in patients who have rosacea.

Angular blepharitis affects mainly the medial or lateral canthal areas of the eyelids, which show eczematoid or ulcerative changes of the skin. The condition develops secondarily in association with some forms of bacterial conjunctivitis (especially that caused by Staphylococci or Moraxella).

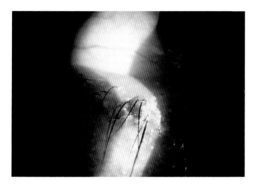

Figure 11-7 Collarette of staphylococcal blepharitis (white flake just inside the right edge of the slit beam).

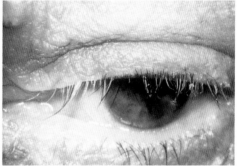

Figure 11-8 Sebaceous material adherent to eyelashes in seborrheic blepharitis (temporal aspect of upper eyelid); note also madarosis (loss of eyelashes) and poliosis (whitening of eyelashes) from prior staphylococcal blepharitis.

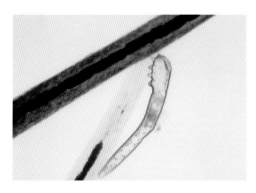

Figure 11-9 *Demodex folliculorum* mite near an epilated eyelash from a patient with demodectic blepharitis (unstained, 200×).

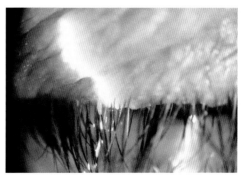

Figure 11-10 Sleeve or cuff in demodectic blepharitis (base of the eyelash, just to left of where the slit-lamp beam appears on the skin of the eyelid).

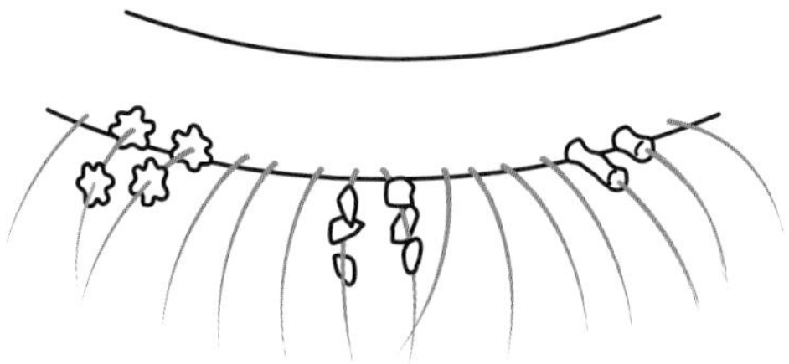

Figure 11-11 Diagrammatic representations of eyelash collarettes (left), seborrheic material (center), and eyelash sleeve (right).

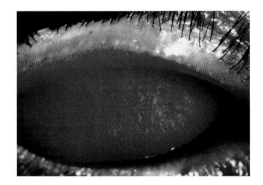

Figure 11-12 Meibomian gland dysfunction in the upper eyelid of a patient with rosacea; fullness, dilation, and irregularity of various meibomian orifices (near the posterior aspect of eyelid margin) are evident.

Malignant Tumors of the Eyelid

The same tumors that affect the skin can occur on the skin of the eyelids. Premalignant lesions include actinic keratosis (hyperkeratotic plaques) and keratoacanthoma (dome-shaped, rapidly growing lesions). Basal cell carcinoma is the most common eyelid malignancy; it most frequently originates from the lower eyelid. It can present as a small translucent nodule with central depression, ulceration, rolled borders, and telangiectasias. Squamous cell carcinoma is less common; it presents with nodular and plaquelike lesions with irregular edges, and chronic scarring. Sebaceous cell carcinoma is a neoplasm that arises from the sebaceous glands and can present as a chronic unilateral blepharoconjunctivitis (see Figure 11-8). It should be considered in any elderly patient with unilateral blepharitis, as it is a highly malignant and potentially lethal tumor.

Conjunctiva

The conjunctiva is best evaluated in a stepwise, anatomically logical fashion, beginning with the palpebral (tarsal) conjunctiva, then proceeding to the limbal conjunctiva and bulbar conjunctiva.

Palpebral Conjunctiva

The conjunctival aspect of the eyelids (palpebral and tarsal conjunctiva) is examined by everting the eyelids (see instructions in Chapter 9). The palpebral conjunctiva can be affected by papillae, follicles, granulomas, membranes and pseudomembranes, and scarring.

Papillae

The palpebral (and the limbal) conjunctiva is normally made adherent to underlying tissues by many tiny, vertically oriented, fibrous septa. *Papillary conjunctivitis* is the term given to any inflammation of the palpebral conjunctiva that leads to the formation of papillae, which are dome-shaped nodules that cause the conjunctiva to have a bumpy appearance (Figures 11-13 and 11-14). Each papilla consists of a central core of hyperemic blood vessels that protrude upward (perpendicular to the tarsal plate) and are surrounded by edema and inflammatory cells, and, in some longstanding cases, fibrosis.

Papillae can be very small (micropapillae), small, medium-sized, or giant. Micropapillae (less than 0.3 mm in diameter) are a normal finding. Small papillae measure 0.3–0.6 mm in diameter and are considered to be abnormal (Figure 11-15). However, they are a nonspecific finding and occur in many different kinds of conjunctival inflammation. They are usually graded on a scale of 1-4 (modified with a plus sign), with 4 being the most severe.

Medium papillae are 0.6–1 mm in diameter. They are an abnormal finding that represent early confluence of small papillae as they enlarge and rupture the intervening fibrous septa (Figure 11-16).

Giant papillae are larger than 1 mm in diameter (Figure 11-17) and occur in vernal conjunctivitis, as a reaction to accumulated deposits on contact lenses or prosthetic eyes, and as a reaction to sutures. Giant papillae represent coalescence of many small or medium papillae and tend to become polygonal as their sides press against one another.

Follicles

The conjunctiva normally contains islands of subepithelial lymphoid tissue. When these enlarge to the extent that they are visible, they are called follicles. Follicles are

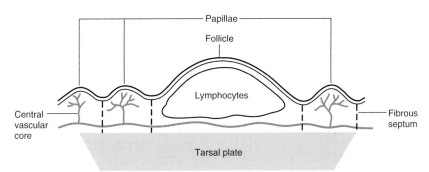

Figure 11-13 Cross-sectional diagrammatic representation of a conjunctival lymphoid follicle and papillae.

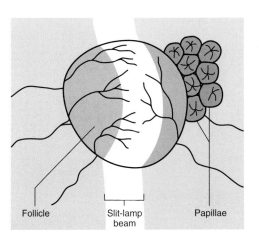

Figure 11-14 Diagrammatic representation of the clinical appearance of a conjunctival follicle and papillae.

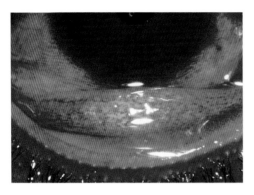

Figure 11-15 Fine papillary reaction of the inferior palpebral conjunctiva.

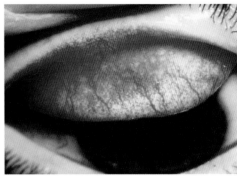

Figure 11-16 Medium-sized papillae of upper palpebral conjunctiva (irregular, pale areas), a reaction to deposits on a soft contact lens. The pallor occurs because the papillae are becoming sufficiently thick and fibrotic as to obscure the vascular cores.

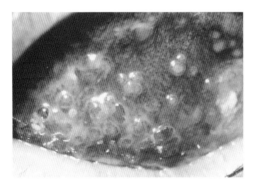

Figure 11-17 Giant papillae of the upper palpebral conjunctiva, a reaction to deposits on an ocular prosthesis.

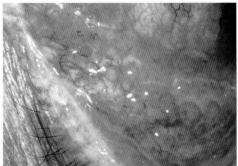

Figure 11-18 Follicular reaction of the lower palpebral conjunctiva to dipivalyl epinephrine eyedrops.

several times larger in diameter than small papillae and consist of masses of lymphocytes, lymphoblasts, and a few macrophages (Figure 11-18). They are like miniature lymph nodes in that they do not contain central vascular cores as do papillae. Follicles enlarge upward from the conjunctival stroma, causing dome-shaped elevations of the conjunctival surface. The normal blood vessels of the conjunctiva are also pushed upward so that they seem to course up onto, and over, the surface of each follicle.

Older children and adolescents often have relatively prominent conjunctival follicles as a normal finding unassociated with inflammation. Follicles that occur with conjunctivitis are usually most prominent in the inferior fornix and the inferior palpebral conjunctiva, except in trachoma.

Pathologic conjunctival follicles constitute a useful clinical finding because they occur in association with only a few specific kinds of conjunctival inflammations, mainly those caused by chlamydia, adenoviruses, herpes simplex (primary infections), molluscum contagiosum, and toxic reactions to certain topical ophthalmic medications.

Granulomas

Granulomatous conjunctivitis is less common than follicular or papillary conjunctivitis and is characterized by the presence of 1 or more conjunctival granulomas that are not merely chalazia (Figure 11-19). Most cases of granulomatous conjunctivitis are caused by the agent of cat-scratch disease (*Bartonella henselae*). Less-common causes include tuberculosis, syphilis, and tularemia. Conjunctival granulomas can develop in patients who have sarcoidosis.

Membranes and pseudomembranes

Certain types of intense conjunctivitis cause transudation of fibrin on the surface of the conjunctiva (Figure 11-20). The material is seen as a white membranous deposit that is adherent to the conjunctiva and that obscures the underlying conjunctival blood vessels.

The layer of fibrin, mixed with an admixture of neutrophils, is referred to as a *pseudomembrane* if it simply lies on the conjunctival surface, in which case the pseudomembrane may be peeled away without bleeding. A true membrane incorporates the conjunctival epithelium and so cannot be removed without causing bleeding. Otherwise, the difference between a membrane and a pseudomembrane is one of degree, the pseudomembrane indicating a lesser intensity of inflammation.

With the exception of ocular diphtheria, which is known to cause a true membrane, the causes of this class of conjunctivitis can lead to the formation of either a membrane or pseudomembrane, depending on the severity of the inflammatory response. The main

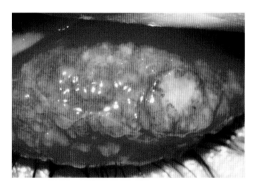

Figure 11-19   Conjunctival granuloma (large, polygonal lesion with central pallor) with adjacent follicles, as a result of cat-scratch disease.

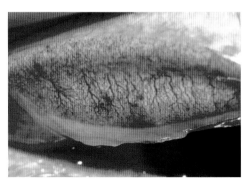

Figure 11-20   Pseudomembranous reaction on upper palpebral conjunctiva in adenoviral conjunctivitis. The pseudomembrane has been partially peeled away, and its edge can be seen folded on itself near the upper border of the tarsal plate (lower part of the photograph).

Figure 11-21 Symblepharon (adhesion between the bulbar conjunctiva and the lower eyelid) occurring in ocular mucous membrane pemphigoid. (© 2014 American Academy of Ophthalmology. Courtesy of Charles S. Bouchard, MD.)

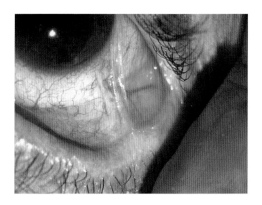

infectious causes are adenovirus, herpes simplex (primary infections), chlamydia (in infants), beta-hemolytic streptococcus, and *Neisseria gonorrhoeae*. Noninfectious causes include ocular cicatricial pemphigoid, chemical burns, acute Stevens-Johnson syndrome (SJS), toxic epidermal necrolysis (TEN), and graft versus host disease (GvHD).

Scarring

Conjunctival scarring can result from a variety of traumatic or inflammatory processes that affect the conjunctival stroma, where fibroblasts reside. Conjunctival scarring is seen as white or gray areas of fibrosis. The more severe degrees of scarring can be associated with contraction of surrounding tissues. Extensive scarring in the inferior conjunctival fornix can lead to foreshortening. Extreme degrees of scarring can cause a band of fibrous tissue, called a *symblepharon*, to develop between the palpebral conjunctiva and the bulbar conjunctiva (Figure 11-21). Ankyloblepharon is when the upper and lower eyelid become fused. Horizontal linear scarring on the upper tarsal conjunctiva, called Arlt line, is characteristic of trachoma.

Foreign bodies

Although foreign bodies can turn up anywhere in the conjunctival sac, they often lodge in the palpebral conjunctiva of the upper eyelid. If vertical abrasions on the cornea are seen, the eyelid should be everted to search for a foreign body. If foreign material is suspected but not found, the conjunctival sac should be swept with a moist cotton swab in an effort to remove any foreign particles. Clinical Protocol 11-1 describes the process.

Conjunctival concretions

Concretions are small, chalky, yellow-white lesions that are often found in the tarsal conjunctiva and are due to degenerating epithelial cells and proteinaceous secretions from conjunctival glands. If they cause symptoms of foreign-body sensation, they can be removed with a 30-gauge needle. Epithelial inclusions cysts can also be seen in the tarsal conjunctiva.

Limbal Conjunctiva

The limbal conjunctiva can be affected by ciliary (limbal) flush, papillae, follicles, and Horner-Trantas dots.

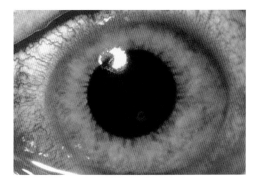

Figure 11-22 Ciliary flush (best seen here along the superior limbus); closely spaced radial vessels extend about 1 mm peripherally from the cornea.

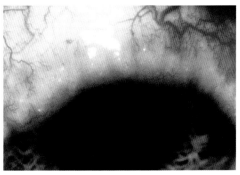

Figure 11-23 Limbal papillae with several Horner-Trantas dots (small white dots), in allergic (vernal) conjunctivitis.

Ciliary (limbal) flush

The anterior ciliary blood vessels form a perilimbal plexus within the conjunctiva and episclera. When hyperemic, these vessels can be seen to extend outward from the limbus for 1–2 mm in a radial pattern. Hyperemia of this plexus is seen as a red to violaceous circumcorneal ring of dilated blood vessels (Figure 11-22). It indicates corneal, episcleral, scleral, or intraocular inflammation.

Limbal papillae and Horner-Trantas dots

The limbal conjunctiva, like the palpebral conjunctiva, has anchoring fibrous septa, so papillae (including giant papillae) can form in the limbal conjunctiva as well. In extreme cases, limbal giant papillae take on the appearance of a gelatinous mass overlying the entire limbal area.

In some cases of chronic allergic conjunctivitis, focal collections of degenerated eosinophils and epithelial cells may be seen at the limbus. (Figure 11-23). These gelatinous limbal papillae, called *Horner-Trantas dots,* are yellow-white, usually about 1–2 mm in diameter, and characteristic of vernal conjunctivitis.

Limbal follicles

Follicles sometimes develop in the limbal area, but they are not common. They have the same appearance as follicles elsewhere. They are most likely to occur with chlamydial infections or toxic follicular reactions to topical ophthalmic medications. Limbal follicles are common in trachoma; with healing, they leave round, often depressed, limbal scars known as *Herbert pits.* Nontrachomatous follicles do not undergo necrosis and thus do not form Herbert pits.

Bulbar Conjunctiva

Although both the bulbar and the palpebral conjunctiva can exude secretions and discharge, pathology is more apparent in the more extensive bulbar tissue. In addition to secretions, the bulbar conjunctiva can manifest chemosis, lymphangiectasia and lymphedema, telangiectasia, hyperemia, epithelial defects and ulcers, and a variety of less common abnormalities.

Secretions and discharge

The characteristics of conjunctival secretions are many and variable and can be diagnostically valuable to the examiner.

Watery discharge on the conjunctiva is actually a secretion rather than a discharge (exudate) because it represents reflex tear flow from the lacrimal gland. The term *tearing* is used when the excess tears merely accumulate within the conjunctival sac; the term *epiphora* is used if the tears spill over the margin of the eyelid onto the face.

Tearing and epiphora can be caused by any irritation of the ocular surface, including inflammatory disease or foreign bodies. Other causes include cold wind, yawning, sneezing, gagging, irritating fumes, or lacrimal-outflow obstruction. The last usually manifests epiphora.

Mucoid discharge is also a secretion. The conjunctival goblet cells secrete mucus (mucin) continuously, but in such small amounts as to be unnoticeable under normal conditions.

Serous discharge consists of proteinaceous fluid that is more viscous than aqueous tears. In its pure form, serous discharge is acellular; it occurs in mild inflammations of the conjunctiva.

Conjunctival mucus is seen as a nearly clear, sticky material on the ocular surface (Figure 11-24). It most often appears in the form of strands that are several millimeters to centimeters long, although amorphous globs can also be seen. The mucus is most often found in the inferior conjunctival fornix or in the area of the semilunar fold and caruncle. Mucus is a nonspecific finding and excessive production can be brought about by any irritation of the ocular surface. Mucus is regularly found with ocular allergies and in dry eyes.

Mucopurulent discharge consists of neutrophils mixed with mucus and so represents a combination of a secretion and a discharge. Mucopurulent discharge has the same appearance as mucus, except that the neutrophils give the mucus a white appearance (Figure 11-25). This type of discharge tends to accumulate during sleep and so is likely to be most noticeable early in the morning; if the patient cleanses it from the eye at that time, it might be difficult to detect at an examination later in the day, as this kind of discharge is often scant. (In this situation, the examiner may conclude that some mucopurulence has been present if the patient has a history of the eyelids being sealed shut upon awakening in the mornings). Mucopurulent discharge is most common with simple bacterial conjunctivitis.

Truly purulent discharge consists mainly or entirely of neutrophils and is usually copious (Figure 11-26). If wiped away, it often reappears within 5 or 10 minutes. Purulent discharge is usually white, but the color can be altered by microbial pigments (yellow

Figure 11-24 Mucous secretion in kerato-conjunctivitis sicca, here stained with rose bengal dye (curvilinear strand nasal to limbus). Note also the rose bengal staining of the conjunctiva and cornea in the interpalpebral area of exposure (typical of the dry eye).

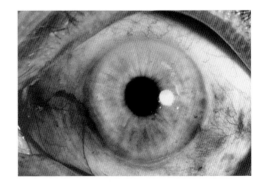

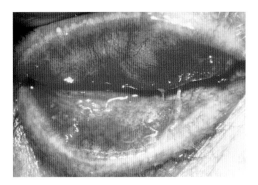

Figure 11-25 Mucopurulent discharge in bacterial conjunctivitis.

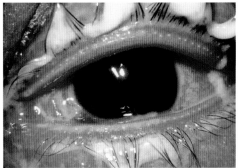

Figure 11-26 Purulent discharge in gonococcal conjunctivitis.

in the case of *Staphylococcus aureus* or greenish-white with pseudomonas). Purulence occurs most often with gonococcal or meningococcal conjunctivitis.

Chemosis

Chemosis is edema of, or beneath, the conjunctiva (Figure 11-27). It appears as a thickening and ballooning of the tissue. Because the bulbar conjunctiva lacks anchoring septa, the swelling can be diffuse, but it is most prominent in the area of the palpebral fissure where the pressure of the eyelids does not restrict the swelling. The color of the edematous conjunctiva can be normal, but it sometimes takes on a slightly yellowish hue.

Chemosis is most often caused by allergy, although it can be caused by a variety of inflammatory conditions, including conjunctivitis, episcleritis, scleritis, uveitis, endophthalmitis, and orbital cellulitis.

Lymphangiectasia

One or more lymphatic channels of the conjunctiva can become dilated (lymphangiectasia) to produce the appearance of clear, slightly elevated structures separated by translucent septate walls. The channel is often sacculated, and so resembles a segment of intestine. Lymphangiectasia is often idiopathic, but it is sometimes related to trauma.

Lymphedema of the conjunctiva results from obstruction of lymphatic outflow and leads to a straw-colored swelling. The problem is generally caused by scarring or, in rare cases, a tumor in the orbit.

Telangiectasia

Telangiectasias appear as corkscrew-shaped, irregularly dilated vessels and can occur in the bulbar conjunctiva, palpebral conjunctiva, or on the eyelid. They may be idiopathic or associated with blood dyscrasias such as sickle cell disease. They can also occur as part of rare syndromes such as ataxia telangiectasia, Fabry disease, Sturge-Weber syndrome, and hereditary hemorrhagic telangiectasia.

Hyperemia

Increased blood flow with associated dilation of blood vessels (hyperemia) in the conjunctiva produces diffuse redness that is usually most prominent peripherally, and tends to fade as the limbus is approached (Figure 11-28). This is because the conjunctival blood

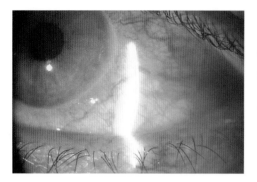

Figure 11-27 Chemosis (conjunctival edema) due to allergic reaction to topical ophthalmic medication. (© 2014 American Academy of Ophthalmology.)

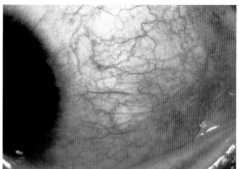

Figure 11-28 Hyperemia of the bulbar conjunctiva in bacterial conjunctivitis.

supply is most prominent in, and enters from, the peripheral bulbar conjunctiva. This blood supply is distinct from the one that produces a ciliary flush.

Papillae do not develop in the bulbar conjunctiva because of the absence of fibrous septa. Conjunctival hyperemia is an entirely nonspecific finding that can occur with any ocular inflammation, dryness, or environmental irritant.

Epithelial defects

Conjunctival epithelial defects most commonly occur after trauma and chemical burns. Epithelial defects are detected by the absence of normal conjunctival luster and by an actual depression in a particular area, which is often surrounded by some hyperemia. Staining with fluorescein (discussed later in this chapter) can also make evident a defect.

Other Conjunctival Abnormalities

A detailed discussion of other possible abnormalities of the conjunctiva is beyond the scope of this book, but such discussions can be found in Section 8, *External Disease and Cornea*, of the Basic and Clinical Science Course of the American Academy of Ophthalmology as well as in many other textbooks. The most important additional abnormalities are listed below. A few of these abnormalities tend to occur only in certain locations, but many of them can occur in either bulbar or palpebral conjunctiva.

- Pigmentations and deposits (accumulation or deposition of melanin, drugs, or systemic or topical heavy metals)
- Dermoid tumors (choristomas, or benign congenital tumors)
- Pinguecula (yellowish, often slightly elevated limbal lesion that result from ultraviolet exposure)
- Pterygium (triangular fibrovascular bulbar conjunctival growth that extends onto the cornea; associated with pinguecula)
- Phlyctenules (nodular inflammation of the conjunctiva or cornea secondary to a hypersensitivity reaction to an antigen, most commonly *Staphylococcus aureus* or *Mycobacterium tuberculosis*)

- Keratinization (dry, lackluster, pearly gray alteration of the conjunctival or corneal epithelial surface, sometimes covered with superficial foamy sebaceous matter)
- Benign tumors, including nevi, papilloma, and lymphoid hyperplasia
- Malignant tumors, including conjunctival or corneal intraepithelial neoplasia, squamous cell carcinoma, sebaceous carcinoma (secondarily affecting the conjunctiva), melanomas, or lymphomas

Episclera and Sclera

Most episcleral and scleral abnormalities are easily observed even with a penlight. A number of differences help the clinician distinguish between conjunctival and scleral or episcleral signs. The episclera and sclera have a blood supply deeper than and separate from that of the conjunctiva. Blood vessels in the conjunctiva are generally finer and less tortuous than the deeper vessels. Furthermore, conjunctival hyperemia has a red appearance, whereas deeper (episcleral and scleral) hyperemia is often violaceous. Conjunctival vessels can be moved by massaging the conjunctiva through the eyelid or directly with a cotton swab; the deeper vessels do not move with such maneuvers. Finally, topical vasoconstricting agents affect conjunctival and episcleral vessels much more than the deeper scleral vessels.

Episcleritis

Episcleritis is an immunologically mediated inflammation of the tissue that lies between the deep conjunctival stroma and the sclera (Figure 11-29). It is typically benign, short lived, and not associated with tenderness, ciliary pain, or flare and cell in the anterior chamber. While most cases of episcleritis are idiopathic, a minority of patients may have an underlying systemic disorder.

Episcleritis occurs in 3 forms, depending on the distribution and extent of the deep hyperemia: diffuse (which involves much or all of the episclera), sectoral, and nodular (see Figure 11-29).

Scleritis

Scleritis is an immunologically mediated inflammation of the sclera itself. Deep hyperemia is seen, along with extreme tenderness and a deep, boring pain. Scleritis is more painful than episcleritis and is not associated with blanching of vessels with application of topical vasoconstrictors. It is likely to have a more prolonged course than episcleritis and can cause damage in the form of scleral thinning, which gives a bluish appearance to the sclera.

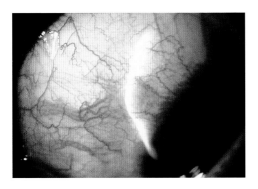

Figure 11-29 Nodular episcleritis. The lesion is nodular but superficial to the sclera; this is also an example of sectoral episcleritis, in that it affects only the superonasal aspect of the left eye.

Unlike episcleritis, scleritis is associated with an underlying systemic disease in about one-half of afflicted patients. The most common causes are autoimmune collagen-vascular (connective tissue) diseases, granulomatous diseases such as syphilis or tuberculosis, or gout or hyperuricemia. Roughly 50% of cases are idiopathic and occur in patients who are otherwise apparently healthy.

Posterior scleritis can occur, but it will not be discussed in this chapter on the anterior segment examination. Anterior scleritis can be diffuse (Figure 11-30), sectoral, nodular (Figure 11-31), or necrotizing. Necrotizing scleritis with inflammation (ischemic scleritis) occurs in patients who have systemic autoimmune vasculitis; it is characterized by severe inflammation and scleral necrosis (Figure 11-32). The affected area often appears to be ischemic in that there are foci of blanched, avascular tissue in or around other nearby areas of severe hyperemia. Necrotizing scleritis without inflammation (scleromalacia perforans, Figure 11-33)

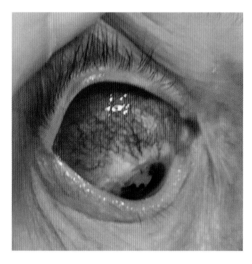

Figure 11-30 Diffuse scleritis. (Courtesy of Fasika A. Woreta, MD.)

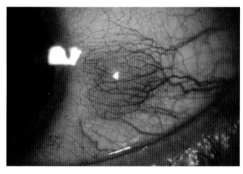

Figure 11-31 Nodular scleritis. (Courtesy of Fasika A. Woreta, MD.)

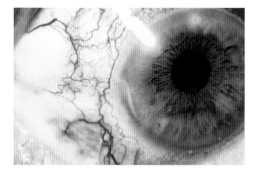

Figure 11-32 Nodular and necrotizing (ischemic) scleritis with inflammation occurring in severe rheumatoid disease with ocular and systemic vasculitis. Note areas of avascularity and the bluish area of scleral thinning and necrosis (lower part of photograph).

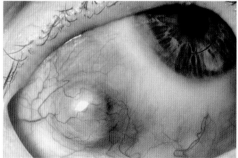

Figure 11-33 Necrotizing scleritis without (evident) inflammation (scleromalacia perforans) resulting from longstanding rheumatoid disease. Note bluish, nodular staphyloma in the presence of a relatively uninflamed eye.

occurs almost exclusively in patients who have chronic rheumatoid arthritis. There is little or no noticeable, or symptomatic, scleritis, yet the sclera gradually thins so as to produce bulging areas of scleral thinning. Because these areas of thinning are lined with uveal tissue, they have a bluish appearance and are referred to as staphylomas (in reference to their grapelike appearance).

The inflammation of scleritis can involve secondarily the corneal stroma, and produce cellular infiltrate adjacent to the scleritis (sclerokeratitis).

Pigmentations

Loops of the long posterior ciliary nerve within the sclera are known as Axenfeld nerve loops. These loops appear as blue-black spots 3 mm posterior to the limbus, and are normal variants.

Congenital melanosis oculi (ocular melanocytosis) is an anomaly that produces deep, slate-gray patches of scleral and episcleral pigmentation, nearly always unilaterally. Associated findings can include ipsilateral hyperpigmentation of the iris, the fundus, and the periocular skin (nevus of Ota; oculodermal melanocytosis).

Brown or brown-black pigmentation is produced by pigmented tumors of the uveal tract (for example, ciliary body melanomas), which occasionally erode into the sclera or episclera and can be associated with dilated episcleral vessels, referred to as *sentinel vessels*.

Involutional Hyaline Plaques

Involutional hyaline and calcific plaques of the sclera are sometimes seen in elderly patients. The plaques develop in the areas of insertion of the medial and lateral (and in rare cases, the inferior) rectus muscles. They have a gray-brown or yellow-brown translucent appearance (Figure 11-34).

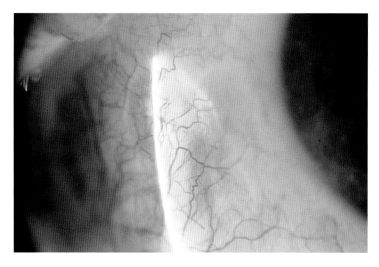

Figure 11-34 Involutional hyaline scleral plaque.

Tear Film

The tear film consists of 3 layers—an anterior lipid layer, a middle aqueous layer, and a posterior mucin layer. The lipid layer originates from the sebaceous glands of the eyelids and serves to retard evaporation of the watery aqueous component. The middle aqueous layer of the tear film originates from the main lacrimal gland and the conjunctival accessory lacrimal glands. The innermost layer, mucin, is produced by the conjunctival goblet cells and serves to stabilize the tear film and to make the hydrophobic epithelial surface wettable.

Closure of the eyelids (blinking) spreads the tear film over the ocular surface. Evaporation then begins, and causes progressive thinning of the tear film. When it becomes so thin that its surface tension can no longer maintain an intact film, it breaks up in focal areas and produces momentary dry spots. These stimulate another blink, and the cycle begins again.

Schirmer testing is used to evaluate tear production and is usually performed as part of the external examination (see Chapter 9). In the anterior segment examination, the tear film is evaluated with the slit lamp for its overall wetness, presence of meniscus, and breakup time as well as a few minor abnormalities.

Overall Wetness

The general presence or absence of moisture on the ocular surface can be evaluated with diffuse illumination. The normal tear film has a glistening appearance, while the severely dry eye has a matte appearance.

Tear Meniscus

When viewed in cross-section with a thin slit-lamp beam (optical section), the tear film forms a roughly triangular meniscus, or "lake," between the margin of the lower eyelid and the place where the eyelid margin apposes the globe (Figure 11-35). Absence of a tear meniscus, or a tear meniscus height of less than 0.25 mm, is indicative of tear deficiency.

Figure 11-35 Normally the tear film forms a roughly triangular meniscus along the posterior margin of the eyelid; this is reduced or absent in the dry eye, and increased (higher and more convex) in the wet eye.

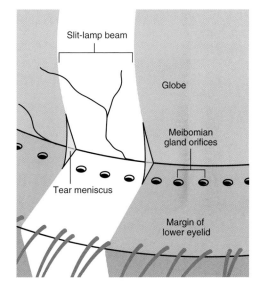

A higher-than-normal meniscus occurs with conditions of tearing or epiphora. The best way to become familiar with the appearance of a normal meniscus is to observe it in a number of patients whose tear films are normal.

Tear Film Breakup Time

The tear film breaks up between blinks. Applying fluorescein dye to the ocular surface and measuring the time between the last blink and the appearance of the first dry spot provides information about the adequacy of the supply of tears. A tear breakup time of less than 10 seconds is considered abnormal. Clinical Protocol 11-2 provides instructions for measuring tear film breakup time.

Other Tear Film Abnormalities

Various kinds of debris can be seen in the tear film. The most common examples are particles of mascara or other cosmetics and clumps of mucus. Soapy deposits are formed when excessive sebaceous oil produces a thicker-than-normal oily layer of tear film. Sebaceous material can lead to the accumulation in the tear film of foamy material that has a yellow-white, bubbly appearance known as *meibomian foam*.

Cornea

The cornea consists of 5 layers, listed here from anterior to posterior:

- epithelium and epithelial basement membrane (the most superficial layers of the cornea)
- Bowman layer (the most superficial part of the corneal stroma)
- stroma (multiple lamellae of collagen fibers, which account for 90% of the cornea's thickness)
- Descemet membrane (the collagenous basement membrane of the corneal endothelium)
- endothelium (a single layer of endothelial cells that act as metabolic pumps to regulate corneal water content)

Diffuse illumination and sclerotic scatter (see Chapter 10) are useful screening techniques for beginning the slit-lamp examination of the cornea and for detecting areas that require closer scrutiny. Such areas are then examined with a small- to medium-sized parallelepiped and with the thin, optical section. The latter is especially useful for accurately determining the level of any abnormality.

Epithelium

Epithelial defects are best seen with fluorescein staining and will be discussed in the section on special stains later in this chapter. Corneal ulcers present with an epithelial defect and white stromal infiltrate that is visible prior to staining with fluorescein. Epithelial filaments are teardrop-shaped tags of degenerated epithelial cells and mucus and occur with severe dry eyes.

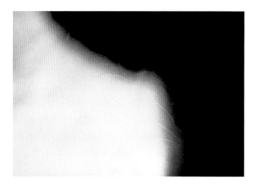

Figure 11-36 Fingerprint lines representing anterior-membrane corneal dystrophy (strips of excessive epithelial basement-membrane collagen beneath, or within, the corneal epithelium).

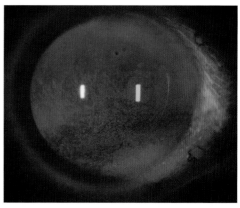

Figure 11-37 Punctate epithelial erosions (PEE) as shown by punctate staining with fluorescein. (Courtesy of Fasika Woreta, MD)

Fingerprint and map lines are curvilinear, translucent, or slightly opaque abnormalities within the epithelium and have the appearance of a fingerprint or a map of an island (Figure 11-36). They occur in primary anterior-membrane corneal dystrophy (also known as *epithelial basement-membrane* or *map-dot-fingerprint dystrophy*) and sometimes after trauma.

Intraepithelial cysts can range from microcysts a fraction of a millimeter in diameter to macrocysts of 1 mm or more. They can be clear (as in Meesmann corneal dystrophy) or opaque, and white to tan if filled with cellular debris (as in the dots of map-dot-fingerprint dystrophy).

Punctate epithelial erosions (PEEs) occur in a large variety of corneal inflammations and surface disturbances. PEEs are evidence of ocular dryness that results in pinpoint breakdown of the epithelium (Figure 11-37). Punctate epithelial keratitis (PEK) and superficial punctate keratitis (SPK) are the result of small foci of inflammation, usually lymphocytes, within the epithelium. The examiner sees small white opacities that do not stain with fluorescein, which are characteristic of Thygeson superficial punctate keratitis (TSPK).

Epithelial edema occurs when stromal edema secondarily involves the epithelium, so it is associated with stromal thickening (discussed in "Stroma," below). Early epithelial edema manifests by the appearance of tiny, clear bubbles of fluid within the epithelium. Retroillumination and indirect lateral illumination are useful for detecting early microcysts. More severe edema leads to the formation of bullae (bullous keratopathy), in which areas of epithelium detach from the underlying tissue (Figure 11-38).

Cornea verticillata describes a whorl-like pattern of deposits in the corneal epithelium as a result of use of certain medications (eg, amiodarone; see Figure 10-11) or in the rare metabolic disorder Fabry disease.

People with skin pigmentation often have circumcorneal melanin pigmentation of the limbus, called complexion-associated melanosis (CAM). Brownish-yellow, curvilinear deposits of iron can be seen in the basal layer of the corneal epithelium. A horizontally oriented iron line (Hudson-Stähli line) develops with advancing age at the junction of the upper two-thirds and lower one-third of the cornea. The other corneal iron lines associated with epithelial irregularities are the Fleischer ring (seen at the base of the cone in keratoconus), Ferry line (seen below a filtering bleb), and Stocker line (seen at the head of a pterygium) (Figure 11-39).

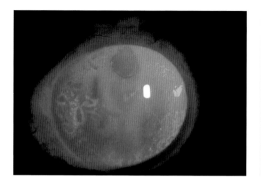

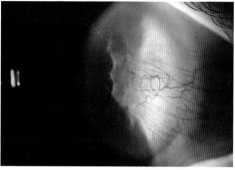

Figure 11-38 Corneal edema in postoperative endothelial dysfunction, made evident by staining of the tear film with fluorescein. Mild epithelial edema (bedewing) is seen in the superonasal and superotemporal areas, and bullous keratopathy is seen at the 12 o'clock position, 3-5 o'clock positions, and 8-10 o'clock positions.

Figure 11-39 A Stocker line is the brown iron line in the cornea anterior to the head of the pterygium. (Courtesy of Preston H. Blomquist, MD.)

Bowman Layer

Although sometimes referred to as Bowman membrane, Bowman layer is not a true or separate membrane, but a superficial area of modified stroma in which the collagen fibers are slightly more irregular than those that lie deeper. As a result, Bowman layer is normally slightly more reflective of light than the stroma when it is viewed with the slit lamp; clinically, this gives the layer a subtly granular appearance.

Superficial corneal vascularization, usually with fibrosis, is called pannus (Latin for "cloth") if it extends further than 2 mm into the cornea, or micropannus if the reach is shorter (Figure 11-40). This kind of vascularization develops at the level of superficial Bowman layer. The vessels tend to branch dichotomously. Superficial corneal vascularization occurs as a response to superficial necrosis or hypoxia and so is seen in association with many different pathologic processes.

Calcium deposits in the cornea are found at the level of Bowman layer and sometimes secondarily involve the epithelium. The deposits usually begin just inside the nasal and temporal limbus in the interpalpebral zone of exposure and, in many cases, eventually extend across the entire cornea (calcific band-shaped keratopathy). The deposits are white and, at first, finely granular. Later, the flecks of calcium become confluent and form solid plaques. The calcium tends not to accumulate around corneal nerves that are coursing through Bowman layer to the epithelium, so that the plaques typically have small clear areas ("Swiss-cheese holes"). Calcium deposits develop most often as a degenerative change or as a result of hypercalcemia.

Any disturbance of Bowman layer can cause fibrosis (scarring). Fibrosis of Bowman layer occurs spontaneously in Reis-Bücklers corneal dystrophy, a hereditary disorder. Focal breaks in this layer are typical of keratoconus.

Stroma

The stroma accounts for 90% of the corneal thickness. It consists of multiple lamellae of collagen fibers surrounded by proteoglycan ground substance. Scattered keratocytes

Figure 11-40 Extensive pannus occurring with hypersensitivity to a preservative in contact lens solution.

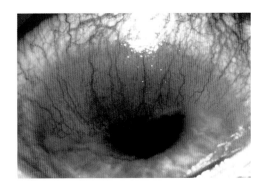

(modified fibroblasts) are also present. The normal, regular arrangement of the collagen fibers is necessary for maintenance of corneal transparency. Any disturbance of the regularity results in some loss of corneal transparency.

White limbal girdle of Vogt is an elastotic stromal change that appears with age, just inside the limbus. It is seen as a yellow-white line, concentric with the limbus, and extends from about the 2 o'clock–4 o'clock positions and the 8 o'clock–10 o'clock positions. A lucid interval may appear between the limbus and the girdle.

Inflammatory cells can infiltrate the stroma in response to infection or to sterile, immunologically mediated diseases. The infiltrate can be purulent (neutrophils), nonpurulent (lymphocytes), or granulomatous (epithelioid cells and multinucleated giant cells).

Marginal infiltrates are a particular kind of sterile, neutrophilic infiltration (Figure 11-41). They are similar to phlyctenules but typically occur inside the limbus, are more apt to be multiple, and are followed by less scarring and vascularization. Whereas phlyctenules are type-IV (cell-mediated) lesions, marginal infiltrates are type-III (antigen-antibody–mediated) infiltrates. They represent a hypersensitivity reaction against staphylococcal antigens.

Stromal vascularization is deeper than pannus. Stromal vessels are usually relatively straight and roughly parallel, like the bristles of a broom, and they show less branching than do superficial vessels. Stromal vascularization is also known as *interstitial vascularization*. The term *interstitial keratitis* (IK) is often used to describe such vessel ingrowth associated with stromal inflammation (Figure 11-42).

Like its superficial counterpart, stromal vascularization is indicative of stromal necrosis or hypoxia and has many possible causes. It is especially common with purulent keratitis and may occur in association with tuberculosis or congenital syphilis. After a disease process has become inactive, the vessels sometimes appear to become devoid of blood; these are called *ghost vessels* and are seen as clear tubules coursing through the stroma.

Normal corneal thickness is 0.54–0.56 mm (540–560 µm), but edematous corneas often have thicknesses of 0.7 mm or more. Increased thickness of the stroma is not always visually detectable if the edema is mild, but corneal thickness can be measured with a *pachymeter*.

Corneal thickness is nearly proportional to corneal water content and so is useful for determining whether corneal edema is present. Early stromal edema can often be detected biomicroscopically by noticing fine, undulating striae in the deep stroma and Descemet membrane, which results from the cornea expanding posteriorly with thickening. After

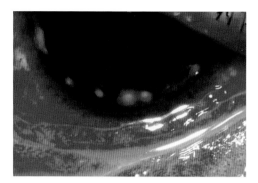

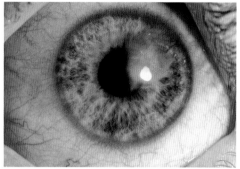

Figure 11-41 Marginal infiltrates (antigen-antibody-mediated reactions to microbial antigens) in staphylococcal conjunctivitis.

Figure 11-42 Interstitial keratitis: cellular infiltration, vascularization, and edema of the corneal stroma in congenital syphilis.

looking for stromal edema with a slit-lamp beam of any width, the examiner can try to ascertain whether the thin, optical-section beam is thicker than normal. This method of detecting corneal edema is usually possible only when the edema is substantial and the examiner has gained experience in evaluating corneal thickness by having examined a number of patients with normal corneal thickness.

The methods above are useful for detecting edema of the corneal stroma. Stromal edema eventually extends into the corneal epithelium and produces vesicular, or even bullous, foci of edema on the corneal surface. Instilling fluorescein onto the eye helps the examiner appreciate epithelial edema because the dye will pool around the bases of elevated blebs of edema (*negative staining*) (see Figure 11-38). Stromal edema causes the stroma to become more relucent and silvery and to lose some of its transparency. Corneal edema in the presence of very high intraocular pressure (IOP; as with acute angle-closure glaucoma) presents with extensive epithelial edema (which has a steamy appearance) and normal (or nearly normal) corneal thickness; the stroma is compressed by the high pressure, which forces much of the fluid into the epithelium. Corneal edema generally indicates dysfunction of the corneal endothelium, usually from dystrophy, inflammation, or trauma.

Stromal thinning can occur in the ectatic corneal dystrophies, such as keratoconus, keratoglobus, and pellucid marginal degeneration; infections; and autoimmune diseases. Stromal thinning is sometimes so extreme that little remains in a particular area other than Descemet membrane, which then tends to bulge forward (a descemetocele).

Corneal metabolic deposits are numerous and can occur with local (corneal) or systemic diseases. The most commonly seen metabolic deposits occur in the 3 classic stromal corneal dystrophies: macular dystrophy (glycosaminoglycan), lattice dystrophy (amyloid), and granular dystrophy (protein of uncertain character). Corneal arcus is deposition of lipid in the corneal stroma. In Schnyder corneal dystrophy, crystals in the anterior stroma are evident on slit-lamp examination.

Corneal nerves are seen as thin, white, dichotomously branching lines in the anterior two-thirds of the corneal stroma. Similar lines seen in the posterior one-third of the stroma are likely to be ghost vessels rather than corneal nerves. Corneal nerves can sometimes become enlarged and more prominent than usual, most commonly from age, keratoconus, and neurofibromatosis.

Descemet Membrane

Descemet membrane (DM), the collagenous basement membrane of the endothelium, is best examined with direct focal illumination and retroillumination. DM wrinkles when the cornea is edematous or if ocular hypotony is present. Trauma (including birth injuries from forceps), necrosis, ectatic corneal dystrophies (keratoconus, keratoglobus), and congenital glaucoma can cause the membrane to rupture. When this occurs, sudden and severe corneal edema (acute corneal hydrops) might ensue and persist until the defect heals (in several weeks to months).

Excessive production of DM collagen can be caused by trauma or corneal dystrophies. Healed ruptures leave behind 1 or more thickened ridges of the membrane, referred to as *Haab striae* in the specific case of congenital glaucoma.

Focal areas of thickening of DM, known as guttata, occur in the early stages of Fuchs corneal dystrophy. The appearance is classically that of beaten metal. A few corneal guttae are normally found with aging in the corneal periphery and are called *Hassall-Henle bodies*.

DM normally terminates beneath the opaque limbus, so that the ridgelike termination (Schwalbe ring) is not visible without gonioscopy (see "Gonioscopy" later in this chapter). Schwalbe ring can be displaced anteriorly into the peripheral cornea as the congenital anomaly called *posterior embryotoxon*. The clinical appearance is of an arcuate band of thickened Descemet membrane just inside the limbus (usually nasally or temporally).

Kayser-Fleischer ring is a deposition of copper in peripheral Descemet membrane. It is usually beige to yellow-brown and occurs with Wilson disease.

Endothelium

The endothelium, the most posterior layer of the cornea, consists of a single layer of endothelial cells that act as metabolic pumps to regulate normal corneal water content. The hydrophilic corneal stroma becomes edematous whenever endothelial function is inadequate. The endothelium is best examined by specular reflection, which allows for visualization of individual endothelial cells (see Chapter 10).

Endothelial cells normally have hexagonal shapes and are roughly uniform in size. The cells have very little ability to regenerate, so as cells die, adjacent ones enlarge to fill the gaps. This results in cells that are larger than normal (polymegathism), cells that vary greatly in size (polymegathism), and cells that have varying and abnormal shapes (pleomorphism). Figure 11-43 depicts endothelial cell polymegathism and pleomorphism.

Pigment from the iris, sometimes seen as brown "dust" on the endothelium, can be observed with diffuse, direct illumination. In pigment dispersion syndrome and pigmentary glaucoma, the pigmentation usually takes the form of a vertically oriented spindle just below the center of the cornea (Krukenberg spindle).

Keratic precipitates (KPs) are accumulations of inflammatory cells on the corneal endothelium that occur with intraocular inflammation. KPs can be fine, medium, or large in size and are variable in shape. Large KPs usually occur with granulomatous inflammation and can be larger than 1 mm; they have a greasy, yellowish appearance and are called *mutton-fat KPs* (Figure 11-44). Other KPs are usually white. They can be punctate, round, or stellate. KPs are seen most often on the inferior or central cornea. After inactivation of inflammation, KPs can disappear, become hyalinized (clear), or

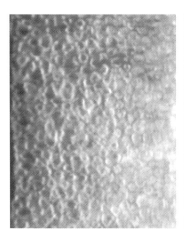 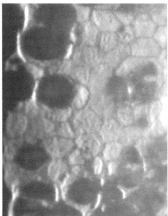

Figure 11-43   Specular microscopy of living corneal endothelium. Normal endothelium is shown on the left. Note the hexagonal shape of the endothelial cells. The corneal endothelium of a patient with Fuchs endothelial dystrophy is shown on the right. Demonstrated are polymegathism (larger cells), pleomorphism (variability in size and shape of cells), and dark areas of endothelial cell loss (guttae). (Courtesy of Preston H. Blomquist, MD.)

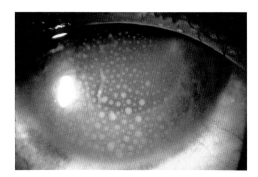

Figure 11-44   Mutton-fat keratic precipitates in granulomatous anterior uveitis. (Reproduced with permission from Johns KJ, *Eye Care Skills: Presentations for Physicians and Other Health Care Professionals,* Version 3.0, American Academy of Ophthalmology, 2009.)

become pigmented. In the case of corneal transplant rejection, a line of lymphocytic KPs can sometimes be seen to advance across the endothelium (Khodadoust rejection line).

Anterior Chamber

The anterior chamber is the area between the cornea and iris and is filled with aqueous humor.

Anterior Chamber Depth

Evaluating the depth of the anterior chamber is important in assessing a patient's risk of or predisposition to angle-closure glaucoma. The depth of the chamber can be evaluated by locating an optical section slit-lamp beam, at an angle of 60°, onto the peripheral cornea just inside the limbus (van Herick method). The chamber is considered to be shallow if the distance between the corneal endothelium and the surface of the iris is less than one-fourth the thickness of the cornea.

This test is useful before instilling dilating eyedrops to ensure that the patient is not predisposed to angle-closure glaucoma, but it is only a screening test and is not a substitute for gonioscopy when glaucoma is suspected. Gonioscopy is discussed in greater detail later in this chapter.

Flare and Cell

Intraocular inflammation produces increased protein and the appearance of inflammatory cells in the anterior chamber. The anterior chamber is normally optically empty, meaning that it appears nearly black as the slit-lamp beam passes through it. However, the beam of light becomes progressively more visible as the protein content of the aqueous humor increases. This visibility of the beam is called *flare*. When inflammatory cells are present, they are seen in the slit-lamp beam as white dots that rise and fall in the convection currents of the anterior chamber and aqueous humor (they rise near the warmer iris and fall near the cooler cornea). Together, these slit-lamp findings are referred to as *flare and cell* and have the appearance of dust particles within a projector's haze of light. Clinical Protocol 11-3 describes the steps in evaluating and recording flare and cell. Table 11-1 summarizes the grading scheme for anterior chamber flare; Table 11-2 includes the scheme for anterior chamber cells. White inflammatory cells should be differentiated from pigment (brown) or erythrocytes (red).

Hyphema and Hypopyon

Blood in the anterior chamber, usually from trauma, is called *hyphema*. If the amount of blood is sufficient, it settles inferiorly, forming a flat-topped layer of blood in the anterior chamber (Figure 11-45). Blood that fills the chamber is called "8-ball hemorrhage."

Purulent (neutrophilic) exudates can occur in the anterior chamber, usually in cases of severe intraocular infections, or with inflammatory conditions such as Behçet disease. As with blood, layering of the white to yellow-white purulent material can occur and is called a *hypopyon* (Figure 11-46). In addition to hypopyon, severe intraocular inflammation may be associated with fibrin in the anterior chamber of a pupillary membrane.

Table 11-1   The SUN Working Group Grading System for Anterior Chamber Flare

Grade	Description
0	None
1+	Faint
2+	Moderate (iris and lens details clear)
3+	Marked (iris and lens details hazy)
4+	Intense (fibrin or plasmoid aqueous)

The Standardization of Uveitis Nomenclature (SUN) Working Group. Standardization of nomenclature for reporting clinical data: results of the First International Workshop. *Am J Ophthalmol.* 2005;140:509–516: Table 4. Copyright 2005, reprinted with permission from Elsevier.

Table 11-2   The SUN Working Group Grading System for Anterior Chamber Cells

Grade	Cells in Field (high-intensity 1×1-mm slit beam)
0	<1
0.5+	1–5
1+	6–15
2+	16–25
3+	26–50
4+	>50

The Standardization of Uveitis Nomenclature (SUN) Working Group. Standardization of nomenclature for reporting clinical data: results of the First International Workshop. *Am J Ophthalmol.* 2005; 140: 509–516: Table 3. Copyright 2005, reprinted with permission from Elsevier.

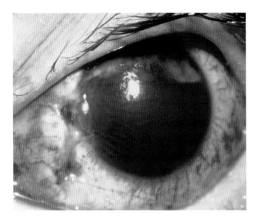

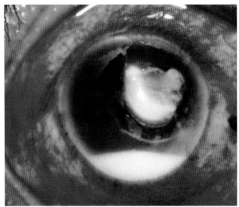

Figure 11-45 Large traumatic hyphema (blood in the anterior chamber).

Figure 11-46 Hypopyon with bacterial keratitis.

Lens material and vitreous

After complicated cataract surgery, lens material or vitreous may be visible in the anterior chamber. Vitreous is usually present as strands to corneal wounds and may cause peaking of the pupil. Inflammation may result from retained lens material.

Epithelial downgrowth and cysts

Traumatic implantation of epithelial cells into the anterior chamber can result in the formation of a cyst as the cells proliferate. Larger cysts can fill a large part of the anterior chamber, indenting and pushing the iris posteriorly. Epithelial downgrowth may also occur after penetrating trauma and can proliferate aggressively over anterior chamber structures such as the angle or endothelium.

Iris

Direct focal illumination is used most often for examining the iris. Indirect illumination is useful for evaluating the interiors of lesions that are not transparent. Transillumination can reveal areas of partial- or full-thickness iris atrophy or other defects of the iris. *Synechiae* are sequelae of inflammation; they are adhesions between the iris and the cornea (anterior synechiae) or between the iris and the crystalline lens (posterior synechiae). Posterior synechiae sometimes involve the entire circumference of the pupillary margin (seclusio pupillae), and so prevent aqueous humor from reaching the anterior chamber. The accumulation of aqueous behind the iris causes it to bow forward (iris bombé), and the angle closes with resultant glaucoma. Iris bombé also can occur when the entire pupil becomes covered by a fibrous membrane (occlusio pupillae).

Nodules

Inflammatory nodules on the iris are most commonly granulomas associated with sarcoidosis. Nodules at the pupillary margin are called *Koeppe nodules,* whereas those on the surface of the iris are called *Busacca nodules.*

Other iris nodules include *Brushfield spots* (white spots on the peripheral iris seen in patients with Down syndrome) and *Lisch nodules* (melanocytic nodules of the iris seen in neurofibromatosis).

Neovascularization

Rubeosis iridis is neovascularization of the iris; it is usually caused by retinal ischemia. The abnormal vessels are fine, irregular, and plentiful (Figure 11-47). They appear on the surface of the iris, first in the area of the pupillary margin and peripherally at the root of the iris. The condition often leads to the formation of extensive peripheral anterior synechiae and secondary angle-closure glaucoma.

Rubeosis iridis is to be differentiated from hyperemia of otherwise normal iris vessels. Hyperemia is manifested by the presence of 1 or more individual cordlike vessels coursing in iris crypts somewhere between the pupillary margin and the peripheral iris. Rubeotic vessels are seen more as tight masses of very fine, tangled vessels.

Tumors

Most tumors of the iris are benign nevi. Iris melanomas may demonstrate growth or significant thickness, and cause ectropion uvea, sectoral cataract, or glaucoma. They are variably pigmented, ranging from tan to brown-black in color (Figure 11-48).

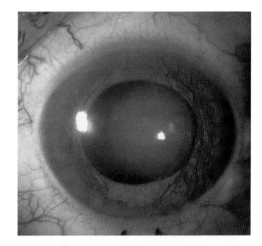

Figure 11-47 Extensive neovascularization of the iris (rubeosis iridis). (Reproduced, with permission, from Johns KJ, *Eye Care Skills: Presentations for Physicians and Other Health Care Professionals,* Version 3.0, American Academy of Ophthalmology, 2009.)

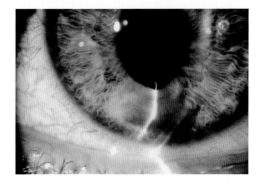

Figure 11-48 Pigmented lesion (melanoma) of the iris.

Persistent Pupillary Membrane Remnants

During embryonic development a membrane is normally present over the pupil. It generally disappears, but remnants sometimes persist. They are usually not extensive, but it is not uncommon to see a few spider web–like strands of this tissue that originate from the iris near the pupillary margin; the other ends can be freely floating or attached elsewhere to the iris, to the anterior lens capsule, or even to the cornea. Stellate deposits of brown pigment are often found on the anterior lens capsule (epicapsular stars) as part of this condition. The posterior capsule of the lens sometimes manifests a small white dot inferonasal to the visual axis (Mittendorf dot); this is a remnant of the lenticular attachment of the embryonic hyaloid artery.

Other Abnormalities

Corectopia, or displacement of the pupil, can be caused by congenital anomalies such as Axenfeld-Rieger syndrome. Iris atrophy also can occur after inflammation or trauma. Iris transillumination defects can be seen with retroillumination from the fundus.

The term *heterochromia* refers to a difference in iris color of the 2 eyes of a patient. Causes include congenital anomaly, iris atrophy (which renders a blue iris darker blue, or a brown iris lighter brown or even blue), or hyperpigmentation (as from a diffuse melanoma of the iris).

Iridodonesis is a quivering of the iris that can be seen with movements of the eye in patients who are aphakic (lacking a crystalline lens) or who have subluxated or luxated lenses. The condition occurs because of the lack of support of the iris by the lens and its zonular attachments.

Crystalline Lens

The lens is an encapsulated structure that contains several lamellae, or layers, that are formed during different periods of development and life (Figure 11-49). The outer layer

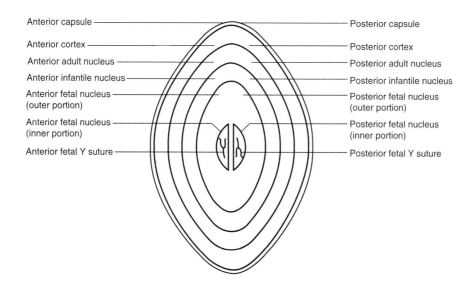

Figure 11-49   Diagrammatic representation of the main layers and nuclei of the crystalline lens as can be seen with the optical section of the slit lamp.

is called the capsule. The next layer, the cortex, continues to grow throughout life. The layer of the lens central to the anterior and posterior cortex is the nucleus.

The lens is best examined after pupillary dilation, usually with the optical section. Diffuse direct illumination and retroillumination are useful for evaluating the posterior capsular and subcapsular area. Beginning anteriorly, the slit-lamp beam passes through the anterior capsule, anterior cortex, anterior adult nucleus, anterior infantile nucleus, anterior fetal nucleus, anterior erect fetal Y suture, posterior inverted fetal Y suture, posterior fetal nucleus, posterior infantile nucleus, posterior adult nucleus, posterior cortex, and posterior lens capsule.

Cataract

A cataract is an opacity of the lens that may or may not be visually significant. Except in the rare instance in which a cataract might cause a threat to the eye (eg, phacomorphic or angle closure glaucoma), the mere presence of a cataract is not a justification for cataract surgery. If the patient cannot function adequately according to their own visual needs, cataract surgery can be recommended after discussion of the risks, benefits, and alternatives. In fact, patients should nearly always be reassured that cataract surgery is not necessary or advisable until such time as they, themselves, decide that they want it in order to see better.

A cataract can involve the lens capsule (capsular cataract) or the lens itself (lenticular cataract). Cataracts can be classified as cortical, nuclear sclerotic, and subcapsular.

Cortical cataracts

Cortical cataracts develop in the anterior and posterior cortex and are mostly associated with age and diabetes mellitus. In age-related cataracts, fluid accumulates among the lens fibrils, producing lamellar separation. This is seen as roughly parallel, relucent lines. These areas then opacify, producing radially oriented cortical spokes (Figure 11-50). Flocculent, snowflakelike opacities can also develop, especially in diabetic patients who have ketoacidosis; these opacities are sometimes reversible with treatment of the ketoacidosis.

Glaukomflecken are gray-white anterior cortical dots that appear after episodes of very high intraocular pressure. They usually indicate a prior acute angle-closure glaucoma attack.

Nuclear cataracts

Nuclear cataract is the most common, and classic, age-related cataract. It may be thought of as a result of the compression of the more central portion of the lens by the ongoing formation throughout life of new, more peripherally located cortical lens fibers (although various biochemical changes are also present). This so-called *nuclear sclerosis* first appears as a progressive yellowing in the center of the lens. (Figure 11-51). Nuclear cataracts are apt to progress slowly, and often require years to affect vision.

Subcapsular cataracts

Subcapsular cataracts are usually found in the central posterior subcapsular area of the lens and appear as silvery and granular, bubbly opacifications in the visual axis (Figure 11-52). Patients with this type of cataract develop symptoms early on and experience more rapid progression of the cataract. Posterior subcapsular cataracts can result from prolonged topical or systemic corticosteroid therapy.

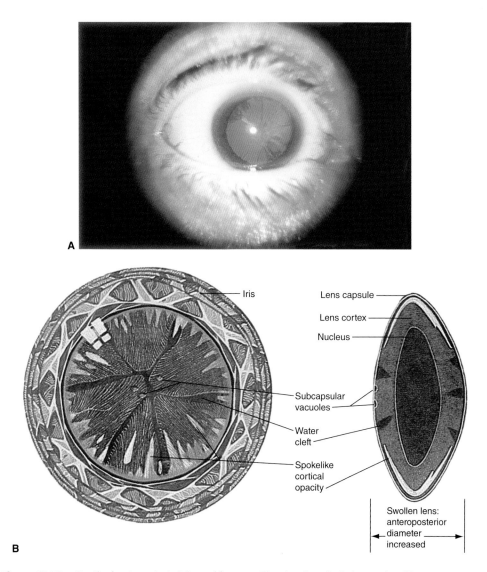

Iris
Lens capsule
Lens cortex
Nucleus
Subcapsular vacuoles
Water cleft
Spokelike cortical opacity
Swollen lens: anteroposterior diameter increased

Figure 11-50 Cortical cataract. **A,** Viewed by retroillumination. **B,** Schematic of immature cortical cataract. (Courtesy of CIBA Pharmaceutical Co, division of CIBA-GEIGY Corp. Reproduced with permission from Clinical Symposia. Illustration by John A. Craig.)

Congenital cataracts

Congenital cataracts can affect the polar areas of the cortex (anterior or posterior), the Y sutures, the fetal or embryonic nuclei, or the capsule (usually anterior). The lamellar (also called *zonular*) form of congenital cataract is common. Lamellar cataracts have opacification of the periphery of a particular zone of the lens, yet the interior of the zone is clear (Figure 11-53).

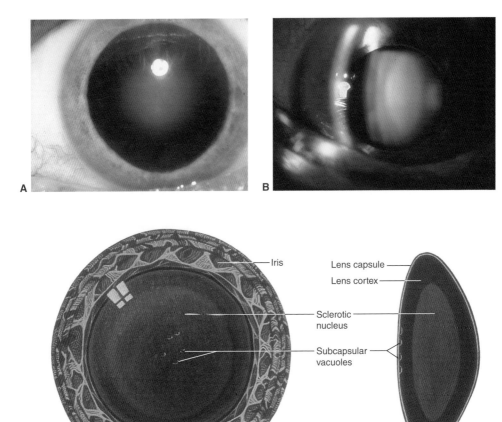

Figure 11-51 Nuclear cataract. **A,** Viewed with diffuse illumination. **B,** Viewed with a slit beam. **C,** Schematic of nuclear cataract. (Courtesy of CIBA Pharmaceutical Co, division of CIBA-GEIGY Corp. Reproduced with permission from Clinical Symposia. Illustration by John A. Craig.)

Soemmering ring

A Soemmering ring is a ring of opacified equatorial (peripheral) lens material that is enclosed in lens capsule. It can result from trauma that causes rupture of the lens capsule and consequent resorption of most of the lens material, or from residual cortex after cataract extraction.

Pseudophakia and aphakia

Patients who have had cataract extraction with implantation of an artificial intraocular lens are said to have *pseudophakia* (Figure 11-54). In uncomplicated cases, the implant is placed in the bag. It is important in pseudophakia to ascertain whether the posterior lens capsule is present and, if so, whether it is clear or opaque. Laser capsulotomy might be indicated if the posterior capsule has become opaque. *Aphakia* is the absence of the lens

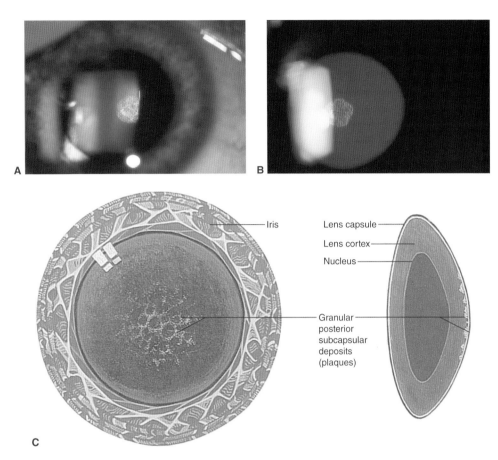

Figure 11-52 Posterior subcapsular cataract. **A,** Viewed at the slit lamp. **B,** Viewed with indirect illumination. **C,** Schematic of posterior subcapsular cataract. (Courtesy of CIBA Pharmaceutical Co, division of CIBA-GEIGY Corp. Reproduced with permission from Clinical Symposia. Illustration by John A. Craig.)

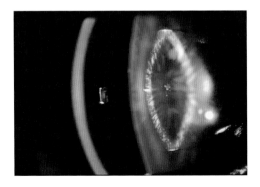

Figure 11-53 Lamellar (or zonular) cataract, affecting mainly 1 layer of the lens (anterior infantile nucleus), although some punctate opacities are also seen in the area of the fetal Y sutures.

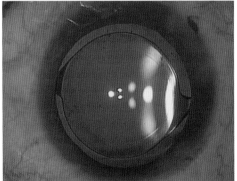

Figure 11-54 Intraoperative photo of posterior chamber intraocular lens implant placed in the capsular bag. (Courtesy of Preston H. Blomquist, MD.)

(and its capsule) and may be seen if the capsular support is compromised and an intraocular lens has not been implanted.

Subluxation and Luxation

The crystalline lens is held in its normal position by multiple fine fibrils that comprise the zonule (zonular fibers) of Zinn (Figure 11-55). The fibers can be disrupted by trauma or systemic disease (most notably Marfan syndrome or homocystinuria); this can result in partial or complete dislocation of the lens from its normal position. In the case of subluxation, the edge of the lens might be visible in the pupil. Complete dislocation (luxation) allows the lens to be displaced into the vitreous or, in rare instances, into the anterior chamber.

Other Conditions

Peters anomaly, a congenital anomaly, manifests a corneal leukoma that is often attached to a cataractous lens by way of a fibrous band that extends across the anterior chamber. The band is sometimes attached to the iris instead of the lens. Pseudoexfoliation (or exfoliation) syndrome causes deposits of a white, fibrillary, dandrufflike material to accumulate on various intraocular tissues, but most prominently on the anterior lens capsule. It appears as a disk of fine, gray-white flecks centrally or paracentrally. The condition is associated with small areas of iris atrophy, deposits of the white material at the pupillary margin, hyperpigmentation of the iris and trabecular meshwork, glaucoma, and fragility

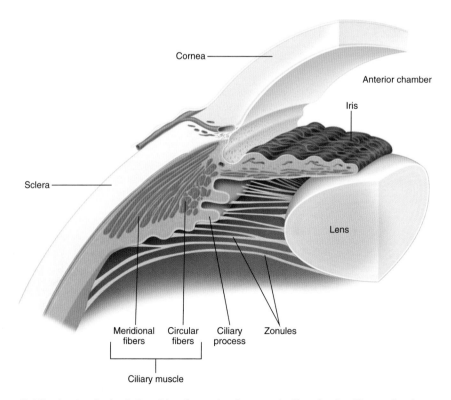

Figure 11-55 Anatomical relationship of zonules, lens, and ciliary body. (Illustration by Mark M. Miller.)

of the zonular fibers. The last accounts for an increased risk of zonular rupture during cataract extraction.

Retrolental Space and Anterior Vitreous

The retrolental space and anterior vitreous can be examined for the presence of cell. In cases of suspected retinal tears, pigment in the anterior vitreous raises the probability of a tear being present (Shafer sign). Inflammatory cells may also be present due to spillover of cells from the anterior chamber or because of inflammation in the vitreous (intermediate uveitis).

Gonioscopy

Gonioscopy is examination of the angle of the anterior chamber (the structures between the peripheral iris and cornea, including the trabecular meshwork, through which aqueous exits the eye). Gonioscopy might not be performed during routine anterior segment examinations. However, gonioscopy should be routinely performed in the evaluation of patients with increased intraocular pressure or glaucoma. It is also used in the evaluation of tumors of the iris and ciliary body and other abnormalities in the area of the angle.

The anatomy and optical properties of the anterior segment of the eye prevent direct visualization of the angle without the use of special (gonioscopy) lenses due to total internal reflection. These lenses, also called *gonioprisms,* either refract light into the angle (Koeppe lens) or reflect light into the angle (Goldmann 3-mirror or Zeiss 4-mirror lens), thereby illuminating it and permitting it to be seen (Figure 11-56). The Goldmann 3-mirror contact lens may also be used to examine the peripheral retina (Figure 11-57).

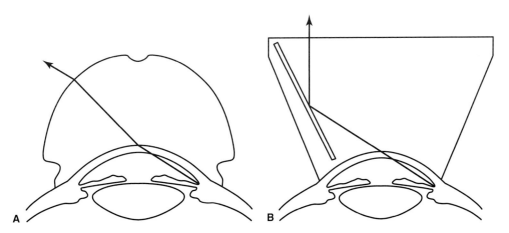

Figure 11-56 Main methods of gonioscopy. **A,** With the Koeppe lens (direct gonioscopy), light rays from the angle are refracted to the eyes of the examiner. **B,** With the Zeiss or Goldmann lens (indirect gonioscopy—more often used), light from the angle is reflected to the examiner by means of a mirror. (Redrawn, with permission, from Stamper RL, ed. *Becker-Shaffer's Diagnosis and Therapy of the Glaucomas,* 8th ed. CV Mosby Co; 2009.)

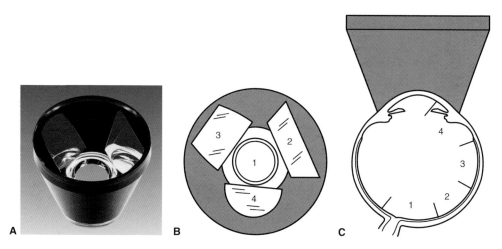

Figure 11-57 Indirect gonioscopy with the Goldmann 3-mirror contact gonioscopy lens. **A,** Photograph of the Goldmann lens. **B, C,** The lens's 3 mirrors are at different angles, which allows for examination of different parts of the internal eye; mirror 4 permits examination of the angle of the anterior chamber and the area of the ciliary body; mirror 3 is used to view the peripheral fundus; mirror 2 is for the mid-peripheral fundus; and lens 1 (not a mirror) affords a view of the posterior pole of the fundus. (Part A courtesy of Haag-Streit AG, Bern, Switzerland.)

Gonioscopy should usually be performed after refraction but prior to dilation of the pupil. Repeating the procedure after dilation can provide additional information (eg, the effect of dilation on the angle), due to a better ability to see the ciliary-body area. Clinical Protocol 11-4 provides instructions for performing gonioscopy.

Figure 11-58 shows a composite drawing of the anatomy of the angle. The trabecular meshwork is bounded superiorly by Schwalbe line (the peripheral termination of Descemet membrane) and inferiorly by the scleral spur (into which the longitudinal muscles of the ciliary body insert). Schwalbe line appears as a thin, opaque, white, linear ridge. The scleral spur is also white and opaque. Between the 2 structures, the trabecular meshwork often appears grayish and somewhat translucent, though it can show varying degrees of pigmentation (including none at all). If pigmentation is light or absent, a slightly darker-gray line can sometimes be seen in the lower area of the trabecular meshwork. This is Schlemm canal, a tubule into which aqueous enters after passing through the trabecular meshwork, and from which it then enters the vascular circulation. Posterior to the scleral spur are often a few normal blood vessels and normal iris processes (fine filaments that extend from the iris to the lower trabecular meshwork). More posterior to this is the *angle recess*, which represents a dipping of the peripheral iris as it inserts into the ciliary body.

The examiner can describe the angle in the patient's record by noting the most posterior structure that can be seen. For example, if only Schwalbe line can be seen, the angle is very narrow, but if the scleral spur can be seen, the angle is open. Usually, however, the width of the angle is graded, most often by the Shaffer method, as described in Table 11-3 and shown in Figure 11-59. The Spaeth grading system adds information about the configuration and insertion of the peripheral iris (Figure 11-60).

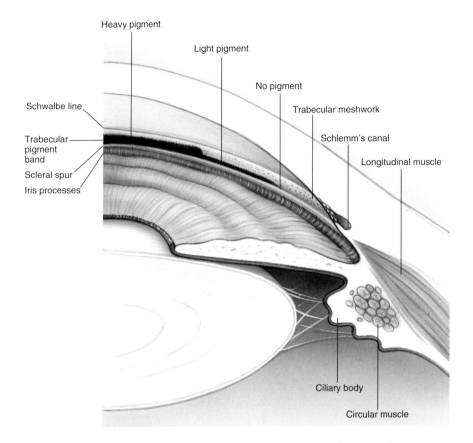

Heavy pigment

Light pigment

No pigment

Schwalbe line

Trabecular meshwork

Trabecular pigment band

Schlemm's canal

Scleral spur

Longitudinal muscle

Iris processes

Ciliary body

Circular muscle

Figure 11-58   Gonioscopic anatomy of the anterior chamber and surrounding structures.

Table 11-3   Shaffer Method for Grading Anterior Chamber Angles

Grade	Description
Grade IV	The angle between the iris and the surface of the trabecular meshwork is 45° (normal).
Grade III	The angle between the iris and the surface of the trabecular meshwork is greater than 20° but less than 45° (normal).
Grade II	The angle between the iris and the surface of the trabecular meshwork is 20°. Angle closure possible.
Grade I	The angle between the iris and the surface of the trabecular meshwork is 10°. Angle closure probable in time.
Slit	The angle between the iris and the surface of the trabecular meshwork is less than 10°. Angle closure very likely.
Grade 0	The iris is against the trabecular meshwork. Angle closure is present.

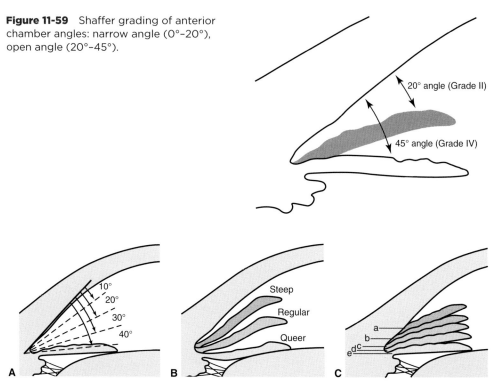

Figure 11-59 Shaffer grading of anterior chamber angles: narrow angle (0°–20°), open angle (20°–45°).

20° angle (Grade II)

45° angle (Grade IV)

10°
20°
30°
40°

Steep
Regular
Queer

a
b
c
d
e

A   B   C

Figure 11-60 Spaeth's gonioscopic classification of the angle of the anterior chamber, based on 3 variables. **A,** Angular width of the angle recess. **B,** Configuration of the peripheral iris. **C,** Insertion of the iris root; a = highest insertion, e = lowest insertion. (Redrawn, with permission, from Shields MB. *Textbook of Glaucoma,* 3rd ed. Williams & Wilkins; 1992.)

Stains

Stains (dyes) instilled into the tear film can facilitate examination of the ocular surface by highlighting certain pathologic changes. The most commonly used stains are fluorescein, rose bengal red (usually referred to simply as "rose bengal"), and lissamine green.

Fluorescein

Fluorescein is available as an eyedrop mixed with a topical anesthetic (Fluress) or as fluorescein-impregnated paper strips. The strips are moistened with an eyedrop of saline solution, artificial tears, or topical ophthalmic anesthetic and then touched to the inside of the lower eyelid. Fluorescein staining is best seen with diffuse slit-lamp illumination with the cobalt-blue filter; the blue light causes the dye to fluoresce a bright green color. The pattern and morphology of staining have diagnostic value (Figure 11-61).

Fluorescein does not stain corneal or conjunctival epithelium but readily enters and stains the stroma in areas in which epithelium is absent (or even in areas in which epithelial cells have loose intercellular junctions). Accordingly, fluorescein is very useful for detecting areas of epithelial deficiency that occur, for example, in cases of corneal abrasion, recurrent corneal erosion, or herpes simplex epithelial (dendritic) keratitis.

Fluorescein is also useful for detecting corneal perforations or wound leaks (Seidel test). The surface is painted with a fluorescein strip moistened with 1–2 eyedrops of sterile saline

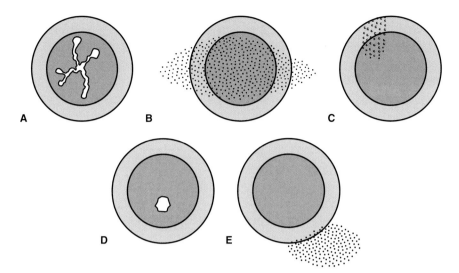

Figure 11-61 Typical patterns of staining with fluorescein or rose bengal and their diagnostic importance. **A,** Dendritiform staining (dichotomously branching lesions, often with terminally bulbous swellings)—typical of herpes simplex keratitis. **B,** Staining in the interpalpebral zone of exposure in the dry eye (usually more so with rose bengal than with fluorescein) in keratoconjunctivitis sicca. **C,** Linear punctate staining in the superior cornea (caused by a foreign body entrapped in the upper palpebral conjunctiva). **D,** Corneal abrasion or erosion (gross epithelial defect), usually just below the center of the cornea. **E,** Eyedrop-induced allergy or toxicity (staining on the inferonasal bulbar conjunctiva of the right eye), where drugs gravitate on their way to the lacrimal-outflow system.

or topical proparacaine. Any leak of aqueous humor onto the ocular surface can be detected by noting a trickle of clear, unstained fluid into the green tear film. Fluorescein is also used for measuring intraocular pressure with the Goldmann tonometer (see Chapter 12). Clinical Protocol 11-2 describes use of the dye for measuring tear film breakup time.

Flare and cell in the anterior chamber should be graded prior to instilling fluorescein, as the dye can enter the chamber and produce a green, false flare. Fluorescein is nonirritating and may be instilled without topical anesthetic.

Rose Bengal

Rose bengal is available as a 1% eyedrop or as an impregnated paper strip. The strip is used the same way the fluorescein strip is. Unlike fluorescein, rose bengal stains abnormal and devitalized epithelial cells. Therefore, it is useful in the evaluation of conditions such as dry eye, in which epithelial cells are present but abnormal. Rose bengal also stains mucus and keratin.

Rose bengal staining is best performed with diffuse slit-lamp illumination with the green (red-free) filter (see Figure 10-4). Stained areas are red with either green or white light. Rose bengal is somewhat irritating and should not be used without a topical anesthetic agent instilled first.

Lissamine Green

Lissamine green is available as a 1% solution or in impregnated paper strips. Like rose bengal it stains devitalized epithelial cells and so is helpful for evaluating dry eyes.

Abnormal cells stain green, and examination may be done with white or blue light. Lissamine green is less irritating than rose bengal.

Pitfalls and Pointers

* Resist any tendency to limit the anterior segment examination to a cursory scanning of the cornea and anterior chamber with only a single kind of illumination. Examine other important tissues (eg, eyelids and conjunctiva) and use various methods of illumination, as doing so can provide valuable information.

* It is often useful to examine the anterior segment (at least that portion posterior to the iris) after pupillary dilation. Otherwise, abnormalities of the lens, retrolental space, and anterior vitreous might be missed or inadequately evaluated.

Suggested Resources

Alward WLM, Longmuir RA. *Color Atlas of Gonioscopy.* 2nd ed. American Academy of Ophthalmology; 2008. (In addition, Dr. Alward created a website, www.gonioscopy.org, which uses videography to demonstrate gonioscopy technique, angle grading, and examples of diagnoses.)

Bacterial Keratitis [Preferred Practice Pattern]. American Academy of Ophthalmology; 2018. Accessed September 28, 2020. https://www.aao.org/preferred-practice-pattern/bacterial-keratitis-ppp-2018

Blepharitis [Preferred Practice Pattern]. American Academy of Ophthalmology; 2018. Accessed September 28, 2020. https://www.aao.org/preferred-practice-pattern/blepharitis-ppp-2018

Conjunctivitis [Preferred Practice Pattern]. American Academy of Ophthalmology; 2018. Accessed September 28, 2020. https://www.aao.org/preferred-practice-pattern/conjunctivitis-ppp-2018

Dry Eye Syndrome [Preferred Practice Pattern]. American Academy of Ophthalmology; 2018. Accessed September 28, 2020. https://www.aao.org/preferred-practice-pattern/dry-eye-syndrome-ppp-2018

External Disease and Cornea. Basic and Clinical Science Course, Section 8. American Academy of Ophthalmology; published annually.

Glaucoma. Basic and Clinical Science Course, Section 10. American Academy of Ophthalmology; published annually.

Lens and Cataract. Basic and Clinical Science Course, Section 11. American Academy of Ophthalmology; published annually.

Orbit, Eyelids, and Lacrimal System. Basic and Clinical Science Course, Section 7. American Academy of Ophthalmology; published annually.

CLINICAL PROTOCOL 11-1

Sweeping the Conjunctival Sac for Foreign Bodies

1. With the patient seated or lying supine, instill a few eyedrops of topical anesthetic. If the patient is seated, the neck should be extended, with the back of the head on a headrest.
2. Separate the eyelids with your thumb and index finger of 1 hand or with an eyelid speculum.
3. Moisten a cotton swab with topical anesthetic, sterile saline solution, or artificial tears. A dry swab is apt to leave cotton fibers on the eye.
4. Wipe away any visible strands of mucus by twirling the swab so as to allow the mucus to coil around it; the strands will adhere readily to the swab but will often break if an attempt is made merely to pull them away from the eye. The strands are most often found at the inner or outer canthal areas or in the lower fornix.
5. Sweep the cotton swab across the upper and lower conjunctival fornices to remove any remaining debris, everting the superior eyelid if necessary.
6. As an additional measure, the conjunctival sac may be irrigated with any sterile, isotonic solution.

CLINICAL PROTOCOL 11-2

Measuring Tear Film Breakup Time

1. Stain the patient's tear film by touching a moistened, fluorescein-impregnated paper strip to the lower palpebral conjunctiva. Fluorescein eyedrops are not used because they add volume to the tear film.
2. Position the patient at the slit lamp and adjust the instrument for diffuse illumination through the cobalt-blue filter.
3. Ask the patient to look straight ahead and to blink.
4. While observing the eye through the slit-lamp oculars, count to yourself the number of seconds that elapse between the blink and the appearance of the first dry spot. The dry spot will appear blue-black (because of the dark blue illumination) when the green-stained tear film pulls away from the area of breakup.
5. Repeat the test at least once more for each eye, because a single measurement might be falsely high or low. The normal tear breakup time (TBUT) is at least 10 seconds.

CLINICAL PROTOCOL 11-3

Evaluating Flare and Cell

1. With the room lights darkened, set the slit lamp for a 1×1-mm beam with illumination at full brightness.

2. Situate the patient comfortably at the slit lamp and direct the beam at an angle of 45°–60° onto the midperipheral temporal cornea and the nasal iris.

3. Use the dark pupil as background for viewing, and grade the intensity of gray-white flare (see Table 11-1). High magnification (16× or above) should be used for evaluation.

4. Without changing the slit-lamp settings, examine for the presence of cells (white dots that rise and fall in the anterior chamber) and grade the presence of cells (see Table 11-2).

CLINICAL PROTOCOL 11-4

Performing Gonioscopy

1. Instill topical anesthetic into the patient's eyes.

2. Assume standard patient and examiner positions at the slit-lamp biomicroscope (see Chapter 10).

3. Set the slit-lamp magnification to 10×.

4. If you are using a Goldmann 3-mirror lens, put in the concave part of the goniolens a small amount of gonioscopy gel, such as methylcellulose, and take care to avoid creating any air bubbles, which interfere with good visualization. Make a habit of storing the bottle of gel upside down so air bubbles do not accumulate near the bottle's tip. Gonioscopy gel is not necessary with use of a Zeiss 4-mirror goniolens.

5. Instruct the patient to look up. Spread the patient's eyelids apart with your thumb and forefinger (see Figure 1 in Clinical Protocol 13-4).

6. Place the 4-mirror lens on the eye and stabilize it. The right hand should be used to hold the mirror for the right eye and the left hand for the left. Instruct the patient to look ahead (see Figure 2 in Clinical Protocol 13-4).

7. Instruct the patient to continue to look straight ahead. Release the patient's eyelids, allowing the goniolens to hold the eyelids apart. Switch hands, if necessary, to hold the contact lens in your hand closer to the eye being examined (eg, your left hand for the patient's right eye), so that your arm does not interfere with use of the slit lamp.

8. Use the joystick to focus the slit lamp toward the patient and direct a broad, dim beam onto the semilunar-shaped mirror of the Zeiss or Goldmann goniolens or directly into the Koeppe goniolens.

    a. Remember that with a Goldmann or Zeiss lens you are viewing the chamber angle by means of a mirror, so you are seeing the inferior angle if, for example, the mirror is at the 12 o'clock position, and you are viewing the 10 o'clock angle if the mirror is at the 4 o'clock position. To see all areas of the angle, simply rotate the goniolens on the ocular surface.

    b. First obtain an overview of the angle with the broad, dim beam. Ascertain the most posterior angle structure visible without tilting the goniolens; this affords an idea of whether the angle is narrow, as some more posterior structures might be seen by tilting, or pushing on, the goniolens.

9. If you are having difficulty locating Schwalbe line, narrow the beam to an optical section (medium brightness). The thin beam produces 2 curvilinear lines that represent the anterior and posterior surfaces of the cornea; Schwalbe line is located where the 2 corneal lines of light meet at the anterior aspect of the anterior chamber angle.

10. Grade the width of the angle (see Table 11-3 and Figures 11-58 and 11-59). Remove the goniolens from the patient's eye and record the angle width in the patient's record. Record also any other notable features of the angle (eg, pigment, synechiae, neovascularization). A simple diagram in the patient's record is useful if the angle is not uniform; draw a circle and write down the grade of angle width at the 12-, 3-, 6-, and 9 o'clock positions.

11. Repeat steps 2–10 for the other eye.

12. After the examination of both eyes is complete, clean the goniolens with alcohol.

12 Tonometry

▶ *This chapter includes related videos, which can be accessed by scanning the QR codes provided in the text or going to aao.org/PracticalOphthalmologyvideo.*

Tonometry is the measurement of intraocular pressure (IOP). It is performed as part of a thorough ocular examination to help detect ocular hypertension and glaucoma and to diagnose ocular hypotony (low IOP) in conditions such as iritis, retinal detachment, postoperative wound leaks, and occult perforations of the globe. When measuring IOP, one must consider the effect of central corneal thickness (CCT) on that measurement.

This chapter discusses measurement conventions and population means associated with IOP and CCT. In addition, it presents the variety of devices and methods currently available for measuring IOP and provides instruction for doing so.

IOP Measurement Conventions and Population Means

By convention, IOP is measured in millimeters of mercury (mm Hg). Intraocular pressure, like many biologic parameters, varies in the population as a whole. In large epidemiologic studies, mean IOP is 16 mm Hg, with a standard deviation of 3 mm Hg. Although there is no strict cutoff between normal and abnormal intraocular pressures, most people have IOPs between 10 and 21 mm Hg. Variables such as the time of day, age, and genetic factors influence IOP.

Types of Tonometers

Several types of ophthalmic instruments are used to perform tonometry. The instruments can be categorized into 2 groups based on the way they determine IOP. *Applanation tonometers* measure the force needed to flatten, or applanate, a small area of the central cornea. The greater the force needed to applanate a known area of the cornea, the higher the IOP. Applanation tonometers are the most commonly used tonometers in clinical practice. *Indentation tonometers* measure the amount of indentation of the cornea produced by a known weight. *Rebound tonometers* (iCare) measure IOP with a probe that lightly bounces against the cornea; this allows for measurement of the rebound motion inside the eye. *Rebound tonometers* are portable and do not require corneal anesthesia. The *Dynamic Contour Tonometer* (PASCAL) measures IOP independent of corneal thickness and other biomechanical properties of the cornea; a sensor measures changes in electrical resistance to calculate a change in intraocular pressure during a period of approximately 5–8 seconds.

Applanation Tonometers

Some of the most common types of applanation tonometers and their characteristics are listed below.

- The *Goldmann applanation tonometer* is the most common tonometer. Usually mounted on the standard slit-lamp biomicroscope, it measures the IOP of a seated patient with high accuracy in most clinical situations. Measurements are less precise for edematous and scarred corneas.

- The *Perkins tonometer* is a handheld, portable applanating device. The technique for its use, its mechanism of action, and its relative accuracy are similar to those of the slit lamp–mounted Goldmann tonometer, and it can be used with either a seated or supine patient. Its portability makes this device useful at the bedside and in the operating room. Because it is not mounted to a stable device, however, the steadiness of both the patient and the examiner are harder to control. Nevertheless, with some practice, the Perkins tonometer is a useful instrument.

- The *pneumatic tonometer,* or *pneumatonometer,* is an electronic pressure-sensing device that consists of a gas-filled chamber covered with a Silastic diaphragm. The gas in the chamber escapes through an exhaust vent. As the diaphragm touches the cornea, the gas vent is reduced in size and the pressure in the chamber rises. The instrument supplies a measurement reading directly in mm Hg. The pneumatic tonometer is portable, can be used with a seated or supine patient, and is especially useful in the presence of corneal scars or corneal edema.

- The *Tono-Pen applanation tonometer* (Reichert Technologies), like many similar portable electronic applanating devices, contains a strain gauge and produces an electrical signal as the tip of the instrument applanates the cornea. This device uses disposable sterile rubber covers for the applanating tip, can be used with a seated or supine patient, and is useful in the presence of corneal scars or edema. Some studies have found that the instrument underestimates IOP in the higher ranges. Although use of the Tono-Pen is easier to learn than Goldmann tonometry, its accuracy is not quite as high.

- The *noncontact (air-puff) tonometer* determines IOP by measuring the time necessary for a given force of air to flatten a given area of the cornea. Because the instrument does not come in contact with the patient's cornea, no anesthetic eyedrops are needed. Readings obtained with these instruments correlate well with those obtained by Goldmann applanation tonometry except at high and low extremes of intraocular pressure. The air-puff tonometer is more commonly used in optometric settings.

Indentation Tonometers

The *Schiøtz tonometer* is an inexpensive, portable, and easy-to-use instrument. The patient must be supine for Schiøtz indentation tonometry, and a conversion table is required to interpret the reading on the tonometer scale. A drawback of this technique is that it assumes that the patient's scleral rigidity is normal and that the corneal curvature approaches that of a standard, which limits accuracy in conditions such as high myopia, prior ocular surgery, and corneal edema. Furthermore, the accuracy of Schiøtz indentation tonometry can be reduced by incorrect technique, inadequate cleaning (the instrument is difficult to clean both adequately and quickly), and improper calibration. The application of a relatively heavy weight to the eye also causes a rise in IOP. Because of a number of practical and theoretical problems, the Schiøtz tonometer is now used much less frequently than in past years.

Although not a device in the usual sense, the examiner's fingertips may be used to indent the globe and roughly estimate intraocular pressure. This is called *tactile tension*. Estimating IOP by digital pressure on the globe may be used with uncooperative patients or in the absence of instrumentation, but it can sometimes be inaccurate even in very experienced hands. In general, digital estimation of IOP is useful only for detecting large differences between a patient's eyes.

Goldmann Applanation Tonometry

The Goldmann applanation tonometer consists of 4 principal operative parts, described below and illustrated in Figure 12-1.

- The tonometer tip, the part of the instrument that comes in contact with the patient's cornea, contains a *biprism* (2 beam-splitting prisms) that converts a circular area of contact between the tonometer tip and the patient's cornea into 2 semicircles.

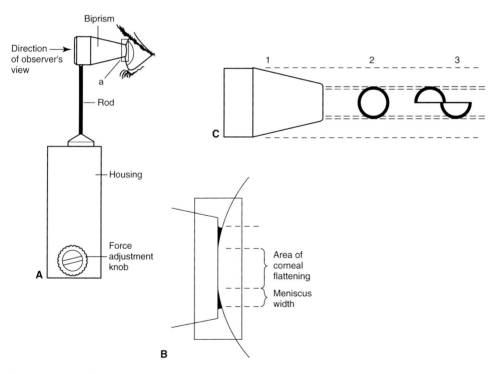

Figure 12-1 Goldmann applanation tonometer and principles of use. **A,** Main features of the instrument, shown in contact with the patient's cornea. **B,** Enlarged area from part A shows tear-film meniscus created by contact between the biprism and cornea. **C,** The view through the biprism (1) reveals circular meniscus (2), which is converted by prisms into 2 semicircles (3). (Redrawn, with permission, from Shields MB, *Textbook of Glaucoma,* 3rd ed. Williams & Wilkins; 1992.)

- A metal rod connects the tonometer tip to the instrument's housing.

- The tonometer housing contains a mechanism that can deliver a measured force, controlled by the force adjustment knob on the housing, to the tonometer tip.

- The force adjustment knob on the housing is used to vary the amount of force needed to applanate the cornea. The force (in dynes) needed to align the semicircles properly can be measured with great accuracy. This end point corresponds to a circular applanated area of the cornea with a diameter of 3.06 mm. The scale reading on the knob is multiplied by 10 to express IOP in mm Hg.

Clinical Protocol 12-1 provides instructions for measuring intraocular pressure with the Goldmann applanation tonometer.

Disinfection of the Applanating Tip

Disinfecting the applanating tonometer tip is critical to prevent the inadvertent spread of ocular pathogens such as adenovirus and herpes simplex virus type 1. Disinfection also eliminates the potential spread of other pathogens, such as hepatitis B and human immunodeficiency virus (HIV). Clinical Protocol 12-2 provides specific instructions for disinfecting the applanating tonometer tip.

Corneal Pachymetry

Corneal pachymetry is the measurement of corneal thickness. It has been used in the evaluation of corneal thickness abnormalities, including thinning disorders such as keratoconus and thickening disorders such as Fuchs endothelial dystrophy. More recently it has been recognized as an important factor in glaucoma management in corneas that may otherwise be without pathology.

There are 2 main methods of pachymetry: optical and ultrasonic. Optical methods of pachymetry use light waves to determine corneal thickness and are advantageous in that they do not require corneal contact. Ultrasonic techniques use sound waves to determine corneal thickness via a transducer in a probe tip that touches the cornea. Currently, ultrasonic pachymetry, also referred to as ultrasound pachymetry, is considered the gold standard, as it has been shown to be more accurate with significantly less variability than optical methods. It also has the advantage of greater portability and ease of use, and has thus become the predominant method of determining corneal thickness. Clinical Protocol 12-3 provides instructions for performing corneal pachymetry.

Corneal thickness varies according to location, and it is commonly measured in microns (µm). The cornea is thickest peripherally and thinnest centrally. It is central corneal thickness (CCT) that has the greatest application for glaucoma management, and it is this value that will be discussed at length here. Population studies have shown a wide range of normal, with mean values for CCT between 537 and 554 µm.

Because of its effect on IOP measurement, pachymetry as a means of measuring CCT is an important component of the ocular examination in patients with ocular hypertension and glaucoma. Tonometry is affected by CCT with all modern methods for IOP measurement, including the Goldmann tonometer, Perkins tonometer, pneumatonometer, Tono-Pen, and the noncontact tonometer. The gold standard for measuring

IOP is the Goldmann tonometer. In designing his applanation tonometer, Goldmann assumed that the average corneal thickness was 520 µm. As stated above, however, CCT varies considerably even among normal corneas. Since applanation tonometry estimates IOP by the amount of force it takes to flatten the central cornea, a deviation from 520 µm may affect the accuracy of the measurement. A high CCT may give an artificially high IOP reading, and a lower CCT may give an artificially low IOP reading, in the context of a normal physiologic cornea.

Several correction factors have been suggested for the effect of CCT on IOP measurement. Some have suggested 0.5 mm Hg correction for every 10 µm difference from 542 µm. Others recommend a correction of 3 mm Hg for every 50 µm of difference from 550 µm. But the relationship between CCT and IOP is not linear, and such correction factors are only rough estimates at best. In addition, the biomechanical properties of corneas—the relative stiffness or pliability (corneal hysteresis)—can vary among individuals and affect IOP measurement. Recent studies show that corneal hysteresis may be an independent risk factor for progression of glaucoma. There is currently no validated correction factor for the effect of CCT on IOP measurement, and any correction should be used with caution and in the context of the overall clinical picture.

CCT is important to take into account in a general sense, however. For example, IOP may be underestimated in the patient who has a very low CCT measurement, progressive optic nerve damage from glaucoma, and IOP that appears to be reasonably well controlled; the patient may indeed benefit from lowering of their IOP. Conversely, in an ocular hypertensive patient with a very high CCT reading, the high IOP may actually be lower than what is measured, and the patient can be considered at lower risk for developing glaucoma than if the CCT reading were lower. It has been estimated that 30%–57% of elevated IOP in ocular hypertensive patients may actually be artifacts.

The Ocular Hypertension Treatment Study (OHTS) found CCT to be a strong independent predictive factor for the development of glaucoma in ocular hypertensive patients. In this population, patients with CCT of less than 555 µm had a significantly greater risk of developing primary open angle glaucoma than those with higher readings. CCT is thus now considered an essential part of the evaluation of ocular hypertensive patients to establish their risk for developing glaucoma.

Pitfalls and Pointers

- Prolonged gonioscopy can alter IOP; during the comprehensive ocular examination, tonometry should precede gonioscopy.

- If you are using your fingers to hold a patient's eyelids open during tonometry, avoid exerting pressure on the globe, which can increase IOP and lead to a falsely high measurement.

- Whenever possible, avoid performing tonometry on patients with infected eyes (or use a Tono-Pen with disposable covers).

- Try to be brief and precise in tonometric testing; excessive repositioning of the tonometer on the patient's cornea can disrupt the corneal epithelium and result in an abrasion.

- A patient's tight collar or breath holding can sometimes falsely elevate the IOP; be sure that your patients loosen any clothing that is restrictive at the neck before they undergo tonometry, and instruct them to avoid holding their breath during IOP measurement.

- The accuracy of Goldmann applanation tonometry is limited in patients with corneas that are irregular (such as in patients with keratoconus), scarred from trauma, or edematous. The pneumatic tonometer and the Tono-Pen are generally considered more accurate in these clinical situations.

- Central corneal pachymetry should be performed in patients with ocular hypertension and glaucoma because IOP readings are affected by the patient's central corneal thickness. A patient's actual IOP is underestimated by applanation tonometry when the central cornea is thin (eg, after refractive surgery); applanation tonometry overestimates the actual IOP in patients with thicker corneas.

Suggested Resources

Allingham RR, Damji KF, Freedman S, Moroi SE, Rhee D, Shields MB, eds. The glaucoma suspect: when to treat? In: *Shields' Textbook of Glaucoma*, 6th ed. Lippincott Williams & Wilkins; 2011:168–175.

Glaucoma. Basic and Clinical Science Course, Section 10. American Academy of Ophthalmology; published annually.

Junk AK, Chen PP, Lin SC, et al. Disinfection of tonometers. A report by the American Academy of Ophthalmology. *Ophthalmology.* 2017;124:1867–1875.

Kass MA, Heuer DK, Higginbotham EJ, et al. The Ocular Hypertension Treatment Study: a randomized trial determines that topical ocular hypotensive medication delays or prevents the onset of primary open-angle glaucoma. *Arch Ophthalmol.* 2002;120:701–713.

Primary Angle Closure [Preferred Practice Pattern]. American Academy of Ophthalmology; 2015. Accessed September 27, 2020. https://www.aao.org/preferred -practice-pattern/primary-angle-closure-ppp-2015

Primary Open-Angle Glaucoma [Preferred Practice Pattern]. American Academy of Ophthalmology; 2015. Accessed September 27, 2020. https://www.aao.org /preferred-practice-pattern/primary-open-angle-glaucoma-ppp-2015

Primary Open-Angle Glaucoma Suspect [Preferred Practice Pattern]. American Academy of Ophthalmology; 2015. Accessed September 27, 2020. https://www.aao .org/preferred-practice-pattern/primary-open-angle-glaucoma-suspect-ppp-2015

CLINICAL PROTOCOL 12-1

Performing Goldmann Applanation Tonometry

1. Insert a clean tonometer tip in the biprism holder. The 180° marking on the tonometer tip should be aligned with the white line on the biprism holder.

2. Instill a topical anesthetic eyedrop and fluorescein dye into each of the patient's eyes. Many clinics use a single solution that contains both the anesthetic and the dye (Fluress; Akorn, Inc.) for this test.

3. Seat the patient at the slit-lamp biomicroscope with the patient's forehead firmly against the headrest and chin comfortably on the chin rest. The patient's eye should be aligned with the black band on the headrest column. Instruct the patient to look straight ahead and to open the eyelids widely. The examiner should be seated facing the patient, behind the slit-lamp oculars. If a patient has a larger body habitus or otherwise cannot bring their forehead and chin to the proper position, you can consider having them stand to position them properly at the slit lamp.

4. Position the cobalt filter in front of the slit-lamp illumination device. The cobalt-blue light causes the fluorescein dye on the patient's eye to fluoresce a bright yellow-green.

5. Set the magnification of the slit lamp at low power, with the light beam at high intensity and shining on the tonometer tip at a wide angle (about 60°).

6. Looking from the side, use the slit-lamp control handle to align the tonometer tip with the patient's right cornea. Adjust the numbers on the tonometer force adjustment knob to read anywhere between 1 and 2 (10 and 20 mm Hg).

7. Instruct the patient to focus on your right ear, blink once (to spread the fluorescein dye), and then to try to avoid blinking, squeezing, or holding their breath. If it is necessary to hold the patient's eyelids open, secure them against the bony orbit; do not apply pressure to the globe.

8. Use the slit-lamp control handle to gently move the biprism forward until it just touches the cornea. Look through the slit-lamp oculars to confirm that the biprism has just touched the cornea: the spot of fluorescein will break into 2 semicircles, 1 above and 1 below a horizontal line. Raise and lower the slit-lamp biomicroscope with the control handle until the semicircles are equal in size. The semicircles can be viewed monocularly through only 1 of the slit-lamp oculars; in most slit lamps the semicircles are viewed through the left ocular.

   If the patient has a large amount of corneal astigmatism, the semicircles seen by the examiner through the instrument ocular will look elliptical rather than circular. An error will be introduced into the pressure determination. In this situation, rotate the tonometer tip so that the dividing line between the semicircles is 45° to the major axis of the ellipse.

9. Slowly and gently turn the force adjustment knob in the direction required to move the semicircles until their inner edges just touch and do not overlap (Figure 1A).

A   B   C

Figure 1 Adjustments for monocular view of fluorescein spots through the slit-lamp oculars. **A,** Correct position. **B,** Incorrect position. **C,** Incorrect position.

    a. If the semicircles are separated, as in Figure 1B, the pressure reading will be too low; if the semicircles overlap, as in Figure 1C, the pressure reading will be too high.

    b. If there is too much fluorescein in the eye or if the examiner is applying pressure to the globe while holding the patient's eye open, the semicircles will appear thick, and an inaccurate pressure reading will result. A small pulsatile motion of the semicircles might be apparent, synchronous with the patient's pulse.

10. With the slit-lamp control handle, pull the tonometer biprism away from the patient's eye. Note the reading on the numbered dial of the force adjustment knob. Multiply the number by 10 to obtain the intraocular pressure in mm Hg, and record the pressure in the patient's medical record.

11. Repeat the procedure for the left eye.

Video 1 demonstrates applanation tonometry.

 VIDEO 1 Applanation Tonometry
Courtesy of Lindreth G. DuBois, MEd, MMSc, CO, COMT.
Access all *Practical Ophthalmology* videos at aao.org /PracticalOphthalmologyvideo.

CLINICAL PROTOCOL 12-2

Disinfecting the Applanating Tip

1. Remove the tonometer tip from the holder after each use.

2. The best way to disinfect the tip of the tonometer is by soaking it in a 10% solution of sodium hypochlorite (household bleach) for no more than 5 minutes. Allowing the tip to soak longer may dissolve the glue and cause cracks.

3. Rinse the tonometer tip with water and dry it with tissue or gauze to remove residual disinfecting solution, which could damage the corneal epithelium. Check the tip for damage prior to reuse.

4. In patients with suspected prion disease, disposable tonometer covers or single-use tonometers should be used.

CLINICAL PROTOCOL 12-3

Performing Corneal Pachymetry

1. Disinfect the tip of the pachymeter probe with an alcohol swab and dry it with a tissue.
2. Instill an eyedrop of topical anesthetic into each of the patient's eyes.
3. Instruct the patient to look straight ahead and to open the eyelids widely.
4. Gently touch the center of the cornea with the probe tip, which should be oriented perpendicular to the cornea. The instrument will beep when a measurement has been registered.

Video 1 demonstrates corneal pachymetry.

VIDEO 1 Corneal Pachymetry
Courtesy of Lindreth G. DuBois, MEd, MMSc, CO, COMT.

13 Posterior Segment Examination

Examination of the posterior segment of the eye (structures posterior to the ciliary body and lens) is important in assessing overall ocular health and in diagnosing and monitoring specific optic nerve, retinal, and systemic disorders. Ophthalmoscopy, or fundoscopy, is the examination of the inner portion of the posterior segment of the eye, also known as the fundus, with the use of an instrument called an ophthalmoscope. The posterior segment can also be visualized with the slit-lamp biomicroscope, with the use of special lenses. Pharmacologic pupillary dilation is usually required to optimize the posterior segment examination.

This chapter introduces the anatomical features and landmarks of the posterior segment and the diverse instruments and methods used to examine them. Effective examination of the posterior segment requires considerable skill and experience. Although this chapter presents instruction in many specific aspects of ophthalmoscopy and indirect biomicroscopy, the ophthalmology resident best gains proficiency through hands-on practice and by carefully documenting and comparing examination findings with those of a more experienced ophthalmoscopist.

Anatomical Landmarks

The structures of the *ocular fundus* include the optic nerve, retina, retinal pigment epithelium, choroid, and sclera. The *posterior pole* is a roughly defined area that includes the optic disc and the macula (Figure 13-1).

The optic nerve exits the eye through the posterior sclera, with its center just above the horizontal meridian. The *optic disc,* or *optic nerve head,* is a slightly vertically elongated oval and is normally pink. The central depression of the normal optic disc is the physiologic *optic cup.* The dimensions of the optic disc are approximately 1.5 mm horizontally and 1.75 mm vertically, with slight differences depending on a person's sex and race. For purposes of estimating distances and measuring lesion sizes during ophthalmoscopy, the size of the optic disc (1 disc diameter = about 1.5 mm) can be used as a reference. The dimensions and relative location of a fundus lesion can then be estimated with use of disc diameters (DD) or disc areas (DA). Any optical effects that the patient's refractive error might cause will apply to both the fundus lesion and the optic disc.

The retinal nerve fiber layer (RNFL) contains ganglion cell axons that run toward the optic disc, with the temporal fibers following an arcuate course around the fovea. The RNFL is seen as bright striations and is most easily visible where it is thickest, at the vertical poles of the optic disc. While individual nerve fibers are too small to see by ophthalmoscopy, bundles of nerve fibers are normally visible at the inferotemporal and superotemporal arcades. Identification of focal RNFL bundle defects can be an important ophthalmoscopic finding; red-free illumination may be helpful in identifying subtle defects.

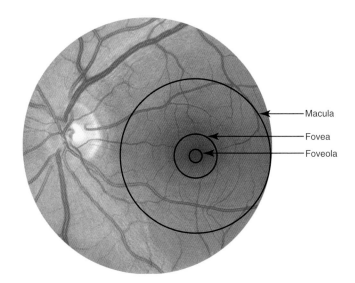

Figure 13-1 Features of the posterior pole.

The *macula* does not have sharp borders. It occupies the area enclosed by the major temporal blood vessels and is approximately 5.5 mm in diameter (about 18° in visual angle). The *fovea* is the central area of the macula, where there is progressive thinning of the inner retinal layers. It measures approximately 1.5 mm (5°) in diameter, centered 4 mm temporal and 0.8 mm inferior to the center of the optic disc. A circular or slightly oval light reflex around the fovea delineates where the retinal sloping begins. In the *foveal avascular zone,* which normally varies from 0.4–0.6 mm (400–600 μm), the retina is critically dependent on the choriocapillaris, the inner layer of the choroid, for its metabolic requirements. The *foveola,* the central foveal area that lies just within the capillary-free foveal avascular zone, contains a central point where light is reflected most brightly; this foveolar light reflex approximately corresponds to the anatomical spot called the *umbo.* Table 13-1 correlates the clinical appearance of these anatomical regions with their histologic features.

The *equator* is the largest circumference of latitude of the eye and is located midway between the corneal apex and the fovea. Because the equator is not an anatomical structure, its position is described by reference to other structures. Externally, the equator of a normal eye lies about 13 mm from the limbus, about twice as far as the rectus muscle insertions. These topographic zones are illustrated in Figure 13-2. Ophthalmoscopically, the equator is about 4 DD posterior to the *ora serrata,* the scalloped perimeter of the retina, and is just anterior to the ampullae of the vortex veins. The retina peripheral to the equator constitutes nearly one-third of the entire retinal surface area.

For diagnostic localization, the fundus can be conveniently divided into quadrants by horizontal and vertical lines centered on the fovea. The long ciliary vessels and nerves lie along the horizontal 3 o'clock (0°) and 9 o'clock (180°) lines and are visible between the equator and the *pars plana.* Short ciliary vessels and nerves may be visible near the superior and inferior vertical meridians. Figure 13-3 shows the principal landmarks of the posterior segment.

Table 13-1   Anatomical Features of the Posterior Pole

Term	Clinical Description	Histologic Definition
Macula	Ill-defined area about 5.5 mm in diameter, centered 4 mm temporal and 0.8 mm inferior to the center of the optic disc; the zone within the temporal vascular arcades might be darker	Central retinal area containing 2 or more ganglion cell layers and xanthophyll pigment (hence, *macula lutea*, or "yellow spot"), often associated with heavily pigmented retinal pigment epithelial cells
Fovea centralis	A central retinal depression approximately 1.5 mm (1 disc diameter) in diameter, surrounded by an oval, halolike light reflex	A depression in the inner retina, where the retina slopes from its thickest dimension toward its thinnest
Foveola	The central foveal area approximately 0.35 mm in diameter that lies just within the angiographic capillary-free zone	The central floor of the fovea where the inner nuclear layer and the ganglion cell layer are absent and all photoreceptors are cones
Umbo	The point underneath the dotlike light reflex in the middle of the fovea	Small central concavity (clivus) of the foveola

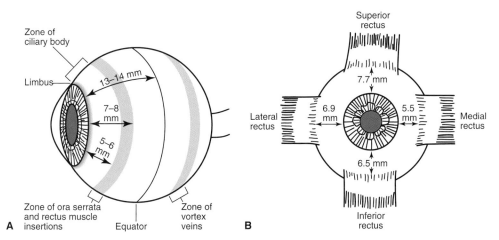

Figure 13-2   Topographic measurements of the globe. **A,** The sclera is divided according to the eye's inner structures into the zone of the ciliary body (5-6 mm from the limbus), the zone of the ora serrata and rectus muscle insertions (a band that extends 8 mm from the limbus), and the equator (about 13 mm from the limbus). The vortex veins exit the globe in various positions; the superior pair is usually 5-8 mm posterior to the equator at the 1 o'clock and 11 o'clock positions, and the inferior pair is 5-6 mm from the equator at the 5 o'clock and 7 o'clock positions. **B,** Although not exactly parallel to the limbus, the rectus muscle insertions form a spiral over the ora serrata; as measured from the limbus, the insertions are as follows: medial rectus, 5.5 mm; inferior rectus, 6.5 mm; lateral rectus, 6.9 mm; and superior rectus, 7.7 mm.

The *ocular media* include the cornea, aqueous humor, crystalline lens, and vitreous humor. The vitreous gel is not uniform and changes with aging. The central vitreous (Cloquet canal) is a semifluid funnel that gradually blends with an intermediate zone (Figure 13-4). The vitreous cortex can be optically denser. The vitreous base extends

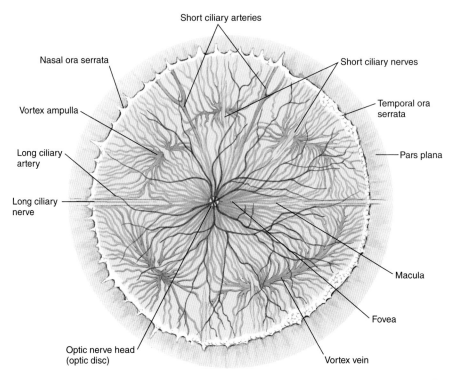

Figure 13-3 Landmarks of the normal posterior segment. (Adapted from Rutnin U, Schepens CL: Fundus appearance in normal eyes. *Am J Ophthalmol.* 1967;64[6]:840–852,1040–1078. Published with permission from Elsevier.

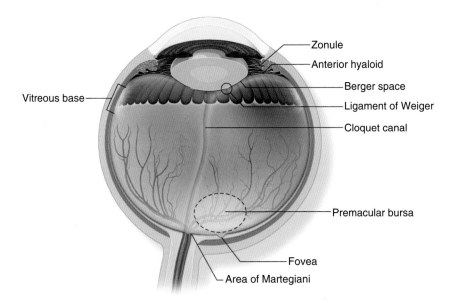

Figure 13-4 Cross-section of the eye with emphasis on the anatomical features of the vitreous. (Illustration by Mark M. Miller.)

on both sides of the ora serrata and is tightly adherent to the underlying retina and pars plana.

Pupillary Dilation

The pupils should be dilated for an adequate posterior segment examination. Visual acuity should be measured prior to pupillary dilation and exposure to the bright lights used for ophthalmoscopy, both of which can temporarily degrade vision. A combination of a sympathomimetic drug (eg, phenylephrine) and a parasympatholytic drug (eg, tropicamide) is preferred for pupillary dilation for ophthalmoscopy because of its rapid onset and short duration. Having the patient close both eyes for 1 minute after instillation can help slow nasolacrimal drainage and reduce systemic absorption. Systemic absorption of phenylephrine can elevate blood pressure, especially in patients with orthostatic hypotension (who have increased sensitivity to α-adrenergic agonists) or who are taking drugs that potentiate adrenergic effects (eg, reserpine, tricyclic antidepressants, cocaine, and monoamine oxidase inhibitors). The 2.5% concentration of phenylephrine is preferred over the stronger 10% concentration, which has been associated with angina, myocardial infarction, and stroke. Adequate dilation is achieved in about 20–45 minutes. Dilation might need to be avoided in a patient who has an iris-supported intraocular lens or a very shallow anterior chamber (to avoid inducing angle-closure glaucoma), or who is under observation by a neurologist or neurosurgeon (eg, for a head injury). Dilation may also be minimized and punctal occlusion used for female patients who are pregnant or lactating.

The dilated pupil gradually returns to normal reactivity after 4–8 hours. Dapiprazole 0.5% (an α-adrenergic antagonist) has been used to reverse mydriasis partially, but it often causes mild conjunctival hyperemia and is no longer available in the United States. Pilocarpine 1% (a cholinergic agonist) is not typically used for pupillary reconstriction or reversal of cycloplegia after diagnostic dilation because of potential increased risk of rhegmatogenous retinal detachment and ciliary pain.

Infants, especially when premature, are more susceptible to the adverse effects of dilating agents. Phenylephrine 10% should never be used because of the potential to induce hypertension. Concentrations of cyclopentolate greater than 0.5% may lead to feeding intolerance.

Table 13-2 lists commonly used dilating drugs according to their purpose. Table 15.4 in Chapter 15 compares the most commonly used dilating agents. Table 13-3 lists a suggested cycloplegic protocol for infants and children.

Table 13-2   Agents for Pupillary Dilation

Reason for Use	Usual Drugs
Cycloplegic refraction	Cyclopentolate 0.5% or 1%, or cyclopentolate 0.2% and phenylephrine 1% combination
Ophthalmoscopy	Phenylephrine 2.5% in combination with either tropicamide 1% or cyclopentolate 0.5%
Preoperative dilation	Cyclopentolate 1% and phenylephrine 2.5% combination
Therapeutic dilation	Scopolamine 0.25%, or homatropine 2% or 5%, or atropine 1%

Table 13-3   Cycloplegic Protocol for Infants and Children

Age	Iris Pigmentation	Eyedrops
Preterm	Light	Cyclopentolate 0.2% and phenylephrine 1% combination
	Dark	Add tropicamide 0.5%
3-12 months	Light	Cyclopentolate 0.5% and phenylephrine 2.5% combination
	Dark	Add tropicamide 1%
>12 months	Light	Cyclopentolate 1% and phenylephrine 2.5% combination
	Dark	Add tropicamide 1%

Instrumentation for Examination

Three instruments are available for examination of the posterior segment: the indirect ophthalmoscope, the slit-lamp biomicroscope, and the direct ophthalmoscope. All work best in a darkened room. Auxiliary handheld lenses are used with the indirect ophthalmoscope and slit-lamp biomicroscope in order to view the posterior segment. A comparison of properties and uses of all 3 instruments and any lenses used with them is presented in Table 13-4. The magnification and field of view vary among the instruments (Figure 13-5). For indirect ophthalmoscopy, the examiner's magnification is estimated by dividing the power of the patient's eye (about 60 D) by the power of the magnifying lens used (eg, with a +20 D handheld condensing lens used in indirect ophthalmoscopy, the magnification is 60/20 = 3×).

Indirect Ophthalmoscope

The indirect ophthalmoscope consists of a headset with a binocular viewing device that optically reduces the examiner's interpupillary distance and an adjustable lighting system wired to a transformer power source. Portable units with rechargeable power packs as well as spectacle-mounted instruments are available.

The indirect ophthalmoscope provides a stereoscopic, wide field of view (40°–50°), allows examination of the retinal periphery, and makes it possible to penetrate hazy media. The instrument can also be used as a magnifying loupe to achieve an erect real image by positioning the examiner's eyes about 10 inches from the patient and focusing the condensing lens on the anterior segment.

For indirect ophthalmoscopy, the examiner positions a convex, handheld magnifying ("condensing") lens close to the patient's eye at an arm's-length distance (Figure 13-6). The examiner tilts their head and adjusts the headset's light beam until an inverted, reversed, magnified image of the fundus is visible at the focal point of the condensing lens. Lenses commonly used in indirect ophthalmoscopy range from +14 D to +30 D and afford magnification between about 4× and 2×. Both +20 D and +28 D lenses are commonly used for routine examination.

Slit-Lamp Biomicroscope

Examination of the posterior segment can be performed on patients seated at the slit-lamp biomicroscope (see Chapter 10 for detailed information about this instrument). As with the indirect ophthalmoscope, the slit lamp affords the examiner stereoscopic

Table 13-4   Comparison of Instruments for Posterior Segment Examination

Technique	Magnification[a]	Field of View	Image	Principal Use
+14 D indirect ophthalmoscopy	4×	40°	Inverted and reversed (real)	Fundus lesion inspection
+20 D indirect ophthalmoscopy	3×	45°	Inverted and reversed (real)	Routine examination
+30 D indirect ophthalmoscopy	2×	50°	Inverted and reversed (real)	Routine examination
+78 D indirect slit-lamp biomicroscopy	10×	30°	Inverted and reversed (real)	Posterior pole and peripheral retinal exam
+90 D indirect slit-lamp biomicroscopy	7.5×	40°	Inverted and reversed (real)	Posterior pole and peripheral retinal exam
Goldmann fundus contact lens biomicroscopy	10×	20°	Erect (virtual)	Optic disc and macula inspection
Direct ophthalmoscopy	15×	5°	Erect (virtual)	Optic disc inspection
Digital Fundus camera	2.5×	30° or 45°	Erect (virtual)	Photodocumentation

[a]Greater magnification is achievable with the slit-lamp biomicroscope and fundus camera.

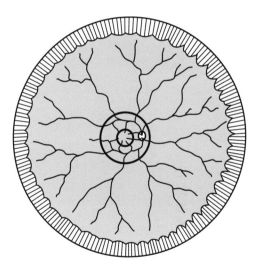

Figure 13-5   Field of view of the posterior segment with ophthalmoscopes and slit lamp with lenses. The outermost edge is the area seen with the indirect ophthalmoscope with a +20 D condensing lens. The inner circle is the area seen with the direct ophthalmoscope. The area that can be seen with the slit lamp and various lenses varies between these 2 dimensions.

vision. Handheld, noncontact, plus-diopter condensing lenses can be used to provide the biomicroscopist an inverted and reversed retinal image, a field of view ranging between 30° and 40°, and magnification between 7.5× and 10×. Slit-lamp examination with a high-plus lens is most useful for examining the optic disc and the macula.

Handheld lenses that are applied to the patient's anesthetized cornea are also used in conjunction with the slit-lamp biomicroscope. A handheld plano-concave fundus contact

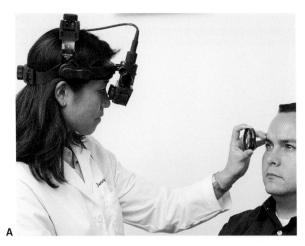

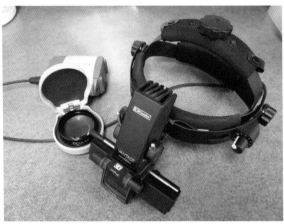

Figure 13-6 Use of the indirect ophthalmoscope. **A,** Examination with an indirect ophthalmoscope. **B,** Indirect ophthalmoscope: power transformer (back), handheld condensing lens and case (left), headset (right). (Courtesy of JoAnn A. Giaconi, MD.)

lens allows direct visualization of the posterior pole with a highly magnified upright image. This lens may be used to examine the microanatomy of the macula and optic disc owing to its excellent axial resolution, and in patients with limited pupillary dilation. Fundus contact lenses with tilted mirrors may be utilized to examine the equatorial and peripheral retina.

Direct Ophthalmoscope

The direct ophthalmoscope is a handheld instrument and is usually battery-powered. It consists of a handle and a head with a light source, a peephole with a range of built-in dial-up lenses and filters, and a reflecting device to aim light into the patient's eye.

The instrument is used to examine the fundus directly (Figure 13-7). It gives greater magnification (15×) than the indirect ophthalmoscope and provides an erect, virtual image of the retina. The field of view is only about 5°, and stereoscopic vision for the examiner is not possible. Approximately one-half of a watt of illumination is provided, several times less than that of the indirect ophthalmoscope and slit lamp. The direct ophthalmoscope is most useful for examining the optic nerve and blood vessels of the posterior pole.

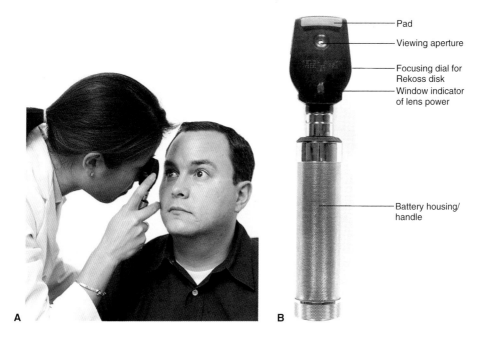

Pad

Viewing aperture

Focusing dial for Rekoss disk

Window indicator of lens power

Battery housing/handle

A   B

Figure 13-7   Use of the direct ophthalmoscope. **A,** Examination with a direct ophthalmoscope. **B,** Direct ophthalmoscope. The dial for selecting the light filter and pattern is on the side of the instrument that faces away in this photograph.

The PanOptic ophthalmoscope (Welch Allyn) provides a field of view (25°) that is 5 times larger than that of the standard direct ophthalmoscope as well as a 26% increase in magnification. It is easier to view the retina through small pupils with the PanOptic ophthalmoscope, and the working distance between practitioner and patient is increased when compared with the standard direct ophthalmoscope.

Indirect Ophthalmoscopy

The indirect ophthalmoscope is widely used for posterior segment examination because of its large field, depth of focus, stereopsis, good illumination, and ease of use with the scleral depressor (a device used to facilitate examination of the retinal periphery). Indirect ophthalmoscopy produces an inverted and reversed real image on the proximal side of a handheld condensing lens, onto which the examiner accommodates. The distance between the image and the observer depends on the examiner's refractive error and correction and on the refractive error of the patient.

Indirect ophthalmoscopy is possible to perform with the patient sitting upright in the examination chair. However, if the examination will take longer than a few minutes or when scleral depression is to be performed, it is easier with the patient supine. A fully reclined examination chair or a padded examination table should provide sufficient height and width for free access around the patient. The examination room should be dimly lit, and the ophthalmologist should be dark adapted.

Headset Adjustment

The indirect ophthalmoscope headset should be positioned comfortably on the examiner's head. The frame-and-prong buckles or adjustment knobs are set to allow most of the headset's weight to be supported by the top cross-strap rather than by the encircling band. The examiner should be able to use the frontalis muscle to raise and lower the headset slightly.

Eyepiece adjustment

The eyepieces should be situated as close as possible to the examiner's eyes, perpendicular to the pupillary plane, without touching the bridge of the nose. A hinged bracket permits the user to adjust the angle of the eyepiece-light housing and simultaneously shift it toward and away from the user's face. Proper positioning will give the housing a slight pantoscopic tilt. A loose eyepiece-light housing will swing freely against the examiner's face, indicating that the screws on the headset bracket must be tightened.

Some examiners do not wear their regular eyeglasses for indirect ophthalmoscopy, because the closer the eyepieces are situated to the examiner's eyes, the larger will be the field of view. A +2 D lens is usually supplied in each of the standard oculars to reduce the amount of accommodation needed to view the image in the condensing lens. For presbyopic examiners who might have trouble accommodating onto the fundus image at one-third meter (33 cm), an intermediate or near add will be needed. Myopic and hyperopic examiners should wear corrective lenses or contact the manufacturer to have the eyepiece power changed to match the spherical equivalent of one's spectacle prescription for an arm's-length distance.

Adjust the interpupillary distance of the oculars by shining the oblong light beam onto your thumb held upright on your outstretched arm. Close the left eye, and adjust the right eyepiece bar by sliding it in or out until the illuminated thumb is horizontally centered in the field of the right eye. Repeat this procedure for the other eyepiece. The examiner should now have a comfortable binocular view with the light horizontally centered at an arm's-length working distance.

Light beam adjustment

The light beam is aligned by using the knurled knob that tilts the reflecting mirror on the headset. With both eyes open, adjust the light beam vertically until the light occupies the upper half of the field of view for an arm's-length working distance. While looking through the eyepieces and the condensing lens, point the light beam onto the thumbnail when the knuckle is in the center of the field. A properly illuminated field will provide diffuse illumination of the upper half of the field, and the image of the bulb's filament should be diffused. In patients with poorly dilated pupils or those sensitive to bright lights, reducing the size of the light beam may improve visibility of the fundus and increase the patient's comfort.

The transformer's power is adjusted by incremental or continuous dialing, depending on the instrument. The 4-volt setting on the transformer is the most useful intensity. A lower setting (eg, 2.5 volts) might be needed for children and light-sensitive patients and for examinations longer than 15 minutes. A higher setting (eg, 6–15 volts) is used for penetrating hazy ocular media and for examining the peripheral fundus.

Limiting the duration of indirect ophthalmoscopy helps to minimize the subjective discomfort felt by the patient. A prolonged examination should use a reduced power setting of the headset light. Any risk of phototoxicity caused by indirect ophthalmoscopy is also minimized if the examiner avoids repeatedly shining the light onto the fovea.

Choosing and Positioning the Condensing Lens

A +20 D lens may be used for a general posterior segment examination with an indirect ophthalmoscope. Higher-powered aspheric lenses (eg, +28 D or +30 D) have less magnification but may be preferred when a wider field is helpful (eg, with large or diffuse retinal abnormalities), when the pupil does not dilate well, and when the examiner views the peripheral fundus through an oblique pupil. Lower-power lenses (eg, +14 D) provide more magnification but a narrower field of view and are reserved for examining the optic nerve and individual lesions. Lenses must be kept spotless and free of dust and finger smudges.

Grasp the edge of the indirect lens between the thumb and index finger, with the more convex side toward you (and the white or silver ring facing the patient). Some ophthalmoscopists will hold the lens in their nondominant hand to reserve their dominant hand for scleral depression and drawing the fundus record (see "Scleral Depression" and "The Fundus Record" later in this chapter). However, a beginning resident may experiment with either hand and use whichever is more comfortable. It may be advantageous to become comfortable holding the lens with either hand. The middle finger of the hand holding the lens may be used to open the upper or lower eyelid, and the thumb of the opposite hand can be used to hold the other eyelid open (Figure 13-8). Depending on where the examiner is standing, the hand holding the lens can be braced against the patient's upper or lower orbital rim to maintain the proper focal distance and to keep the image centered. Figure 13-9 provides instruction and practice in centering an image in a condensing lens. A +20 D condensing lens gives a 2-inch working distance for an emmetropic eye. Clinical Protocol 13-1 summarizes how to obtain a fundus image with the headset and lens.

Two distracting light reflections corresponding to the images of the ophthalmoscope's bulb on the front and back surfaces of the condensing lens are seen when the lens is held exactly perpendicular to the line of sight. Tilt the lens to spread these reflections apart. Some lenses have an antireflective coating to reduce these bothersome reflections.

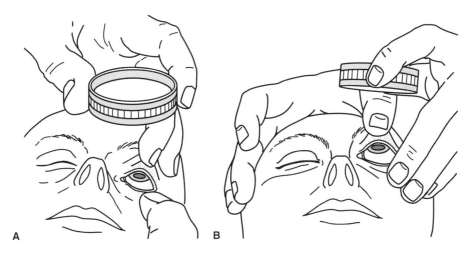

A   B

Figure 13-8 Techniques for holding the condensing lens during indirect ophthalmoscopy while holding the patient's eyelids open. **A,** Elevating the upper eyelid with the third finger of the hand holding the lens while retracting the lower eyelid with the free hand's thumb. **B,** Elevating the upper eyelid with the free hand's thumb while retracting the lower eyelid with the third finger of the hand holding the lens.

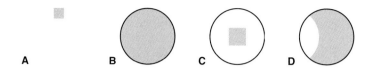

Figure 13-9   Practice and instruction in focusing the condensing lens for indirect ophthalmoscopy. **A,** A small square, such as this, is the target over which you should hold the lens. **B,** Center the square in the lens and move the lens toward or away from the page to make the entire image uniformly fill the lens, as in this example. **C,** If the image in the lens looks like this, you are too far from or too close to the square. **D,** If the image in the lens looks like this, you are too far sideways.

Changing Position to View Different Fundus Areas

Alignment

During indirect ophthalmoscopy, the examiner maintains a viewing axis through the condensing lens while pivoting around the patient's pupil to examine different portions of the fundus (Figure 13-10). Move your head and tilt the lens while using your rigid third finger as a fulcrum. Keeping the pupil centered in the condensing lens will maintain alignment of the light beam and the view returning to both of the examiner's eyes (Figure 13-11). Some examiners prefer to move their torsos and approach the patient from different directions and angles as opposed to examining each portion of the fundus by having the patient look in different directions. Examination of the equatorial and peripheral fundus might require changing the direction of the light beam, switching to a different condensing lens, or tilting the head (Figure 13-12).

Working distance

The ophthalmoscopic examination is performed at arm's length, normally with about 40–50 cm between the examiner's headset and the patient's eye. Difficulty seeing through a small pupil can be partially overcome by withdrawing to a greater examination distance or by using a higher-power lens.

The working distance between the examiner and the lens does not have to be fixed. The distance can be shortened (lens brought closer to examiner) for greater magnification of fundus details, although the field then becomes narrower and binocularity can be lost more easily. The examiner can shift the lens to estimate grossly the relative height of a lesion. Each 1 cm of up or down displacement needed to focus on the lesion's apex or pit is equivalent to about 1 mm of lesion elevation or excavation, respectively.

Sequence of the Examination

For patients who are about to undergo any type of fundus examination, avoid using any ointment or inducing corneal haze, such as by instilling certain topical anesthetics or applying diagnostic contact lenses. Ensure that the patient's pupils are well dilated, and instruct the patient to keep both eyes open. Warn the patient what to expect by explaining that a very bright light will be used, but that it will not be harmful. It is helpful to begin the examination by having the patient lie down in a relaxed position with the plane of the head exactly horizontal. This avoids your having to hold the lens out in front of you in a fatiguing position and facilitates movement around the patient's head to get optimal views. By convention, the right eye is examined first.

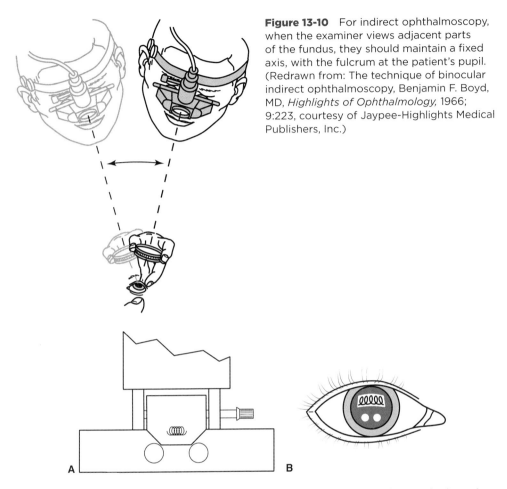

Figure 13-10   For indirect ophthalmoscopy, when the examiner views adjacent parts of the fundus, they should maintain a fixed axis, with the fulcrum at the patient's pupil. (Redrawn from: The technique of binocular indirect ophthalmoscopy, Benjamin F. Boyd, MD, *Highlights of Ophthalmology,* 1966; 9:223, courtesy of Jaypee-Highlights Medical Publishers, Inc.)

A   B

Figure 13-11   Indirect ophthalmoscopy. **A,** Indirect ophthalmoscope with the standard eyepiece oculars set 15 mm apart and the light bulb filament reflected in the tilted mirror. **B,** Examiner's view of the patient's dilated pupil, which shows the relative positions of the light entering the pupil superiorly and the binocular images produced by the light reflected off the fundus.

Many examiners begin indirect ophthalmoscopy without the condensing lens by quickly shining the light of the indirect ophthalmoscope into the patient's eye to get a red reflex in order to discern any changes in the anterior eye or media. The condensing lens is then brought into position (Clinical Protocol 13-1). With experience, the examiner automatically finds the proper spot for the lens. The beginner should hold the condensing lens close to the patient's eye and then withdraw it slowly until a focused image is seen. Keep in mind that the fundus image that the examiner sees is completely inverted; that is, it is upside down and reversed.

The examiner begins the examination of the fundus by identifying the optic disc, then shifting the viewing axis from 1 part of the fundus to another, keeping the axis centered at the patient's pupil. Rather than having the patient look in 1 direction and then observing this view of the fundus, the examiner should follow each meridian from the posterior pole to the periphery by changing the viewing axis. This enables each meridian to be examined completely, following retinal vessels from the optic disc to the equator.

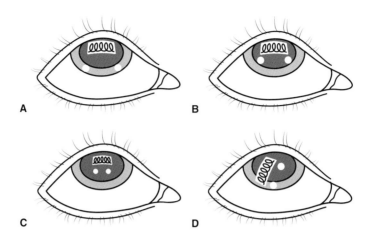

Figure 13-12 Indirect ophthalmoscopy in an eccentric gaze position. When the examiner views the rotated globe, the pupil appears elliptical rather than round, which reduces the effective pupil size. **A,** Problem viewing the superior periphery with the patient's eye in upgaze because the light and viewing axes are too far apart relative to the pupil. **B,** Redirecting the light beam brings it closer into alignment with the viewing axis. **C,** Switching to a higher-power condensing lens (eg, +30 D) reduces the image. **D,** If maneuvers B and C do not work, tilting your head so that light enters a portion of the patient's pupil will permit viewing by 1 eye.

Smooth body–lens coordination will help obtain a continuous, sweeping picture of an entire meridian of the fundus, from the optic disc to the periphery. The superior or nasal periphery is often examined before the inferior and temporal fundus, because the patient experiences less photophobia in the former regions.

When examining the peripheral fundus, the examiner must change position to see through the tilted pupil. Moving your body around the patient's head or tilting your head will permit the light beam to enter and allow you to see the fundus. If only 1 eye's visual axis is aligned with the reflected image, stereoscopic viewing will not be possible.

After each eye has been examined, suspected abnormalities such as optic disc cupping or pallor are evaluated by rapidly alternating views of the patient's eyes with the indirect ophthalmoscope to compare optic nerves and other fundus details. Finally, scleral depression is performed to examine the peripheral fundus and ora serrata of each eye.

Scleral Depression

Scleral depression, or indentation, is done to examine the area between the equator of the fundus (14 mm from the limbus) and the ora serrata (8 mm from the limbus). Scleral depression brings the region around the ora serrata into view, away from the optical distortions produced by the edges of the condensing lens.

A scleral depressor is used for the examination (Figure 13-13). A commonly used type of scleral depressor, made of metal, consists of a thimblelike section with a short, curved stem attached to the closed cap of the thimble; the stem ends in a T-shaped nib (the depressor tip). This type of depressor can be worn over the index or middle finger of the depressing hand, thereby freeing the fingers to help keep the patient's eyelids open. This depressor can also be held between the thumb and the index and middle fingers. The pencil depressor, another type of instrument also made of metal, has a long, slim handle with a T-shaped or olive-shaped knob on its end. The long handle is grasped, as would

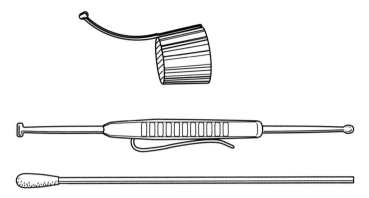

Figure 13-13 Instruments for scleral depression (top to bottom): thimble scleral depressor; pencil-type depressor; cotton-tipped applicator.

be a pencil, between the thumb and first 2 fingers of the hand not holding the condensing lens. This type of depressor allows ready alignment of the instrument with the viewing axis. A cotton-tipped applicator may also be used in a similar way.

To perform scleral depression, the tip of the scleral depressor is placed on the eyelid just past the tarsus, and the examiner applies gentle pressure to indent the sclera. The amount of pressure on the depressor should not exceed that used for tactile tonometry. Clinical Protocol 13-2 includes instructions for examining the posterior segment with scleral depression.

Scleral depression can be uncomfortable for the patient, and some patients even find the procedure painful, particularly if the examiner does not use careful and responsive movements. Patient cooperation can be encouraged by gradual advancement to the limit of the patient's tolerance. Be especially careful not to allow the depressor tip to slip off the eyelids and onto the cornea.

Sequence of scleral depression

Because the ora serrata is most easily visualized superonasally, this area is often examined first in a circumferential sequence. To begin scleral depression, the examiner stands to the right of the patient. The patient is asked to look inferotemporally. The depressor is applied at the upper tarsal margin of the inner portion of the upper eyelid. The patient is then asked to look straight ahead. As the upper eyelid moves up, the instrument's tip is slid along the globe. The examiner then tilts their head to direct the headset's light beam into the patient's pupil, and the left hand brings the condensing lens into position, which enables the examiner to observe the superonasal equatorial fundus. Gentle pressure is then exerted with the scleral depressor. The indented fundus will be seen on the side of the inverted image opposite the scleral depressor, and the condensing lens is brought slightly closer to the examiner to focus on this mound. The patient is then instructed to look superonasally, and the examiner's fingers help keep the patient's eyelids open. The instrument's tip is then slid anteriorly until the superonasal ora serrata is seen.

This entire sequence is repeated in all principal meridians, with the examiner's visual axis and the scleral depressor always kept in alignment. This entails moving around the patient's head and instructing the patient to look in the appropriate direction each

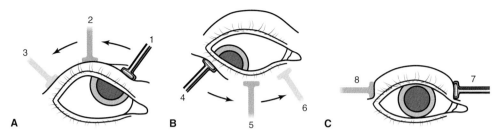

Figure 13-14 Sequence of circumferential scleral indentation through upper and lower eyelids. **A,** Examination of superior periphery. The depressor tip is first placed superonasally (1), then moved superiorly (2) and superotemporally (3). **B,** Examination of inferior periphery. The depressor tip is placed inferotemporally (4), then moved inferiorly (5) and inferonasally (6). **C,** Examination of the periphery in the horizontal meridians by placement of the depressor tip nasally (7) then temporally (8).

time a new section is examined. After you examine the superonasal ora serrata, lift and reposition the depressor superiorly, superotemporally, inferotemporally, inferiorly, and inferonasally to see the entire ora serrata and the posterior one-third of the pars plana (Figure 13-14). The nasal and temporal horizontal meridians are usually examined last because they are often the hardest to examine for the beginning ophthalmologist.

Check with the patient periodically about discomfort. A topical anesthetic eyedrop is used if it becomes necessary to place the depressor directly onto the globe.

Having achieved a circumferential view of the ora serrata and the peripheral fundus, any fundus lesion is reexamined. The examiner locates the lesion on the mound produced by scleral depression and rolls the lesion over the indentation by moving the depressor with fine anteroposterior and sideways movements. Changing the angle of observation of a lesion on the fundus mound will allow the examiner to determine the lesion's relative elevation or depression and will highlight its margins.

Tips on scleral depression

- If the area of indentation cannot be seen, resist the temptation to press harder; instead, move the depressor gently into the line of sight, hugging the border of the tarsus.

- Release the pressure on the depressor if the patient begins to squeeze the eyes forcibly.

- Because the pupil appears oval when you are viewing the retinal periphery, you might have to tilt your head slightly to keep both of your eyes focused on the fundus image. Movement of the lens just off direct alignment achieves a prismatic effect that can help you get a more peripheral view.

- At each location, first hold the depressor stationary by pressing lightly onto the globe, indenting it about 2.5 mm. Then shift the depressor's tip laterally (by half its diameter) and anteroposteriorly. The rolling mound produced by these slight movements can bring out details of fundus lesions and will enhance the contrast around a retinal break.

- The mound produced by scleral depression should be kept in view at all times. Slight movements of the depressor can cause the indented image to disappear from view. To avoid this, always move the depressor in the direction opposite the direction you want the visibly indented area to go, whether laterally, anteroposteriorly, or obliquely. The axis of observation might also have to shift, in the same direction that the examiner wants the visibly indented area to go. These lateral movements maintain a collinear relationship between the eyepieces of the ophthalmoscope, the condensing lens, and the depressor tip; the pupil is their pivot point.

Posterior Segment Examination with the Slit Lamp

This section reviews biomicroscopy with an indirect slit lamp and a fundus contact lens.

Indirect Slit-Lamp Biomicroscopy

High-plus handheld condensing lenses are useful for examining the posterior segment with the slit-lamp biomicroscope. The most commonly used lenses are the +90 D and +78 D lenses, but other lenses are available and range from +60 D to +132 D. The stereo-magnified view provides a good way to examine the optic disc and posterior pole. Both clear and yellow convex lenses are available; the yellow filter absorbs ultraviolet and short-wavelength visible light of less than 480 nm but substantially distorts the color of the fundus image. Almost all condensing lenses used with the slit lamp are double-aspheric lenses, so it does not matter which side is held toward the patient. Lower-powered (eg, +60 D) lenses afford a more magnified view but are harder to focus. Some lenses have adapters that expand the field or increase magnification.

For indirect slit-lamp biomicroscopy, the condensing lens is held in the same way as for indirect ophthalmoscopy; the fingers can be similarly employed to help keep the patient's eyelids open (Figure 13-15). Resting fingers of the lens-holding hand on the brow and forehead rest will also alert the beginning ophthalmoscopist if the patient's head begins to pull back. The width of the slit lamp's light beam can be varied, although the image degrades when the beam width is more than 10 mm. The lens power determines the field of view, and the magnification is varied by changing the magnification setting on the slit lamp. A setting of 10× or 16× is generally selected to begin the examination; higher magnification will not improve resolution. As with other types of posterior segment examinations, the right eye is usually examined first.

Moving the instrument's viewing and illumination arms makes indirect ophthalmoscopy with the slit lamp a dynamic, creative examination. However, the beginning resident should initially become proficient at examining the posterior segment at the slit lamp with coaxial illumination. Light intensity with the slit lamp is often stronger than with the indirect ophthalmoscope. Consequently, the duration of viewing should

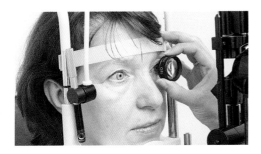

Figure 13-15 Use of a condensing lens to observe the fundus at the slit-lamp biomicroscope.

be kept below 5 minutes per eye to avoid phototoxicity. Clinical Protocol 13-3 includes instructions for examining the posterior segment with the slit-lamp biomicroscope.

Overview of the examination

The optic nerve is first evaluated for cupping and other changes. The peripapillary retina is then examined for the nerve fibers that enter the optic disc circumferentially. Nerve fibers are most easily seen adjacent to the superotemporal and inferotemporal edges of the optic disc and are more obvious with moderately dark fundus pigmentation. Bright linear reflections are normally seen from closely packed bundles; as the nerve fiber layer thins during optic neuropathies, dark slits may be seen. Increasing the light or putting in the red-free filter on the slit-lamp illumination arm can help the examiner to see the nerve fiber layer.

Attention is then turned to the macula. After examination with a beam 4 mm wide, a thin slit is focused onto the fovea. Sideways movement of a narrow slit beam can help to visualize the relative convexity or concavity of a macular lesion. A patient with a suspected macular hole or other lesion is asked whether a thin beam focused directly across the foveola appears complete, has central thinning or break, or has another distortion (Watzke-Allen test). Indirect lateral illumination of the fovea can help identify cystoid macular edema.

The vitreous body is then examined. By this time the examiner should be sufficiently dark adapted to evaluate the posterior vitreous cavity. Mobility of vitreous strands is assessed by having the patient look up and down and then rapidly return to primary position. In upgaze the gel tends to move downward; in downgaze it moves in the opposite direction; and when the eye comes to rest in the straight-ahead position, the undulating fibrils continue to move for about 10 seconds. An angle of greater than 10° between the axis of observation and the line of illumination helps to visualize vitreous opacities. The presence of hemorrhage, pigment (Shafer sign), or vitreous cell may be observed. Use of the green or blue filter can enhance the visibility of vitreous structures.

Contact Lens Biomicroscopy

Used with the slit-lamp biomicroscope, a fundus contact lens is valuable for examining the posterior pole, particularly if the pupil is small. Contact lens biomicroscopy combines stereopsis, high illumination, and high magnification with the advantages of a slit beam. Clinical Protocol 13-4 includes instructions for examining the posterior segment with a fundus contact lens and the slit-lamp biomicroscope.

Several types of contact lenses are available, including the Goldmann fundus lens (with a power of -64 D) and the Goldmann 3-mirror lens. The central portion of the Goldmann 3-mirror lens enables examination of the central and posterior vitreous and the posterior pole. Angled mirrors help to study vitreoretinal relationships at the equator and in the periphery. Each mirror is tilted differently (59°, 67°, 73°) to give views of the peripheral retina, the equatorial fundus, and the area around the posterior pole, respectively. Refer to Figure 11-57 and Chapter 11 for detailed information about the Goldmann 3-mirror lens and gonioscopy.

Wide-field (panfunduscopic) indirect contact lenses with a field of view up to 130° are available for fundus examination and for performing laser photocoagulation, although the fundus image is inverted. It is possible to examine the peripheral fundus by applying scleral depression (a special conical holder with an attached scleral depressor is available for use with the Goldmann 3-mirror lens), although this method is less commonly performed.

Direct Ophthalmoscopy

The direct ophthalmoscope gives approximately 15× magnification (depending on the patient's refractive error) and is most useful for examining the optic disc and posterior pole. The rheostat is generally turned to the brightest light, unless the patient is very light sensitive. Some instruments have a sliding polarizing filter for reducing glare. Besides the open light, filters contain different spot sizes, a streak projection, a calibrated grid, a fixation target, and a red-free filter. These illumination options and their uses are listed in Table 13-5. The grids are meant for localizing and determining the size of fundus lesions but are not normally used because it is customary to describe lesions in terms of disc diameters. The slit aperture is not used much because of difficulties in seeing contour clues monocularly.

The monocular direct ophthalmoscope is particularly useful for viewing through a small pupil to determine the shape and contour of the optic nerve. Even with pupillary dilation, the examiner will not be able to see beyond the equator with the direct ophthalmoscope.

Overview of the Examination

Direct ophthalmoscopy is performed with the eye that corresponds to the eye being examined, putting the examiner cheek to jowl with the patient. Even if you have a strong monocular dominance, you must learn to perform direct ophthalmoscopy with the correct eye and in a comfortably balanced position.

The direct ophthalmoscope is focused by twirling the dial for the Rekoss disk (named after Egbert Rekoss, who invented the rotatable disk of concave and convex

Table 13-5   Illumination Openings of the Direct Ophthalmoscope

Aperture	Description	Use
○	Full spot	Viewing through a large pupil
○	Small spot	Viewing through a small pupil
●	Red-free filter	Help in detecting changes in the nerve fiber layer and identifying microaneurysms and other vascular anomalies
▯	Slit	Evaluating retinal contour
⊞	Reticule or grid	Measuring vessel caliber or diameter of a small retinal lesion (marked in 0.2 mm increments)
◉	Fixation target	Identifying central or eccentric fixation

Table 13-6   Focusing the Direct Ophthalmoscope

Direct Ophthalmoscope[a]	Patient's Refractive Error
−30 D	−15 D
−20 D	−12 D
−10 D	−8 D
−5 D	−4 D
0	plano
+5 D	+6 D
+10 D	+15 D

[a]Comparison of the direct ophthalmoscope's refractive power with the patient's spherical equivalent. This assumes that the examiner's eye is emmetropic or corrected and that the examination distance between the ophthalmoscope and cornea is 20 mm.

lenses that he added to Hermann von Helmholtz's ophthalmoscope in 1852). The optimal focusing lens on the Rekoss disk depends on the patient's refractive error, the examiner's refractive error (including unintended accommodation), and the examination distance (Table 13-6).

To begin a basic direct-ophthalmoscopic examination, the focusing lens is set at 0 (or the examiner's refractive error), and the patient's red reflex is checked from a distance of 2 feet (Figure 13-16A). By focusing the ophthalmoscope on the iris, opacities in the ocular media can be seen as dark shadows. Vitreous floaters are seen as the patient rotates the eye up and down. The technique works best with a dilated pupil. The examiner then approaches the patient's eye without accommodating, perhaps by imagining looking into the distance through a keyhole or by keeping the other eye open to look at a distant wall. The examiner steadies the instrument against the patient's face by resting the ulnar border of the hand holding the instrument against the patient's cheek; the thumb of the free hand raises the upper eyelid (Figure 13-16B). The patient is instructed to stare into the distance. Many lanes and hospital rooms have a target marked on the wall opposite the examining chair or on the ceiling for this purpose.

While holding the patient's eyelids open, the examiner dials the ophthalmoscope's focusing lenses into place to clarify the fundus image. Minus lenses, for example, are used to correct for the patient's myopia and for the examiner's unintended accommodation. With the examiner's eye being emmetropic or corrected, the power of the ophthalmoscope's focusing lens is near the patient's distance refraction for low myopia or hyperopia. Optimal viewing occurs 2–3 cm from the patient's eye.

As the patient stares at a distanced target, the ophthalmoscope is angled about 15° temporal to fixation so that the patient's optic disc is at or near the first visible field. The light beam must remain centered within the pupil, although slight tilting of the ophthalmoscope can avoid troublesome corneal light reflexes. At this point, the examiner is ready to begin examining the fundus. Clinical Protocol 13-5 describes the steps for evaluating the fundus.

The retinal nerve fiber layer bundles are seen as fine, bright striations that fan off the optic disc. The reflectivity of the inner limiting membrane can make the bundles harder to see in children. The green (ie, red-free) filter enhances the visibility of the retinal nerve

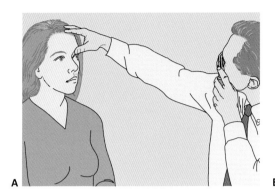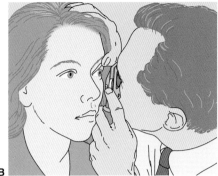

A   B

Figure 13-16 Direct ophthalmoscopy. **A,** Checking the red reflex to detect any opacities in the refractive media. **B,** Focusing on the optic disc.

fiber layer. Examination should begin where the retinal nerve fiber layer is best visualized, at the inferotemporal region close to the optic disc; the examination then proceeds to the superotemporal region, followed by the superonasal and the inferonasal parts. Except for spindle-shaped slits between bundles, localized defects of the retinal nerve fiber layer do not occur in normal eyes.

The Fundus Record

Whether you are performing indirect ophthalmoscopy, slit-lamp examination of the posterior segment, or direct ophthalmoscopy, a detailed and accurate record of the examination is required. Documentation has evolved in recent years, as many ophthalmology practices have transitioned to electronic health record (EHR) systems. Ophthalmologists use a combination of detailed text descriptions of examination findings, integrated EHR fundus and optic nerve drawing modules, and standard hand drawings that may be scanned into the EHR. Digital photography and other imaging modalities are also increasingly used for documentation of fundus lesions and baseline posterior segment findings. Despite these changes, it remains important for ophthalmologists in training to develop proficiency in standard fundus drawing. In addition to its importance in specific clinical situations, the practice of creating detailed and accurate visual representations of the fundus helps hone the resident's examination skills. Furthermore, individual patients' historical records and medical records from colleagues will continue to include standard drawings that must be accurately interpreted.

The retinal drawing is made inside a circle centered on the fovea that shows the relative positions of the optic disc, major retinal blood vessels, and ora serrata. Standard preprinted fundus charts, or vitreoretinal charts, display 3 concentric circles that represent the equator, the ora serrata, and the anterior limit of the pars plana (Figure 13-17). Roman numerals indicate the fundus meridians in clock hours. Labeled horizontal and vertical cross-section schematics are provided for recording changes in the vitreous body. A separate chart may be used for recording the appearance of the optic disc (Figure 13-18).

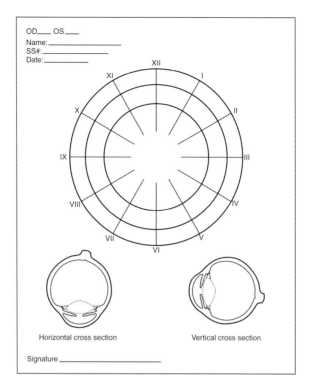

Figure 13-17 Vitreoretinal drawing chart. The inner circle identifies the relative location of the equator, the middle circle represents the ora serrata, and the outer circle locates the ciliary processes (anterior limit of the pars plana). The roman numerals indicate the fundus meridians in clock hours. The labeled horizontal and vertical cross-sections are used for recording changes in the vitreous body.

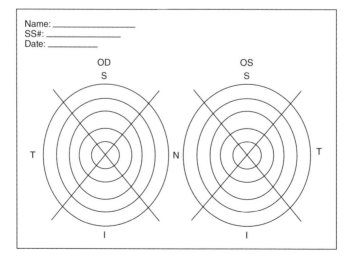

Figure 13-18 Optic disc drawing chart. The concentric circles (actually ovals) and quadrant dividing lines serve as guides when the examiner draws the borders of the optic cup. These circles represent 0.2, 0.4, 0.6, 0.8, and 1.0 cup diameter: disc diameter ratios and outline areas of approximately 4%, 16%, 36%, 64%, and 100%, respectively.

The spherically shaped fundus cannot be easily mapped in an anatomically correct way on a flat drawing. For example, the equator of the eye always has a larger circumference than the ora serrata, but the opposite is shown on the standard fundus record. As a result, lesions anterior to the equator are exaggerated in size on the fundus record.

The image obtained by the indirect ophthalmoscope is vertically inverted and laterally reversed. Drawing the inverted, reversed image takes practice. When examining a supine patient, the beginning resident can place the chart on the patient's chest so that the 12 o'clock meridian points toward the patient's feet, thereby preparing the resident to make an inverted drawing of an inverted image (Figure 13-19). After making many drawings, the experienced examiner will learn to correct mentally for the inverted image (Figure 13-20). Clinical Protocol 13-6 summarizes the steps of making the fundus drawing. Standard color coding for drawing the fundus makes it easier for examiners to interpret or compare fundus drawings. Table 13-7 lists the colors and the entities they are used to represent; Figure 13-21 shows a sample drawing.

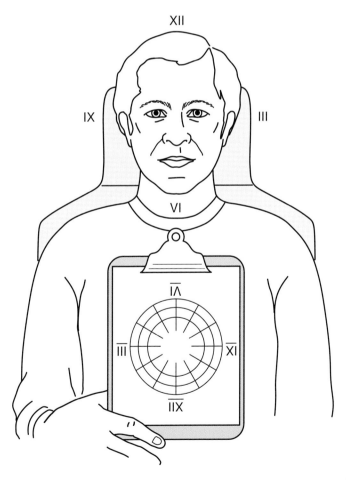

Figure 13-19   The vitreoretinal drawing chart is inverted on the supine patient's chest so that the examiner can draw the image that is seen in the condensing lens on the chart.

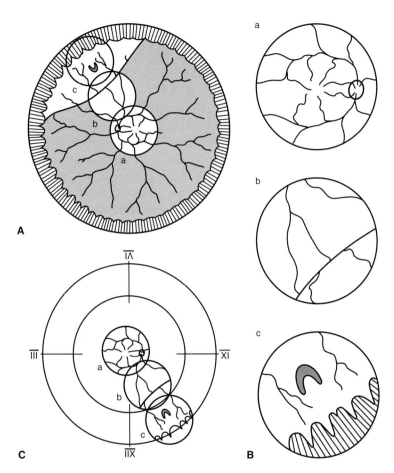

Figure 13-20 Transposing indirect ophthalmoscopic fundus views of a left eye to a vitreoretinal chart. **A,** The patient's fundus viewed directly as if the anterior segment were removed. **B,** Three corresponding views as seen by the examiner (a, b, c). **C,** Each image is drawn as seen directly onto the inverted chart.

Table 13-7   Color Code for Fundus Drawing

Color	Representations
Red	Retinal arterioles, attached retina[a], retinal hemorrhage, microaneurysms, retinal break or hole
Blue	Retinal venules, detached retina, outline of retinal break or hole
Orange	Elevated neovascularization
Purple	Flat neovascularization
Yellow	Exudate, edema
Green	Vitreous opacity (eg, hemorrhage)
Brown	Pigmentation, detached choroid
Black	Ora serrata, drusen, hyperpigmentation

[a]Or use light red or leave uncolored for attached retina.

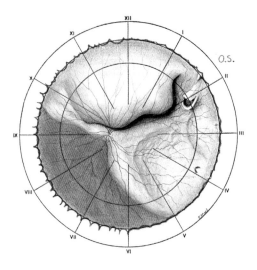

Figure 13-21 Example of a retinal drawing that shows bulbous retinal detachment with peripheral exudates (yellow) and large and small horseshoe tears. (Courtesy of Fred M. Wilson Sr, MD.)

Imaging Studies

Many types of imaging studies are useful in evaluating and documenting vitreoretinal and choroidal findings. These include fundus photography, angiography, ultrasonography, and optical coherence tomography, as discussed below. Radiography, computed tomography (CT), and magnetic resonance imaging (MRI) also contribute information to the diagnosis of ocular abnormalities, but discussion of these techniques is beyond the scope of this book.

Photography

Magnified photographs of the macula and the optic disc (as a single image or a stereoscopic pair) can be useful to document abnormalities of the fundus. In addition to the standard 30° field, wide-angle images can also be created either as a digital montage of smaller images, or acquired with use of newer ultrawide-field fundus imaging systems (multiwavelength laser imaging technology). Clear instructions on the reasons for photography must be given to the ophthalmic photographer so that the correct fields and magnifications are selected. Corresponding photographs are usually taken of both eyes for comparison.

Angiography

Fluorescein angiography (FA) is a critical test in the evaluation of retinal and choroidal disease. Sodium fluorescein solution is injected intravenously, and the fluorescent properties of the dye are captured (with use of the special filters placed within the fundus camera) as it passes through the retinal and choroidal circulations.

The endothelium of the retinal vasculature and the tight junctions of the retinal pigment epithelium (RPE) maintain the inner and outer blood ocular barriers, respectively, and are normally impermeable to the dye. The circulation time, or transit time, of the dye can be measured as it sequentially passes through the retinal arterial, capillary, and venous systems. Delayed arm-to-eye and arteriovenous transit time can result from retinal vascular occlusive disease as well as from more proximal carotid or intracranial vascular stenosis or cardiac disease. Retinal microvascular diseases such as diabetic and hypertensive retinopathy have characteristic angiographic findings, including abnormal leakage of the dye.

FA imaging of the choroid is limited by partial blockage of fluorescence due to overlying RPE, and the free extravasation of small fluorescein molecules through the highly fenestrated choriocapillaris, which obscures details of larger underlying choroidal vessels. However, various choroidal diseases that cause abnormalities of the RPE and result in subretinal exudation can be identified with FA, including choroidal neovascular membranes, central serous chorioretinopathy, and inflammatory choroidopathies.

Indocyanine green (ICG) angiography is helpful in elucidating choroidal disease because the dye is almost completely bound to plasma proteins and has limited diffusion through the small fenestrations of the choroid. ICG fluoresces in the near-infrared range of the light spectrum, which more easily passes through the RPE and allows deeper imaging of choroidal anatomy and pathologic processes. Several conditions are more accurately characterized with the addition of ICG angiography; these include polypoidal choroidal vasculopathy, choroidal inflammatory or infiltrative disease, central serous chorioretinopathy (in some cases), and choroidal neovascularization in the presence of overlying blood or when the membrane is occult and difficult to identify with FA.

Ultrasonography

Diagnostic ultrasonography, or echography, is a useful technique when media opacification prevents adequate ophthalmoscopy of the posterior segment. Two formats are available: an "A-scan" is a 1-dimensional display used to characterize tissues, and a "B-scan" is a 2-dimensional display used for architectural information (Figure 13-22).

B-scan echography is often performed through the eyelids with methylcellulose as a coupling gel (Figure 13-23). Increased resolution is made possible by placement of the probe directly on the anesthetized globe or by use of water-bath immersion. The B-scan image is a cross-sectional display of the globe and orbit. Moving the probe allows the examiner to create a 3-dimensional mental image. The mobility of intraocular abnormalities is noted during imaging. Images of the display screen are often acquired.

A-scan ultrasonography is used to measure the echographic amplitudes of the tissue interfaces along a linear wave front. The horizontal baseline of the graphic display represents distance, and the vertical dimension plots echo intensity.

Ultrasonographic technology is critical in the clinical evaluation of various choroidal tumors, including choroidal melanoma.

Optical Coherence Tomography

Optical coherence tomography (OCT) is a noninvasive, noncontact imaging technology that uses interferometry and low-coherence laser light to create micrometer-resolution cross-sectional images (tomograms) of the retina. A 2-dimensional image of the backscattered light from the different layers of the retina is produced, which appears similar to those of histopathologic specimens. Newer Fourier-domain, or spectral-domain, technology delivers greater detail with shorter acquisition time than time-domain OCT scanners (Figure 13-24). OCT angiography (OCTA) is an emerging technology capable of noninvasively imaging the retinal vasculature, including the deep, middle, and superficial layers of the macular capillary system.

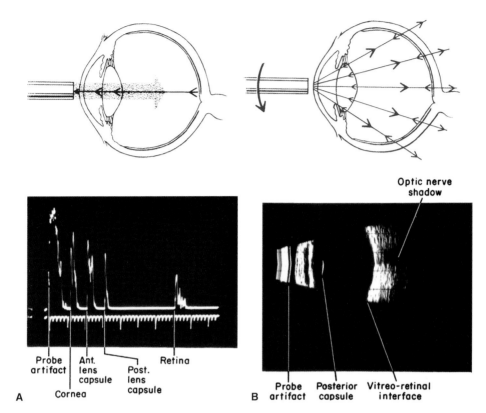

Figure 13-22   Ultrasonography of the eye. **A,** In A-scanning, a beam of ultrahigh-frequency sound waves enters the eye (top) and is reflected by ocular tissue interfaces at different amplitudes (bottom). **B,** In B-scan echography, the transducer moves back and forth in a plane (top), and the display shows the echo pattern for the tissue interfaces as dots (bottom). (Top figures reprinted, with permission, from Michels RG, Wilkinson CP, Rice TA. *Retinal Detachment.* St Louis: Mosby-Year Book; 1990.)

OCT is an outstanding tool for evaluating the vitreomacular and retinal-RPE interfaces. It is very useful in diagnosing epiretinal membranes as well as impending, early, or late macular holes and their response to surgical treatment. OCT imaging has also greatly increased the accuracy in diagnosing and monitoring macular edema due to various diseases such as diabetic retinopathy and retinal venous occlusive disease. A retinal thickness map can be created by determining the distance between the inner and outer retinal boundaries. Macular volume can be assessed and followed over time to determine efficacy of therapy for these retinal vascular diseases.

In addition, OCT can shed light on subretinal diseases such as choroidal neovascularization and its sequelae. Spectral-domain OCT imaging is more sensitive in detecting early or subtle exudation from choroidal neovascularization (CNV) than the most expert ophthalmoscopist. Therefore, OCT imaging should be obtained in the context of any new visual complaints or macular examination findings in patients with AMD or other conditions associated with an increased risk of CNV. Untreated CNV can lead to rapid and irreversible loss of central vision.

Figure 13-23 Application of an ultrasound probe to the eye with a cross-sectional image displayed on the screen. (Courtesy of Preston H. Blomquist, MD.)

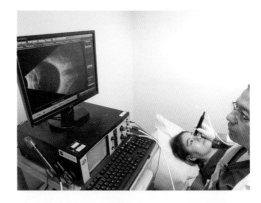

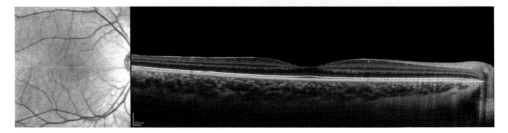

Figure 13-24 Optical coherence tomography of a normal macula. (Courtesy of Andrew J. Barkmeier, MD.)

In glaucomatous optic nerve damage, the retinal nerve fiber layer thins as nerve fibers die, and the optic cup increases in size. OCT can measure the absolute thickness of the retinal nerve fiber layer around the optic disc. The measurements can be compared to age-matched normal values and followed serially over time to detect clinical progression of glaucoma. A *scanning laser polarimeter* can also be used to assess the retinal nerve fiber layer. A combination of a scanning laser ophthalmoscope and a polarization modulator and detector, the scanning laser polarimeter takes advantage of the birefringent properties of the retinal nerve fiber layer to measure its relative thickness. A *confocal scanning laser ophthalmoscope* can create a 3-dimensional image of the optic nerve head. While these instruments show great promise, one cannot rely solely on optic nerve head and retinal nerve fiber layer imaging devices to diagnose and follow glaucoma. Detailed and careful clinical observation and comparison with baseline stereophotographs of the discs remain important to the examination of the glaucoma patient.

The Normal Fundus and Its Common Variations

To be comprehensive in performing ophthalmoscopy, the examiner should note a variety of characteristics of every principal structure of the entire posterior segment. Table 13-8 lists the major features that should be recorded during a stepwise examination of the posterior segment. Embryonic remnants and other normal developmental variations should be noted. Various age-related changes are often found, and while most do not require treatment, these too should be drawn or described (Table 13-9).

Optic Disc

The optic disc is described by its color and topography. The nasal half tends to look pinker and slightly less distinct than the temporal rim. Myelinated nerve fibers are white, featherlike bundles that usually extend in one or more directions from the optic disc. They can also occur separate from the disc. Hyaline bodies (improperly but commonly called *drusen*) of the optic nerve are calcified sphingomyelin concretions that are sometimes found within the optic nerve head. The presence of either myelinated nerve fibers or hyaline bodies should be recorded on the optic disc drawing or described in the chart.

Optic cup

The physiologic optic cup is the slight indentation at the center of the optic disc, through which the major retinal vessels enter and exit the eye. Normal cups occupy 30%–50% of the area of the optic disc. Genetic variations lead to some normal cups filling almost 70% of the disc's area. Asymmetry of the cup–disc ratio of more than 0.2 between the 2 eyes occurs in less than 1% of individuals with normal eyes.

Because determination of the cup–disc ratio by ophthalmoscopy can be inaccurate and may vary from observer to observer, examiners must strive for internal consistency in their

Table 13-8   Major Features of the Posterior Segment

Structure	Characteristics to Note
Optic disc	Cup: cup–disc ratio, cup shape and depth, visibility of lamina cribrosa Rim: shape or area, pallor, border demarcation Surrounding area: juxtapapillary chorioretinal status, visibility of nerve fiber layer Blood vessels: venous pulsations, caliber and patency, hemorrhages and exudates, neovascularization
Retina	Blood vessels: caliber and patency of arterioles and venules, AV crossings, neovascularization, atypical branching patterns Hemorrhages: subretinal, intraretinal, preretinal Fluid: subretinal, intraretinal, exudates, fibrin
Background	Pale areas: composition, size, number Red areas: depth, hue, and border Dark areas: elevation, size, location
Macula	Foveal light reflex, color and opacities
Vitreous	Clarity, uniformity

Table 13-9   Normal Degenerative Changes of the Aging Eye

Location	Alteration
Posterior pole	Loss of foveal light reflex, drusen
Retinal vessels	Narrowing, increased light reflex
Equator	Drusen, reticular pigmentary degeneration
Periphery	Chorioretinal degeneration, paving-stone degeneration
Vitreous humor	Liquefaction, floaters, posterior vitreous detachment

assessments as well as have a low threshold to obtain color photographs for documentation. OCT RNFL analysis can also be helpful in accurately assessing the nerve for glaucomatous damage. In addition to the cup–disc ratio, other measurements may be recorded.

Scleral rim

A physiologic scleral rim is seen when the choroid and RPE do not reach the optic disc. Its outer border is formed by the edge of the RPE and the inner border by the scleral canal of the optic nerve. If either of these pigmented layers is thickened, a pigment crescent (conus) is seen. A darkly pigmented area is caused by the RPE extending farther than usual, and a lightly pigmented area is seen if the RPE stops short and exposes the choroid. Other normal variants include slightly blurred disc borders, which result from a narrowed scleral aperture in hyperopic eyes and from a tilted disc in myopic eyes.

Posterior Pole

The macula has a diameter of about 18°, and its central zone, the fovea, a diameter of 5°. The yellow color of the macula lutea is not visible with white light but can be seen with bright illumination through a red-free interference filter. A healthy nerve fiber layer is slightly opaque and has parallel striations in an arcuate pattern above and below the macula. The central point of the foveola often has a reflex that is an inverted image of the light source. Loss of the foveal light reflex is a common age-related change of the posterior pole, as are atrophic spots on the retinal pigment epithelium (RPE).

Retinal Blood Vessels

Retinal blood vessels radiate from the optic disc, dividing dichotomously into a pattern of branches unique to each individual. While the inner retinal layers are usually supplied by the central retinal artery and its branches, cilioretinal arteries derived from the ciliary circulation are present in about 20% of all eyes and can supply circulation to a portion of the inner retina between the optic nerve and fovea. The width of the central retinal artery (or at least the visible blood column, because the vascular wall is normally transparent) is about 0.1 mm.

Retinal venules

Under normal conditions of intraocular pressure and aortic and carotid artery sufficiency, retinal arterial pulsations are not seen, but retinal venous pulsations are common. During systole, the retinal arterial pulse pressure is briefly transmitted to the intraocular pressure. When the intraocular pressure exceeds the retinal venous pressure during diastole, the retinal veins collapse. Spontaneous retinal vein pulsations are seen at the optic disc in 80% of normal people. When present, these pulsations indicate that retinal venous pressure and intracranial pressure are normal.

Retinal arterioles

The caliber and light reflectivity of the retinal arterioles are noted. A chronic rise in blood pressure produces narrowing of the retinal arterioles. In arteriolosclerosis, an age-related process that thickens arteriolar walls, the light reflex takes up more of the arteriolar width because the width of the bright stripe down the center of the blood column is proportional to the thickness of the vessel wall. Vessels with a wide light reflex are said to exhibit *copper-wiring*. When the light reflex is obscured and the fibrotic arteriole is a thin white stripe, they are referred to as silver-wire arterioles.

Vascular crossings

Retinal arteries generally remain at 1 level and the vein passes underneath; compression of the venule is then seen as arteriovenous (AV) nicking in hypertensive individuals. When the vein passes over the artery, a humping effect is seen.

Fundus Background

Physiologic color variations are commonly encountered in the background of the normal fundus. In a lightly pigmented (blond or albinotic) fundus, retinal and choroidal blood vessels are seen on a virtually white background. The fundus of a darkly pigmented person has an even, dark color, especially at the posterior pole. Nonuniform distribution of choroidal melanin, as occurs in some myopic fundi, produces a streaked or tessellated fundus background.

The venous tributaries of the choroid drain into the *vortex ampullae,* of which there are usually 4 (at the 1, 5, 7, and 11 o'clock positions) but sometimes more. A circle connecting the vortex ampullae corresponds roughly to the equator of the globe. The long posterior ciliary nerves are broad, yellow lines along the horizontal meridians. The long posterior ciliary arteries are usually inferior to the temporal nerve and superior to the nasal nerve.

Drusen

Drusen are small yellowish excrescences at Bruch membrane. Drusen are more common at the equator, especially nasally, than in the posterior pole. Macular drusen are more often found in the elderly. Patients with an increasing number or size (>63 μm) of drusen are diagnosed with age-related macular degeneration (AMD). AMD carries a risk of severe vision loss from development of choroidal neovascularization (wet or exudative or neovascular AMD) or from progressive RPE and retinal atrophy (geographic atrophy).

Pigmentary changes and nevus

Congenital hypertrophy of the retinal pigment epithelium appears as a well-circumscribed, densely black, flat spot; grouped lesions are sometimes called *bear tracks*. Reticular pigmentary degeneration is an age-related degeneration of the retinal pigment epithelium. Also called honeycomb degeneration, it forms a fishnet or honeycomb pattern that is most prominent along the nasal equator.

A choroidal nevus is a dark, minimally elevated lesion that can have associated drusen and does not typically grow.

Peripheral Fundus

The ora serrata is characterized by about 50 dentate processes that point posteriorly and by ora bays that are formed between the processes. These serrations of the peripheral retina are generally most pronounced nasally, sometimes with meridional ridges or folds. The transition from the deep nasal ora bays to the shallow temporal bays occurs at approximately 5 o'clock and 11 o'clock in the right eye and at 1 o'clock and 7 o'clock in the left eye.

A pigmented zone (demonstrable by transillumination of the globe) is located along the ora serrata. This area of retinochoroidal adhesion is 3–4 mm wide in the temporal periphery and 1 mm wide in the nasal periphery, and represents the normal fusion of the retina and the retinal pigment epithelium.

Several changes of the fundus periphery can be found (Figure 13-25). *Lattice degeneration* is a spindle-shaped area of retinal thinning that can have white, sclerotic blood vessels. Cortical vitreous is tightly adherent to the border of these lesions. Lattice degeneration is present in 6%–8% of individuals and is associated with an increased risk of retinal tears and detachment.

One or more pearls at the ora serrata might be identified. These ora pearls are drusen that look like shiny white spherules near the ora serrata. They have no clinical importance despite their remarkable appearance.

Cystoid degeneration appears as an area of granular tissue. This belt of agglomerated cysts occurs at the extreme retinal border, especially temporally. Cystoid degeneration can coalesce to form senile retinoschisis, a benign splitting of the retina. Pars plana cysts

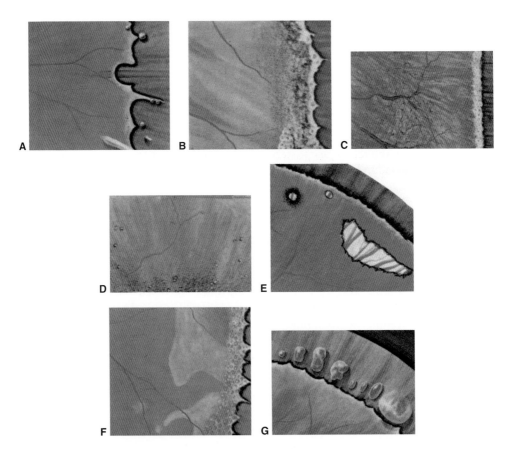

Figure 13-25   Normal variations of the fundus equator and periphery. **A,** Ora pearls. **B,** Chorioretinal degeneration. **C,** Reticular pigmentary degeneration. **D,** Equatorial drusen. **E,** Paving-stone degeneration. **F,** White with/without pressure. **G,** Pars plana cysts. (Reproduced from Rutnin U, Schepens CL. Fundus appearance in normal eyes. *Am J Ophthalmol.* 1967;64[6]:840–852, 1040–1078. Published with permission from Elsevier.)

are transparent, elevated cysts that measure 1 or 2 disc diameters. Pars plana cysts are usually multiple, bilateral, and limited to the posterior half of the temporal pars plana. They are difficult to visualize without anterior scleral depression.

White with pressure is a term used to describe a blanched color of a flat area of the peripheral retina during scleral depression. This condition is usually caused by preretinal vitreous opacification. *White without pressure* is a related phenomenon that is visible without scleral indentation.

Paving-stone degeneration, also known as *peripheral chorioretinal degeneration* and *cobblestone degeneration,* consists of clusters of nummular, atrophic, depigmented spots in the periphery. Because there is loss of the outer retina, the retinal pigment epithelium, and the choriocapillaris, a patch of white sclera is visible, with baring of the choroidal vessels. Clumps of pigment can border the margin of these circumscribed areas. Coalescent patches form an elongated zone with a scalloped margin parallel to the ora serrata.

Vitreous Humor

Light reflexes off of the internal limiting membrane are more apparent in children and younger adults. With reduced illumination, a glimmering halo that encircles the macula can be seen.

Remnants of the fetal hyaloid artery may include an epipapillary membrane or veil, referred to as *Bergmeister papilla.* The hyaloid canal passes from the optic nerve head to the lens, and a residual point of attachment often can be seen as a dot on the posterior capsule (Mittendorf dot).

Neither the anterior nor the posterior limit of the vitreous base can be seen in an eye with a normal vitreous humor. With a posterior vitreous detachment, a white line is sometimes seen on the retina just posterior to the ora serrata at the posterior limit of the vitreous base. The boundary of the vitreous base varies among individuals but normally extends about 2–3 mm on either side of the ora serrata.

Age-related liquefaction (syneresis), which typically begins in the central posterior vitreous, produces optically clear cavities. Liquid vitreous is then able to enter the space posterior to the vitreous cortex, which results in *posterior vitreous detachment,* a separation between the posterior vitreous cortex and the internal limiting membrane. Acute posterior vitreous detachment can cause floaters and flashes of light (photopsia). The incidence typically increases after age 50. *Asteroid hyalopathy* consists of small white spheres of calcium-phosphate-phospholipid crystals that do not usually impair vision.

Pitfalls and Pointers

- Other imaging problems and their causes are summarized in Table 13-10. Model eyes are available for training and practice, and a teaching mirror shows the beginner exactly what is supposed to be seen. Skill in the art and interpretation of indirect ophthalmoscopy takes daily practice with patients.

- Ophthalmoscopy is uncomfortable for the patient. A considerate examiner uses the minimum required light intensity, area of retinal illumination, and overall length of examination to achieve a detailed and thorough examination. Beginning the examination at the equator and periphery can give the patient a chance to adapt to the light before the posterior pole is examined. Allowing the patient to blink at regular

Table 13-10 Common Problems During Indirect Ophthalmoscopy

Problem	Reason
Large portion of the image is dark or distorted	Faulty lateral or vertical lens positioning
Image is too small	Condensing lens too near or too far from the eye
Central reflections obscure the image	No lens tilt
Irregular reflections and haziness	Dirty lens
Dull image	Light not properly centered in the pupil
Peculiar meshwork of vessels	Looking at conjunctiva
Image suddenly lost	Patient moved eye
Inability to go from 1 fundus area to another	Moving the viewing axis in the wrong direction

intervals and to have brief rest periods is important for both visualization and patient comfort. As the examiner changes position, the light should not be shining unnecessarily into the eye.

- Often a quick look at the posterior pole is all an examiner will be able to achieve in small children. Turning down the illumination brightness, keeping the child in the parent's lap, and avoiding any touching of the child's face can facilitate indirect ophthalmoscopy. For children who continue to move their eyes, try using only a bright, handheld flashlight, such as a Finnoff transilluminator. While sighting down the light beam that is directed at the child's dilated pupil, interpose a condensing lens to view the posterior pole.

- During scleral depression, inability to see the indented area is often wrongly interpreted as insufficient pressure. As the examiner pushes harder, the patient moves the eye, making it impossible to find the retinal periphery. If the area of scleral depression cannot be seen, the examiner should realign the axis of view or the depressor.

- To avoid confusion in localizing a fundus lesion, recall that a fundus lesion is located in terms of meridians of the clock. Its placement along an anteroposterior meridian is estimated in disc diameters in relation to the ora serrata, equator, and fovea. Keeping the axis of observation fixed with the lens withdrawn, the examiner guesses what portion of the far side of the inside of the eyeball would be illuminated by the light passing through the pupil. The examiner then confirms the anteroposterior location by placing the scleral depressor on the lesion and looking to see how far back the depressor is from the limbus. The ora serrata is 8 mm behind the limbus, and the equator is usually 12–14 mm from the limbus.

- Although the direct ophthalmoscope is simple to use and provides an upright, high-magnification image of the retina, its lack of stereopsis, small field of view, and poor view of the retinal periphery limit its utility. Many ophthalmologists will use slit-lamp biomicroscopy with a +78 D or +90 D handheld condensing lens to examine the macula and disc in lieu of direct ophthalmoscopy, especially when the pupil is dilated.

- Although bradycardia from the oculocardiac reflex is uncommon during routine examination, vasovagal syncope can result from application of a fundus contact lens. The contact lens should be held, but not pushed, against the eye and removed if the patient begins to feel faint.

Suggested Resources

Retinal conditions

Age-Related Macular Degeneration [Preferred Practice Pattern]. American Academy of Ophthalmology; 2019. Accessed September 27, 2020. https://www.aao.org/preferred-practice-pattern/age-related-macular-degeneration-ppp

Diabetic Retinopathy [Preferred Practice Pattern]. American Academy of Ophthalmology; 2019. Accessed September 27, 2020. https://www.aao.org/preferred-practice-pattern/diabetic-retinopathy-ppp

Posterior Vitreous Detachment, Retinal Breaks, and Lattice Degeneration [Preferred Practice Pattern]. American Academy of Ophthalmology; 2019. Accessed September 27, 2020. https://www.aao.org/preferred-practice-pattern/posterior-vitreous-detachment-retinal-breaks-latti

Indirect ophthalmoscopy

Friberg TR. Examination of the retina: ophthalmoscopy and fundus biomicroscopy. In: Albert DM, Miller JW, Azar DT, Blodi BA, eds. *Albert & Jakobiec's Principles and Practice of Ophthalmology*. 3rd ed. WB Saunders Co; 2008.

Regillo CD, Benson WE, Edmunds W. *Retinal Detachment: Diagnosis and Management*. 3rd ed. Lippincott Williams & Wilkins; 1998.

Rubin ML. The optics of indirect ophthalmoscopy. *Surv Ophthalmol.* 1964;9:449–464.

Direct ophthalmoscopy

Orient JM. *Sapira's Art and Science of Bedside Diagnosis*. 5th ed. Lippincott Williams & Wilkins; 2018.

Fluorescein angiography

Berkow JW, Flower RW, Orth DH, Kelley JS. *Fluorescein and Indocyanine Green Angiography: Technique and Interpretation*. Ophthalmology Monograph 5. 2nd ed. American Academy of Ophthalmology; 1997.

Optical coherence tomography

Chen TC, Hoguet A, Junk AK, et al. Spectral-domain OCT: helping the clinician diagnose glaucoma. A report by the American Academy of Ophthalmology Ophthalmic Technology Assessment Committee Glaucoma Panel. *Ophthalmology.* 2018;125(11):1817–1827.

McDonald HR, Williams GA, Scott IU, et al. Laser scanning imaging for macular disease: a report by the American Academy of Ophthalmology. *Ophthalmology.* 2007;114(6):1221–1228.

CLINICAL PROTOCOL 13-1

Obtaining a Fundus Image in Indirect Ophthalmoscopy

1. Ask the reclining, well-dilated patient to gaze steadily at a distant target on the ceiling. Having the patient look just above and beyond your shoulder (your right shoulder when examining the patient's right eye) will help to align your view onto the posterior pole. Patients with poor vision may be asked to extend an arm and to stare at their outstretched thumb.

2. While you are standing above the patient, direct the headset's light by tilting your head so that it illuminates the fundus when focused through the condensing lens.

3. While you are holding the condensing lens in the standard manner, position it just in front of the patient's eye and center the pupil in it.

4. Pull the lens slowly away from the patient's eye by flexing your wrist and by bending the fingers holding the lens (Figure 1) until you see a stereoscopic, focused image of the fundus in midair in front of the condensing lens (Figure 2). For a +20 D condensing lens, the image is seen when the lens is positioned about 5 cm in front of the patient's eye.

5. Accommodate on this image with both eyes, and maintain it by keeping the headset's light in the patient's pupil.

6. If light reflections from the front and back surfaces of the condensing lens are centered (Figure 3A), tilt the lens slightly to move them apart (Figure 3B).

7. Shift the field of view by moving your head and the condensing lens in unison along a fixed axis. Use the extended finger of the hand that is

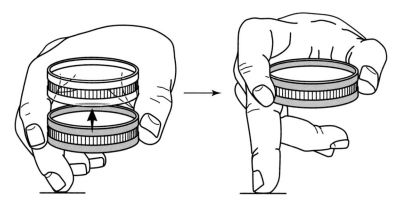

Figure 1 The lens is pulled slowly away from the patient's eye. (Redrawn from: The technique of binocular indirect ophthalmoscopy, Benjamin F. Boyd, MD, *Highlights of Ophthalmology,* 1966;9:213, courtesy of Jaypee-Highlights Medical Publishers, Inc.)

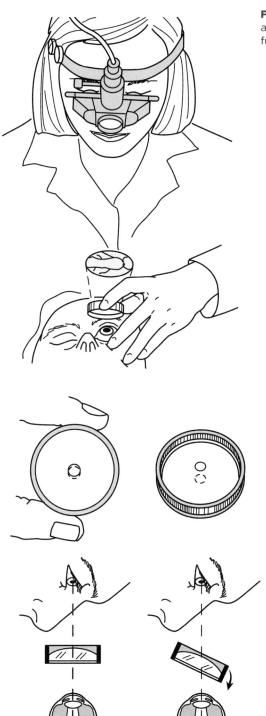

Figure 2 The lens is stopped midair when a stereoscopic, focused image of the fundus is visible.

Figure 3 Positions of light reflections on the pupil. If the reflections are centered **(A)**, the examiner tilts the lens slightly **(B)** to move the reflections apart. (Modified from: The technique of binocular indirect ophthalmoscopy, Benjamin F. Boyd, MD, *Highlights of Ophthalmology,* 1966;9:219, courtesy of Jaypee-Highlights Medical Publishers, Inc.)

A   B

Figure 4 Keeping the viewing axis centered. (Redrawn from: The technique of binocular indirect ophthalmoscopy, Benjamin F. Boyd, MD, *Highlights of Ophthalmology,* 1966;9:222, courtesy of Jaypee-Highlights Medical Publishers, Inc.)

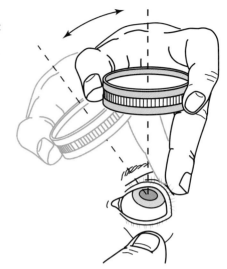

holding the condensing lens as a pivot to keep your viewing axis centered on the patient's pupil (Figure 4).

8. Mentally note that the image of the patient's fundus is inverted and reversed.

CLINICAL PROTOCOL 13-2

Performing Scleral Depression

1. While you are standing opposite the area to be examined, instruct the reclining patient to look toward you. It can also help in positioning to have the patient turn their head away from the direction of the zone of regard.

2. Increase the voltage setting on the ophthalmoscope transformer to the highest setting that the patient can tolerate, in order to compensate for the reduced light entering the eye obliquely through the pupil.

3. Rest the tip of the scleral depressor lightly at the skin crease of the eyelid (Figure 1). Align the shaft of the instrument with your visual axis and keep the depressor nearly parallel to the surface of the patient's eye (Figure 2A).

4. Instruct the patient to move the eyes toward the tip of the scleral depressor (Figure 2B). Often it is necessary only that the patient resume a straight-ahead, primary position rather than gaze excessively far in the meridian being examined.

5. Press the depressor gently. This action creates a mound in the fundus (Figure 2C).

6. As for indirect ophthalmoscopy of the posterior pole, keep the ophthalmoscope's light beam in the upper half of the field and first obtain a red reflex, then interpose the condensing lens (Figure 3).

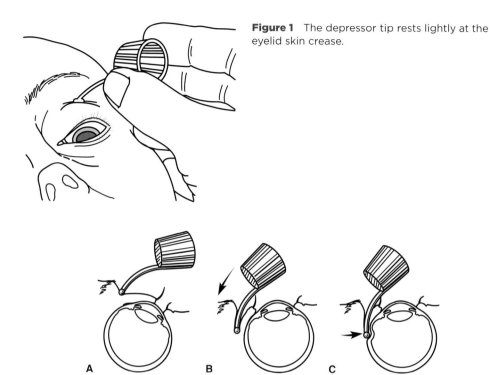

Figure 1 The depressor tip rests lightly at the eyelid skin crease.

A   B   C

Figure 2   Scleral depressor. **A,** The depressor tip is held nearly parallel to the patient's eye. **B,** The patient moves the eyes toward the tip. **C,** The examiner gently presses the depressor. (Figure 2 from: The technique of binocular indirect ophthalmoscopy, Benjamin F. Boyd, MD, *Highlights of Ophthalmology,* 1966;9:243, courtesy of Jaypee-Highlights Medical Publishers, Inc.)

7. While you keep the depressor tangential to the globe and pressed against the equator, a grayish mound should come into view in the lower part of the red reflex; this indicates that the depressor tip is aligned with the axis of observation (Figure 4).

8. Modify the lens position to bring the bulging, indented part of the peripheral fundus into clear focus. The inverted image of the indentation will be opposite the location of the scleral depression.

9. To view the ora serrata, instruct the patient to look slightly farther in the direction of the tip of the scleral depressor. While you keep the fundus image focused, slide the depressor's tip anteriorly until the ora serrata is visualized (Figure 5A).

10. To view the equatorial fundus, keep the scleral depressor stationary and instruct the patient to shift their gaze toward primary position (Figure 5B).

Figure 3   Technique for indirect ophthalmoscopy.

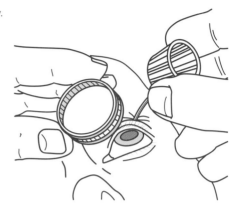

Figure 4   Visualizing a grayish mound to indicate correct alignment of the depressor tip.

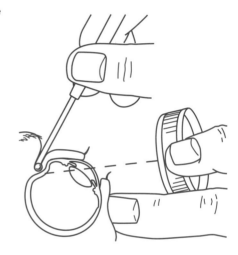

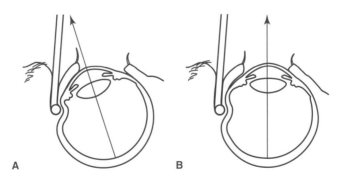

Figure 5   Depressor tip position for visualizing the ora serrata **(A)** and equatorial fundus **(B)**.

CLINICAL PROTOCOL 13-3

Performing Indirect Slit-Lamp Biomicroscopy

1. Assume standard patient and examiner positions at the slit-lamp bio-microscope (see Chapter 10).

2. Ensure that the patient's pupils are well dilated.

3. Set the slit-lamp magnification to 10× or 16×.

4. Focus and center a slit beam about 4 mm wide onto the corneal surface at the central (nearly coaxial) position. Use the brightest (below supra-maximal) light intensity that the patient can easily tolerate.

5. Hold the +78 D or +90 D condensing lens stationary between thumb and forefinger, approximately 5–10 mm from the patient's cornea, while bracing your hand against the headrest frame or the patient's cheek and resting your elbow comfortably on a support. This permits you to see the anterior segment to make sure that the pupil is centered in the lens. The third and fourth fingers help open the patient's eyelids.

6. While you keep the slit beam centered on both the condensing lens and the cornea, grasp the slit-lamp joystick with your free hand and pull the slit lamp away from the patient until the patient's red reflex becomes visible; then stop.

7. Move the condensing lens toward yourself until the red reflex becomes a focused fundus image. The distance between the lens and the patient's cornea will be shorter for higher-powered lenses. If you encounter bothersome light reflection, tilt the condensing lens about 6° and/or angle the slit beam.

8. Ask the patient to fixate steadily just past your ear. This should bring the optic disc into view. Get the optic disc into the center of the fundus image either by realigning the viewing arm or directing the patient's gaze appropriately.

9. Figure 1 shows a suggested sequence of examination. Begin at the optic disc (1), then proceed temporally across the posterior pole to make a circumferential sweep around the posterior pole (2 through 6), and end at the macula (7). This sequence requires redirecting the patient's gaze in these directions with verbal instructions or a target such as a fixation light or your fingertip. Direct the patient's gaze into primary position with a fixation target after the central fundus examination is complete.

10. To examine the vitreous cavity, angle the slit beam about 10°–20° from the axis of observation. Move the condensing lens slightly toward yourself to examine the vitreous. Having the patient follow a target that moves a few degrees can help you to see strands of the vitreous humor. To help visualize opacities or the Weiss ring of a posterior vitreous detachment, move the slit-lamp joystick and illumination arm to produce alternating direct illumination and retroillumination. Vitreous examination can also be enhanced by a small circular rotation of the condensing lens in 1 plane.

Figure 1 Suggested sequence of examination for slit-lamp biomicroscopy.

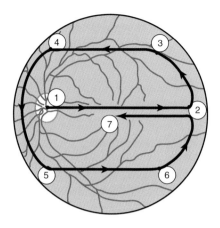

11. To examine the peripheral vitreous and fundus, use the coaxial slit lamp position and ask the patient to look in the direction of each meridian being observed (typically up, up and right, right, down and right, etc.).

CLINICAL PROTOCOL 13-4

Performing Contact Lens Biomicroscopy

1. Instill topical anesthetic onto the eye.
2. Assume standard patient and examiner positions at the slit-lamp biomicroscope (see Chapter 10).
3. Ensure that the patient's pupils are well dilated.
4. Set the slit-lamp magnification to 10× or 16×.
5. Put into the concave part of the contact lens a small amount of gonioscopy gel, such as methylcellulose solution, while taking care to avoid creating any air bubbles. Explain to the patient, in a reassuring way, what is to be done.
6. Instruct the patient to look up and to keep their head all the way forward and in contact with the forehead rest. Spread the patient's eyelids apart with your thumb and forefinger.
7. Hold the contact lens between the thumb and index finger and place the lower edge of the contact lens on the patient's exposed lower globe (Figures 1A, 1B).
8. Angle the contact lens onto the globe from below and instruct the patient to look straight ahead (Figures 2A, 2B). Release the patient's eyelids and allow the contact lens to hold the eyelids apart. Switch hands, if necessary, to hold the contact lens in your hand closer to the patient's eye (eg, your left hand for the patient's right eye) so that your arm does not interfere with use of the slit lamp.
9. If any air bubbles are caught between the contact lens and the cornea, slightly tilt the lens to allow them to float out. Allow the contact lens to sit gently on the cornea, and avoid unnecessary pressure on the lens by your fingers, which are keeping the lens steady.

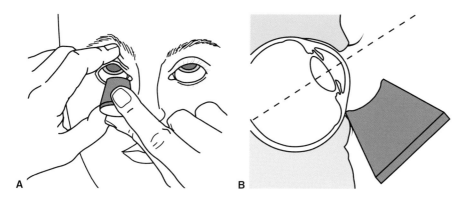

Figure 1   Position of contact lens on the lower globe **(A)**, with side view shown **(B)**.

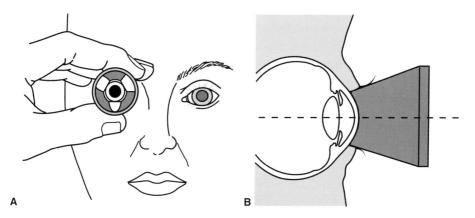

Figure 2   Contact lens in place, with the patient's eyes in straight-ahead position **(A)**, with side view shown **(B)**.

10. Use the joystick to focus the slit lamp toward the patient. Begin with the illumination arm in the coaxial position and examine the posterior pole. Tilt the lens slightly to maneuver light reflections from the lens surface away from the central viewing area.

11. If a 3-mirror lens is used, position the light source on the same side as the side of the eye being examined so that the light beam bounces off the mirror. Begin with the largest, least-angled mirror to examine the area around the posterior pole.

12. To examine the adjacent fundus area, twirl the lens on the eye with a dialing motion for 1 or 2 clock hours. Realign the slit beam to view the new fundus area.

13. After circumferential examination of the fundus with 1 mirror, repeat with the other 2 mirrors to examine the equatorial and peripheral fundus. The lens might need to be rocked or rotated to see all parts of the fundus.

14. Remove the lens by tilting it off the cornea. Clean and disinfect the contact lens before reuse.

CLINICAL PROTOCOL 13-5

Evaluating the Fundus with the Direct Ophthalmoscope

1. Find the optic disc by following a retinal blood vessel. The arrows formed by vascular bifurcations point to the optic disc. Depending on the patient's refraction, the entire disc or only a portion of it will be visible in any one view.

2. Examine the peripapillary retina. Use a red-free absorption filter to examine arcuate nerve fiber layer defects that occur in glaucoma and other optic neuropathies.

3. From the optic disc, follow the blood vessels outward to examine the superonasal (1), inferonasal (2), inferotemporal (3), and superotemporal (4) areas around the posterior pole (Figure 1). Note the vascular color, caliber, bifurcations, crossings, and the surrounding background.

4. Use the red-free light to highlight the refractile changes in the vascular wall caused by arteriolosclerosis, especially at points of arteriovenous compression.

5. Examine the macula (5) for irregularities. Use a slit beam to detect distortions of the retinal surface. Level differences can be seen by a blurring of a portion of the light stripe; lacking stereopsis, estimating the convexity or concavity of a fundus lesion with the slit beam of the monocular direct ophthalmoscope is difficult.

6. If choroidal or retinal pigment epithelial abnormalities are suspected, direct the ophthalmoscope adjacent to the fundus detail under study. Allow proximal illumination to help you to distinguish between translucent and opaque lesions.

7. Approximate the height of an elevated lesion (eg, choroidal tumor or disc edema) with use of the focusing dial.

   a. First focus on flat retina, then refocus on the lesion surface.

   b. Subtract the 2 dioptric values to deduce the level difference (in a phakic or pseudophakic eye, 3 diopters = 1 mm).

Figure 1 Suggested sequence of examination for fundus evaluation with use of the direct ophthalmoscope.

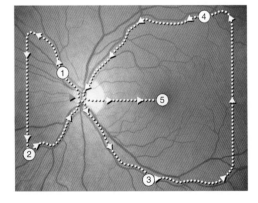

CLINICAL PROTOCOL 13-6

Drawing the Indirect Ophthalmoscopic Fundus

1. Invert the vitreoretinal chart on the patient's chest.
2. View, then draw, an initial landmark, such as the superonasal blood vessels of the posterior pole.
3. Follow the vessels anteriorly and continue to draw their bifurcations and branches in 1 quadrant.
4. Repeat for the remaining quadrants.
5. Using scleral depression, locate the blood vessels already drawn in each meridian and sketch their terminal branches.
6. Draw the ora serrata.
7. Reexamine any fundus lesion and sketch its borders and details in relationship to the blood vessels and other landmarks already drawn.

14 Ophthalmic Emergencies

This chapter gives a brief overview of common emergencies encountered by beginning ophthalmology residents on call, including how to evaluate patients in the emergency department. Opinions differ with regard to certain aspects of therapeutics (such as the management of hyphema), but the information given should serve as a useful base upon which to build further knowledge as your training progresses.

The diagnosis and management of ophthalmic emergencies require a disciplined, methodical approach to ensure proper care and to avoid mistakes. The need for a quick examination of a patient experiencing a medical emergency should not preclude thoroughness. Proper documentation, timely treatment, and meticulous attention to detail are necessary for optimal medical care as well as for medicolegal reasons (see Chapter 3). If you are uncertain of how to handle an ophthalmic emergency, you are obligated quickly to seek the help of an experienced ophthalmologist and to obtain appropriate consultations from other medical specialists as the situation demands.

Emergency Equipment and General Evaluation

Ideally, a patient who arrives in the emergency department is evaluated in an examining room equipped with a visual acuity chart and slit lamp, or else, if the patient is stable, they are transported to the eye clinic. Portable equipment must be made available for evaluation of patients with ophthalmic emergencies who are not able to sit at a slit lamp. It is helpful for beginning residents to prepare a call bag that contains essential equipment and supplies, including the following:

- light source (eg, muscle light)
- near-vision card
- pinhole occluder
- +2.50 D lens
- small toys or other pediatric fixation targets
- fluorescein strips
- cobalt-blue filter (for light source)
- Desmarres eyelid retractor
- pH strips
- Fox eye shields and a roll of surgical tape
- certain ophthalmic medications, such as proparacaine and mydriatic eyedrops
- exophthalmometer
- color-vision plates

In addition, an indirect ophthalmoscope (with a cobalt-blue filter) and handheld tonometer (Tono-Pen or iCare) should be available.

Evaluation of patients with eye emergencies begins with a thorough history. Always inquire about the patient's baseline visual acuity. Knowing that a patient who presents with blunt trauma and 20/200 vision also has a history of amblyopia may drastically change the clinical picture. However, never defer treatment of a true ocular emergency (chemical burn, central retinal artery occlusion, or acute angle-closure glaucoma) to take the history. In all emergency cases, the history should be tailored to suit the nature of the disorder. For splash injuries, identification of the chemical is important, and information from a material safety data sheet (MSDS) can help guide treatment after initial irrigation. If surgical intervention is a possibility, ask about the patient's last oral intake and withhold further oral intake until a therapeutic decision is made. Also, ask about the date of the patient's last tetanus booster in all cases of penetrating or perforating trauma.

The ophthalmic examination should be based on the history and symptoms of the patient. The first step is to accurately measure visual acuity, as this is important for counseling regarding prognosis in certain emergencies. To assess acuity in the emergency setting, it is useful to have a pinhole occluder on hand to help account for refractive errors, a +2.50 D lens to help account for presbyopia, and a near reading card. If the patient's vision is greatly impaired, the ability to count fingers, see hand motion, or detect light with or without projection should be documented. If a patient has no light perception, this should be documented with the brightest light source possible and confirmed by a second examiner. The pertinent aspects of the external, motility, confrontation visual fields, pupillary, and anterior segment examinations; tonometry; and ophthalmoscopy are then performed in that order. If significant head trauma exists, defer dilation of the pupils to preserve the pupillary reaction for serial neurologic evaluations, and until the patient is cleared by the neurology or neurosurgery department. Maneuvers that apply pressure to the globe, such as scleral depression, gonioscopy, and ultrasonography, should not be performed on patients with potential open-globe injuries. In the presence of significant swelling, a Desmarres retractor may be used to gently open the eyelids without putting pressure on the globe. External or slit-lamp photography can aid in documenting the extent of the injury.

Pediatric Evaluation

Special techniques are needed for the evaluation of children in the emergency setting. Patience, tact, and sensitivity to the concerns of parents are essential. To avoid prompting crying spells in pediatric patients, try to gather as much information as possible by careful observation without touching the child. Avoid a demeanor and gestures that might feel threatening to the child—keep a low profile during the evaluation, if possible, and move about slowly and deliberately. Toys and interesting fixation targets can simplify pediatric examinations, and infants might be easier to evaluate if given a pacifier or small amount of sweet solution (oral sucrose).

A papoose board, parent, or nurse may be needed help to restrain an uncooperative child for a brief examination. If the globe is open, however, the papoose board should not be used; it can provoke straining and elevated intraocular pressure, which could lead to extrusion of ocular contents. A swaddle may be used for infants. Conscious sedation may be provided in the emergency department setting, but should be considered only if an examination or procedure can be completed in under 30 minutes. Once an open-globe injury is identified and the patient is committed to going to the operating room, further examination may be deferred until the child is under anesthesia in order to prevent further straining and elevated intraocular pressure.

Examination of the anterior segment and fundus may be facilitated by the use of a pediatric eyelid speculum and, for small children and infants who cannot be placed at the slit lamp, a portable slit lamp.

Ocular Trauma in the Emergency Setting

Patients with ocular trauma seen in the emergency department might have other, nonocular injuries as well. Priority must be given to treatment of life-threatening conditions, and communication among the various physicians involved is helpful in establishing the best sequence of treatment for multiple injuries. A protective eye shield should be taped in place until the patient is stabilized; attention can then be turned to the ocular trauma. The most common traumatic ocular disorders and their treatments are detailed below.

Corneal Abrasion

Corneal abrasions are defects in the epithelial layer of the cornea and are most commonly due to trauma from a fingernail scratch or contact lens. Corneal abrasions are generally accompanied by significant pain, foreign-body sensation, tearing, blepharospasm, and decreased vision if the abrasion is central. A corneal erosion is a spontaneous epithelial defect that is frequently recurrent and can occur at the site of a prior corneal injury or in association with corneal dystrophies such as anterior basement membrane dystrophy.

Evaluation is made easier by instilling an eyedrop of topical anesthetic, the response to which is often dramatic. Once the patient is comfortable, vision can then be more accurately assessed and the eye more thoroughly examined at the slit lamp. The diagnosis is facilitated by fluorescein dye, which stains the part of the cornea devoid of epithelium.

It is critical to distinguish between a typical corneal abrasion and a corneal ulcer. A corneal ulcer is an infection of the cornea that is associated with an epithelial defect, and generally presents as a white opacity. In patients with vertical corneal abrasions, rule out a foreign body embedded in the tarsal conjunctiva of the upper or lower eyelid by eversion of the eyelids and sweeping of the fornices. The vertical pattern results from the foreign body rubbing the corneal epithelium with each blink. Clinical Protocol 9-6 presents complete instructions for eyelid eversion; Clinical Protocol 11-1 includes instructions for sweeping the conjunctival sac and fornices.

Treatment

The treatment of a typical corneal abrasion is as follows:

1. Instill an eyedrop of topical anesthetic onto the affected eye.
2. Rule out a foreign body in the affected eye. Inspect the fornices.
3. Instill an eyedrop of a cycloplegic agent (eg, cyclopentolate 1% or homatropine 5%) to relieve the discomfort caused by ciliary spasm.
4. For abrasions smaller than 3–4 mm in diameter, patching the eye is not necessary. Instead, prescribe a topical antibiotic ointment to be used 3 times daily until the abrasion is healed.

5. For abrasions larger than 4 mm in diameter, a patch may be applied over the closed eyelids to reduce discomfort caused by the eyelids moving against the cornea. This technique is described in Clinical Protocol 14-1. Usually a topical antibiotic ointment is applied to the ocular surface prior to patching.

   a. Allow the patch to remain in place until reexamination in about 24 hours. A patch should not be worn for more than 24 hours because of the risk of infection. If the patient experiences worsening symptoms while patched, they may remove the patch before reevaluation. Discontinue patching if the abrasion is mostly healed.

   b. Never patch an eye if any type of infection is suspected. Patients with abrasions related to contact lens wear or vegetation (eg, a tree branch) should not be patched due to the risk of infection.

6. Alternatively, apply a bandage soft contact lens. A prophylactic antibiotic eyedrop is used in conjunction with the bandage contact lens. Bandage soft contact lenses should be avoided for patients at high risk for infection, such as those mentioned in step 5b, above.

7. For abrasions associated with contact lens wear, remove the contact lens if the patient is still wearing it and inspect with the slit lamp both the contact lens and the cornea for defects. Treat the abrasion as described in the above steps for a typical abrasion. Due to the high risk of infection, a careful slit lamp examination to assess for the presence of any infiltrate should be performed, and there should be a low threshold to treat with topical antibiotics.

Corneal Foreign Body

A corneal foreign body is an object that is superficially adherent or embedded into the cornea. Common corneal foreign bodies include metal, wood, dirt, vegetable matter, glass, and plastic. Knowing the composition of the foreign body is important because metallic foreign bodies embedded in the cornea can leave a rust ring, and vegetable foreign bodies such as wood pose a greater risk of microbial keratitis (Figure 14-1). High-velocity foreign bodies (eg, from striking metal on metal) have the potential to penetrate the globe, and the cornea should be examined carefully for signs of an entry wound. The slit-lamp biomicroscope is used to determine the depth of corneal foreign bodies. The upper and lower eyelids should be everted to exclude the possibility of

Figure 14-1 A metallic corneal foreign body, surrounded by a visible rust ring and corneal haze.

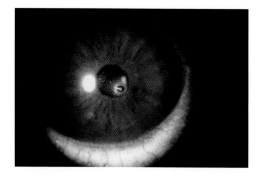

foreign bodies in the tarsal conjunctiva or the fornices. If there is any suspicion of associated microbial keratitis, the cornea should be scraped and cultured as for a corneal ulcer.

Treatment

Treatment depends on the nature, location, and depth of the corneal foreign body. Superficial foreign bodies that appear to have penetrated no deeper than the superficial stroma may be removed in the clinic or emergency department, as described in Clinical Protocol 14-2. If the foreign body is embedded deep in the cornea or if corneal perforation is suspected, treat the patient in the sterile setting of an operating room equipped to handle corneal perforations. The patient should wear a rigid fenestrated aluminum (Fox) shield until it is time for surgery (Clinical Protocol 14-1).

Eyelid Laceration

All patients with eyelid lacerations should be meticulously evaluated for the possibility of concurrent injuries, such as canalicular lacerations, occult trauma to the globe, and orbital wall fractures. Inquire about the object that caused the laceration, the time and severity of the injury, and any associated symptoms and signs.

Treatment

Any ocular conditions associated with an eyelid laceration (eg, open-globe injury) should be treated as required. Eyelid lacerations need not be repaired immediately and are best done by a physician experienced in such repairs. The repair may be delayed for 12–24 hours, especially if the wound is contaminated or is a result of a human bite. Because of the rich vascular supply of the eyelids, infections are uncommon and debridement should be minimal, if necessary at all. Tissue on pedicles and flaps should not be removed. Ensure that the patient's tetanus prophylaxis is up to date.

Closed-Globe Injuries

Closed-globe injures typically result from a direct blow to the eye by a blunt object. Ophthalmic sequelae include subconjunctival hemorrhage, hyphema (see below in this section), cataract or lens dislocation, orbital wall fractures (see "Orbital Fracture," below), iridodialysis, angle recession and subsequent glaucoma, iris sphincter rupture, traumatic iritis, posterior segment alterations, and traumatic optic neuropathy. Significant blunt trauma can also lead to globe rupture, which will be discussed in the Open-Globe Injuries section, below.

When significant swelling is present, gently retract the eyelids manually or with an eyelid retractor to expose the globe. Inspect the ocular surface for signs of rupture. Assess the pupil for traumatic mydriasis-associated sphincter rupture, miosis associated with traumatic iritis, and the presence of an afferent pupillary defect indicative of traumatic optic neuropathy. Evaluate the anterior segment with the slit lamp, and look for hyphema, traumatic iritis or microhyphema, and trauma cataract or subluxation of the lens. Perform a motility examination. An isolated elevation deficit suggests inferior orbital blowout fracture; mild to moderate generalized limitation of eye movements can accompany orbital edema or hematoma. Crepitus on palpation of the eyelid or cheek supports the diagnosis of an orbital fracture.

Although acute swelling of the eyelids might preclude it, gonioscopy should be performed at an appropriate time to rule out angle recession, which places the patient at risk for glaucoma in the future. A widened ciliary body will be evident, and comparison to the other angle is useful in detecting pathology. Intraocular pressure should be checked with a Tono-Pen or iCare; this may be challenging (Figure 14-2). Intraocular pressure can be artificially elevated from forced opening of the eyelids to obtain the measurement. Pressure in the low teens or less in the setting of blunt ocular trauma suggests the possibility of a ruptured globe. A low pressure reading could also be indicative of a cyclodialysis cleft, which would be evident on gonioscopy A thorough fundus examination is required, but scleral depression should be deferred in patients with hyphema or suspected scleral rupture. Posterior segment findings associated with blunt ocular trauma include commotio retinae (whitening of the retina, which causes a cherry-red spot when the fovea is involved), choroidal rupture (crescent-shaped breaks in Bruch membrane concentric to the optic disc), vitreous hemorrhage, retinal hemorrhage, and retinal detachment.

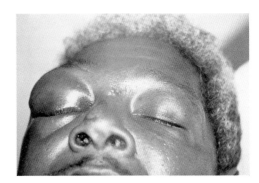

Figure 14-2 Marked orbital swelling after blunt trauma can make the ocular examination difficult or impossible.

Treatment

Treatment of closed-globe injuries depends on the nature of the findings, as detailed throughout this chapter. The physician may recommend supportive measures such as intermittent ice packs to the orbit for the first few days after the injury (if the globe is intact), elevation of the head of the bed, and medical pain management.

Traumatic Hyphema

Hyphema denotes blood in the anterior chamber (Figure 14-3). The bleeding can occur spontaneously (eg, in patients with iris neovascularization or juvenile xanthogranuloma), after intraocular surgery, or after trauma. Traumatic hyphemas vary in clinical manifestations and potential complications. Ranging in size from microscopic to complete,

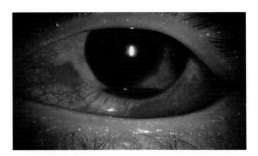

Figure 14-3 Hyphema (blood in the anterior chamber). (Courtesy of Fasika A. Woreta, MD.)

hyphemas might subside with medical management or they may require washout. The height of the blood (in mm) should be recorded. Hyphemas are frequently associated with other signs of blunt ocular trauma, including corneal abrasions, traumatic iritis, angle recession, pupillary sphincter rupture, and posterior segment abnormalities.

Elevated intraocular pressure is commonly seen at presentation, especially in patients with large hyphemas or in those with sickle cell trait or disease.

A sickle cell preparation should be obtained in patients of African or Mediterranean descent. If a history of bleeding disorders exists, laboratory workup, including coagulation markers and platelet count, should be obtained.

Treatment

The treatment of traumatic hyphema is controversial. Generally, a protective eye shield, moderate restriction of physical activity, avoidance of nonsteroidal anti-inflammatory drugs or aspirin, and elevation of the head of the bed during the first 5 days from onset are reasonable recommendations. Topical steroids and cycloplegia are also generally prescribed.

Patients with hyphema should be examined daily for at least the first 5 days due to the risk of elevated intraocular pressure and rebleeding. If the intraocular pressure is elevated, glaucoma medications may be started as needed. Topical beta-blockers (eg, timolol maleate) and carbonic anhydrase inhibitors, either in topical form (eg, dorzolamide) or systemic form (eg, acetazolamide, methazolamide), can lower the pressure sufficiently in some patients. Methazolamide is preferable to acetazolamide in patients with sickle cell disease or trait to avoid the side effect of metabolic acidosis, which can trigger sickling of red blood cells and exacerbate the intraocular hypertension by blocking the trabecular meshwork.

Rebleeding may occur within the first week after trauma; rebleeding tends to be more severe than the initial bleeding and is more likely to be associated with elevated intraocular pressure. Given that the majority of patients are managed as outpatients, they should be instructed to return immediately for reevaluation if a sudden decrease in vision or increase in pain occurs.

Surgical intervention is indicated in selected cases, including those with prolonged elevations of intraocular pressure refractory to medical management, corneal blood staining, or an intraocular pressure above 30 mm Hg for 24 hours in patients with sickle cell trait or disease.

Orbital Fracture

Blunt head trauma is often associated with fractures of bones in the orbital and periorbital areas. Fractures that affect the orbital floor but spare the orbital rim (blowout fractures) are the most common. The thin medial wall of the orbit, the lamina papyracea, is the second-most frequently fractured structure. Much greater force is needed to fracture the orbital rim than the thin walls of the orbit. Blowout fractures are caused by objects larger than the diameter of the orbital opening, such as a fist, a dashboard, or a baseball, striking the anterior orbit. Smaller objects may rupture the globe.

Symptoms and signs of orbital floor blowout fractures include ecchymosis and edema of the eyelids and cheek, orbital and eyelid emphysema, limitation of upgaze or downgaze (with associated diplopia), enophthalmos, and loss of sensation in the distribution of the inferior orbital nerve (ipsilateral cheek and upper lip). Limited extraocular movements can result from restrictive strabismus caused by entrapment of extraocular muscles between fractured bones, generalized edema and soft tissue injury, or from damage to the ocular motor nerves. Careful examination of the globe is necessary to rule out concomitant ocular injuries. Forced duction testing of the inferior rectus muscle with toothed forceps may show restriction of passive eye movement. Baseline exophthalmometry measurements should be obtained (see Clinical Protocol 9-3). Computed tomography of the orbits and brain (including axial and coronal cuts) with 1–2 mm cuts should be obtained to confirm the diagnosis and guide surgical management.

Treatment

The physician should consider prescribing nasal decongestants for 1–2 weeks and intermittent applications of ice packs for the first few days after the trauma. Advise the patient not to blow the nose vigorously in order to avoid orbital emphysema. Consider broad-spectrum antibiotic prophylaxis, particularly if sinus infections coexist. Indications for surgical repair of blowout fractures are controversial. Oral steroids in some cases may decrease edema and prevent fibrosis of the involved extraocular muscle. General indications include diplopia in the primary or reading position, significant enophthalmos, entrapment of extraocular muscles, or a large fracture.

The timing of orbital fracture repair is variable. In many cases, repair is not considered a surgical emergency and usually can safely be delayed for a week or longer. The exception is the "white-eyed" fracture in children, in which the inferior rectus muscle is entrapped due to the elasticity of the orbital bones in children. On attempted upgaze, the child may experience nausea, vomiting, and bradycardia due to activation of the oculocardiac reflex. These patients require immediate surgical intervention.

Open-Globe Injuries

Open-globe injures can be classified into ruptures after blunt trauma and lacerations after injury with a sharp object. Anteroposterior compression of the globe with equatorial expansion leads to rupture under weak points such as the insertion of the rectus muscles, limbus, or site of prior surgery.

Signs of an open-globe injury include low intraocular pressure compared to that of the fellow eye, change in depth of the anterior chamber (it may be either shallow or deep), displacement of or change in shape of the pupil, prolapse of ocular tissue, and marked bloody chemosis of the conjunctiva. Another sign of likely laceration of the globe is total (or large) hyphema with low or normal intraocular pressure; total hyphemas in intact globes are nearly always associated with elevated pressure.

A Seidel test can be performed to detect the presence of a full-thickness laceration. In this test, a fluorescein strip moistened with a few drops of sterile saline or topical proparcaine eyedrops is applied directly over the suspected site of perforation while the examiner observes the site through the biomicroscope with the cobalt-blue light. If a leak exists, the dye will be diluted by the aqueous and will appear as a green stream within the dark-orange concentrated dye.

It is important to recognize the presence of vitreous or uveal tissue on the ocular surface. Do not mistake vitreous for mucus and try to wipe it away vigorously; if in doubt, defer the determination to someone more experienced or until the patient is in the operating room.

Once the presence of an open globe is identified, avoid applying pressure to the globe during examination (eg, tonometry, scleral depression, gonioscopy, ultrasonography) or by patching. Because the patient will require surgery, keep them NPO (*nil per os*); that is, do not allow them food or water, and apply a Fox shield over the eye. The physician should always consider the possibility of an intraocular foreign body (IOFB) in any patient with a globe laceration. Signs such as a corneal entry wound, focal iris transillumination defect, or focal cataract should raise suspicion. A computed tomography (CT) scan with thin cuts (1–2 mm) should be performed in all cases of suspected IOFBs. In general, contrast dye is not needed when acute traumatic ocular and orbital injuries are imaged. Magnetic resonance imagining (MRI) is contraindicated with a suspected metallic IOFB. Ultrasonography can also be helpful in diagnosing occult globe ruptures or small IOFBs.

Treatment

In the emergency-department setting, consider the administration of antiemetics to suppress nausea and vomiting. Sedatives and analgesics may be administered judiciously. Tetanus prophylaxis should be administered if needed. A rigid shield (without an underlying eye pad) should be placed over the eye. Give appropriate prophylactic parenteral antibiotics. Definitive repair is then performed in the operating room. In cases of massive disruptive injury to the globe, informed consent for possible primary enucleation should be obtained from the patient or the family after thorough explanation and counseling. However, every attempt should be made to preserve the eye if there is even a remote chance of any vision. Patients should be counseled about a poor visual prognosis with severe globe injury as well as the need for additional operations, including enucleation.

Retrobulbar Hemorrhage

Retrobulbar hemorrhage (RBH) is rare but sight-threatening emergency that can occur after significant trauma. This is a true compartment syndrome, in which the accumulation of blood in the retrobulbar space can lead to increased intraocular pressure, compression of the optic nerve, and a compromise in ocular perfusion that leads to permanent damage unless there is rapid intervention. Signs of RBH include significant periorbital ecchymosis, proptosis, decreased vision, a relative afferent pupillary defect, and elevated IOP.

Treatment

Emergency lateral canthotomy and cantholysis is the mainstay of treatment and should be performed as soon as the diagnosis is made in order to prevent irreversible vision loss.

Ocular Infections in the Emergency Setting

Ocular infections encountered in the emergency department range from mild (viral or bacterial conjunctivitis) to vision threatening (corneal ulcers and endophthalmitis). This section discusses certain acute ocular infections that are commonly encountered in the emergency setting.

Acute Conjunctivitis

Patients with acute conjunctivitis commonly present to the emergency department physician with red eyes, discharge, and ocular irritation. The specific clinical signs and symptoms of the individual disorders are discussed in Chapter 11. Viral conjunctivitis, the most common type, presents with conjunctival injection, watery or mucoid discharge, and ipsilateral preauricular lymphadenopathy. Acute bacterial conjunctivitis is generally characterized by more of a mucopurulent discharge.

Treatment

Patients with viral conjunctivitis should be considered contagious for the first 10 days after onset and given appropriate instructions to avoid viral spread. Generally, viral conjunctivitis requires only supportive treatment with cold compresses and artificial tears to provide symptomatic relief.

Bacterial conjunctivitis responds to topical antibiotic treatment. Exceptions are gonococcal and chlamydial conjunctivitis, which require systemic antibiotics supplemented by topical eyedrops; these are discussed in the following sections.

Ophthalmia Neonatorum

Ophthalmia neonatorum, or neonatal conjunctivitis, describes an acute conjunctivitis that occurs within the first month of life (Figure 14-4) and can be caused by a chemical, bacterial, or viral process. Infectious causes include *Chlamydia trachomatis* (the most common), *Staphylococcus aureus, Streptococcus pneumoniae, Neisseria gonorrhoeae,* and herpes simplex virus (HSV). Affected neonates show conjunctival infection, eyelid edema, and chemosis. In gonococcal conjunctivitis, the discharge is more purulent and can lead to rapid corneal ulceration and perforation if untreated. The mother should be questioned about previous sexually transmitted disease.

Conjunctival cultures should be obtained for Gram and Giemsa stains and a chlamydial immunofluorescent antibody test or polymerase chain reaction (PCR) test. Cultures should be obtained on blood and chocolate agar. Viral cultures, PCR, and fluorescent antibody tests are ordered as indicated.

Treatment

The initial treatment of ophthalmia neonatorum rests on the clinical impression and the results of the initial stains. A pediatric consultation should be obtained. In neonates with

Figure 14-4 Gonococcal conjunctivitis in an infant (ophthalmia neonatorum).

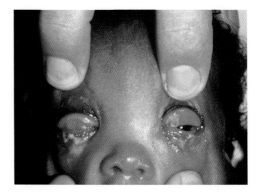

conjunctivitis caused by *Chlamydia trachomatis,* systemic erythromycin therapy is recommended, since pneumonitis and otitis media can coexist. The neonate with gonococcal conjunctivitis should be hospitalized and treated with systemic antibiotics (IV or IM ceftriaxone) with frequent irrigation and topical antibiotics. The mother and her sexual partner should also be treated. Sexual abuse of a child may be suspected with certain infections, and appropriate authorities should be alerted with the approval of the attending physician.

Microbial Keratitis

Corneal ulcers can be caused by bacteria, fungi, viruses, or amoebae. Bacterial infection is common and can be sight-threatening. Patients usually present with pain, conjunctival injection, photophobia, and decreased vision. A light-blocking white infiltrate is present on examination. There is typically a corneal epithelial defect (Figure 14-5). The most common risk factor for bacterial keratitis in the United States is contact lens wear; 19%–42% of patients with culture-proven microbial keratitis use contact lenses. The risk of microbial keratitis increases almost 15-fold with use of extended-wear soft contact lenses when compared with daily-wear lenses. *Pseudomonas aeruginosa* is the most common pathogen and can progress rapidly if untreated.

Fungal keratitis is less common than bacterial keratitis; it comprises only 5%–10% of corneal ulcers and can be caused by molds or yeast. Filamentous fungal keratitis occurs more frequently in warmer, more humid areas. Trauma to the cornea from plant and vegetable matter is the leading cause of fungal keratitis. Yeast keratitis is most frequently caused by *Candida* species. Fungal ulcers are also associated with contact lens wear, but are less common than bacterial infections.

Several key features may help distinguish fungal keratitis from bacterial keratitis by appearance alone. Fungal infections tend to be more indolent, while bacterial infections are more fulminant. Fungal ulcers may demonstrate feathery margins and satellite lesions. A deep stromal infiltrate may occur despite an intact corneal epithelium. An endothelial plaque and/or hypopyon may develop if the infected area is large or if the infection is sufficiently deep in the cornea. Microbiologic examination should be performed in ulcers

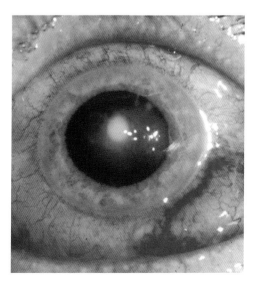

Figure 14-5 Microbial keratitis with suppurative infiltrate, overlying epithelial defect, and thinning of cornea. (Courtesy of Fasika A. Woreta, MD.)

larger than 1 mm, central ulcers, and ulcers with atypical features in which a fungus or parasite is suspected. When the culture is performed, glass sides should also be prepared for Gram staining by the Microbiology Department. Culture media should be inoculated in a sterile matter to grow the causative organism for identification and determination of sensitivities to antibiotics. Typical culture media used are blood agar, chocolate agar, and Sabouraud dextrose agar plates as well as thioglycollate broth. Special media may be considered for atypical ulcers (eg, anaerobic plates, Lowenstein-Jensen agar for suspected mycobacterial infection, or non-nutrient agar with *Escherichia coli* overlay for suspected *Acanthamoeba* infection). For contact lens–associated infections, culture of the contact lens, the lens case, and solutions may help provide a clue to the causative organism. If Acanthamoeba is suspected, glass slides should be sent to a pathologist for special stains to examine for the characteristic cysts.

Treatment

Initial broad-spectrum antibiotic therapy is begun and maintained until the causative pathogen is identified on culture. For severe infections, frequent administration (eg, every 30–60 minutes) of fortified topical antibiotics are used. One popular regimen for initial empiric treatment is vancomycin 25 mg/ml, alternated with tobramycin 14 mg/ml. Modification of therapy is based on clinical response. For less severe ulcers (<2 mm in diameter, not in the central cornea, and not associated with significant thinning), monotherapy with a commercially available fourth-generation topical fluoroquinolone such as moxifloxacin instilled hourly can be considered. Fungal infections are treated with topical antifungal agents; natamycin 5% is recommended for most filamentous fungal infections, while amphotericin B is used to treat yeast infections of the cornea. Oral antifungals may be added in severe fungal keratitis, but liver function tests should be monitored closely.

Patients should be followed closely (eg, daily for severe infections), and admission to the hospital should be considered for those patients who are unable to comply with the need for frequent dosing as an outpatient.

Dendritic Keratitis

Herpes simplex keratitis may present with the distinctive appearance of a dendritic corneal ulcer. It is caused by active replication of the herpes simplex virus, either HSV-1 or HSV-2, which results in destruction of the corneal epithelial cells. Patients typically present with unilateral ocular symptoms, including pain, photophobia, tearing, and decreased vision. Patients may have a history of these ocular symptoms or of herpetic oral or skin lesions.

On examination, preauricular lymphadenopathy, vesicular skin lesions on the eyelid, and decreased corneal sensation may be apparent. If herpetic disease is suspected, corneal sensation should be checked prior to the instillation of topical anesthesia. (Instructions for this are in Clinical Protocol 9-1). The classic dendritic ulcer is linear and branches dichotomously, with each branch terminating in a bulb. The borders of the lesion are heaped with swollen epithelial cells that stain with rose bengal or lissamine green (Figure 14-6). The center of the lesion is devoid of epithelial cells and stains positively with fluorescein.

The diagnosis of HSV epithelial keratitis is usually determined by clinical findings, making laboratory tests unnecessary; however, viral culture, fluorescent antibody

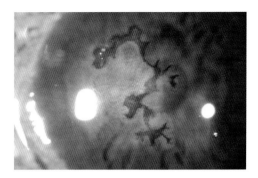

Figure 14-6   Rose bengal staining of herpetic dendritic keratitis. (Courtesy of Preston H. Blomquist, MD.)

testing, PCR, and Tzanck smear testing may be useful in securing the diagnosis in atypical and challenging cases.

Treatment

HSV epithelial keratitis is self-limited and often resolves spontaneously. The aim of treatment is to hasten the resolution and minimize corneal scarring. Acceptable treatment options include topical or oral antivirals. The 2 most common topical antivirals used are ganciclovir 0.15% ophthalmic gel 5 times a day, or trifluridine 1% eyedrops every 2 hours while awake. Trifluridine is toxic to corneal epithelium and should not be used for longer than 2 weeks. Topical ganciclovir is less toxic, but its use is limited by its high cost. The patient can also be treated with oral acyclovir 400 mg 5 times a day or oral valacyclovir 1 g 3 times a day in place of a topical antiviral, with an antibiotic ointment to help with discomfort. Topical corticosteroids can worsen the infection and should be discontinued if the patient was using them at the time of diagnosis. Finally, prophylactic doses of acyclovir (400 mg 2 times a day) or valacyclovir (1 g once a day) can be used in patients who have recurrent disease; these have been shown to decrease the recurrence rate by approximately 40%.

Preseptal and Orbital Cellulitis

Preseptal cellulitis is an infection that involves the soft tissues of the eyelids but does not involve the orbital structures (Figure 14-7). It affects only the eyelids and periorbital tissues anterior to the orbital septum, a fibrous barrier that separates the anterior eyelids and facial tissues from the orbit itself. Patients present with erythema, swelling, and tenderness of the eyelids and surrounding periorbital area. Preseptal cellulitis does not usually require a diagnostic workup.

The presence of proptosis, ophthalmoplegia (limited ocular motility), decreased vision, significant pain on eye movements, or abnormal pupillary reflexes indicates orbital cellulitis, a much more serious infection that involves extension of the infection posterior to the orbital septum and into the orbit (Figure 14-8). It results most commonly from spread of a bacterial infection from adjacent paranasal sinuses, the most common source being the ethmoid sinus.

The diagnostic workup of orbital cellulitis includes a CT scan to assess for subperiosteal abscess, intracranial involvement, and contiguous sinus disease. Blood cultures and cultures from the sinus, if it is drained, should be obtained.

Figure 14-7 Preseptal cellulitis.

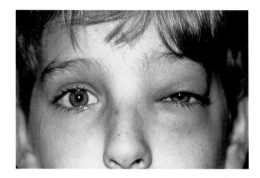

Figure 14-8 Orbital cellulitis.

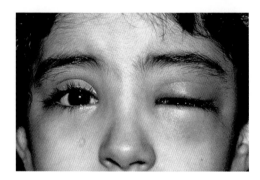

Treatment

Patients with mild preseptal cellulitis can be treated with oral antibiotics on an outpatient basis. Antibiotics are selected to cover the most likely organisms, which include *Staphylococcus aureus, Staphylococcus epidermidis, Streptococcus pyogenes,* and *Streptococcus pneumoniae.* In children who are unvaccinated, one must also consider *Haemophilus influenzae.* Community-acquired methicillin-resistant *S aureus* (CA-MRSA) has emerged in recent years as a major cause of skin- and soft tissue infections in many communities. Empiric treatment of preseptal cellulitis (with trimethoprim-sulfamethoxazole or clindamycin) should always cover CA-MRSA in endemic areas, and eyelid abscesses should be incised and drained. Children younger than 2 years or those with severe preseptal cellulitis should be hospitalized for treatment with intravenous antibiotics.

Because patients are at risk for cavernous sinus thrombosis, meningitis, and brain abscesses, treatment of severe orbital cellulitis should begin urgently. The patient should be admitted to a treatment center, and broad-spectrum intravenous antibiotics should be administered until the precise infectious agent is identified.

Because debridement of the sinuses can be required in severe cases, consultation by an otolaryngologist should be obtained for patients with sinus disease. Drainage of a subperiosteal abscess may be indicated, often in conjunction with sinus drainage.

If the patient with orbital cellulitis is immunocompromised or has diabetes mellitus, particularly with ketoacidosis, mucormycosis, a life-threatening fungal infection, must be seriously considered. Immediate surgical debridement and antifungal therapy is necessary to the save the patient's life. Affected patients can show a black eschar in the nose or on the roof of the mouth.

Endophthalmitis

Endophthalmitis denotes infection within the eye, including vitreous involvement, that spares the sclera. Panophthalmitis is an infection that involves all layers of the eye. These serious infections can be endogenous, exogenous, or post-traumatic. The resident must learn to recognize these disorders because they require immediate treatment if the eye is to be saved. Patients with endophthalmitis typically present with ocular pain, decreased vision, conjunctival injection, anterior chamber inflammation and hypopyon, and vitritis.

The diagnosis rests on clinical grounds and is confirmed with vitreous paracentesis with appropriate stains and cultures. Systemic risk factors for endogenous endophthalmitis include systemic debilitation, indwelling catheters or intravenous drug history, immunodeficiency, and cardiac valvular disease; if endophthalmitis is suspected, an appropriate systemic workup should be initiated. Acute exogenous endophthalmitis classically presents within the first week after intraocular surgery and requires urgent vitreous tap and antibiotic injection to eradicate the infectious agent (typically *Staphylococcus* or *Streptococcus* species). Chronic exogenous endophthalmitis may be caused by bacterial (eg, *Propionibacterium acnes*) or fungal infection.

Treatment

Time is of the essence. Acute exogenous endophthalmitis requires emergency vitreous paracentesis and broad-spectrum antibiotic injection (eg, vancomycin 1 mg/0.1 mL and ceftazidime 2 mg/0.1 mL) with or without steroid injection (dexamethasone 400 µg/0.1 mL). Obtain a consultation with a vitreoretinal surgeon to consider vitrectomy, especially with severe vision loss. The Endophthalmitis Vitrectomy Study found that, for endophthalmitis after cataract surgery or secondary intraocular lens implantation, vitrectomy was superior to intravitreal antibiotic injection only for patients with light perception vision at the initial visit. The recommendations of the Endophthalmitis Vitrectomy Study may not be applicable to other forms of endophthalmitis. Unfortunately, there is a very high risk of blindness with acute endophthalmitis, especially with delayed antibiotic injection.

Other Ocular Emergencies

Ocular emergencies can be arbitrarily subdivided into 2 categories. True ocular emergencies require treatment within minutes (chemical burns, central retinal artery occlusion, and acute angle-closure glaucoma). Urgent conditions require treatment within hours (various forms of ocular trauma and infections). This section describes other conditions often seen in the emergency department.

Acute Angle-Closure Glaucoma

Aqueous humor normally flows from the posterior chamber through the pupil, and then drains through the trabecular meshwork in the anterior chamber angle. Angle-closure glaucoma occurs when the iris becomes apposed to the trabecular meshwork and blocks aqueous humor drainage (Figure 14-9). Pupillary block is the most common cause of acute angle-closure glaucoma. In this condition, the flow of aqueous humor through the pupil is impeded. As a result, aqueous humor accumulates behind the iris and causes the iris to bow forward against the trabecular meshwork. Some patients are anatomically

Figure 14-9 In acute angle-closure glaucoma, the iris root occludes the trabecular meshwork, impeding the flow of aqueous humor. (Reprinted, with permission, from Simmons ST, *Glaucoma. Basic and Clinical Science Course*, Section 10. San Francisco: American Academy of Ophthalmology, 2006–2007.)

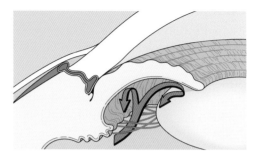

Figure 14-10 Acute angle-closure glaucoma produces corneal edema, a red eye, and a fixed, mid-dilated pupil.

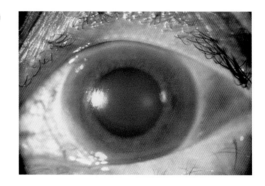

predisposed to developing pupillary block. Predisposing factors include a small, hyperopic eye and a narrow chamber angle. Pupillary block is more likely to occur when the pupil is mid-dilated and can be precipitated by topical mydriatics, systemic anticholinergics, stress, excitement (sympathetic release), or dim illumination.

Because of the acute rise in intraocular pressure (IOP), patients can present with headaches, severe eye pain, nausea, and vomiting. Ocular injection is present, and the cornea is steamy due to epithelial edema (Figure 14-10). This gives the patient the perception of rainbow-colored halos around lights and blurry or smoky vision.

On examination, the pupil is mid-dilated and sluggish, the conjunctiva has significant injection, the anterior chamber is shallow, and the intraocular pressure is significantly elevated. The anterior chamber angle is closed on gonioscopy, and the fellow eye almost always has a narrow angle. Corneal epithelial edema can impede the view of the anterior chamber and preclude gonioscopy or treatment by laser iridotomy. The corneal edema secondary to high IOP manifests as diffuse epithelial edema without stromal thickening, because the high pressure compresses the stroma, unlike edema associated with endothelial cell dysfunction (eg, Fuchs corneal endothelial dystrophy).

Treatment

Medical treatment is used initially to break the acute attack and paves the way for definitive surgical treatment. Stepwise medical treatment is as follows:

1. Instill a round of topical IOP-lowering medications.
2. In cases of recent onset, corneal indentation performed with a 4-mirror lens, which can help break the pupillary block, may be helpful.

3. In phakic patients, instill pilocarpine 1%–2% every 15 minutes 3 times. Only in pseudophakic or aphakic pupillary block: instill topical mydriatic and cycloplegic eyedrops (eg, phenylephrine 2.5% or tropicamide 1%) every 15 minutes 3 times.

4. Administer systemic carbonic anhydrase inhibitors (eg, acetazolamide 250 mg orally or 250–500 mg intravenously).

5. Administer systemic osmotic agents (eg, mannitol 1–2 g/kg intravenously over 45 minutes). Avoid these medications in patients with congestive heart failure or renal failure.

6. Administer systemic analgesics (eg, acetaminophen).

7. Apply topical anesthetic eyedrops, then apply topical glycerin, which can temporarily reduce corneal edema and swelling, and so allow adequate view for examination and laser iridotomy. (Topically applied glycerin is painful because of its hypertonicity, so topical anesthetic eyedrops should be given first.)

Definitive treatment consists of laser iridotomy or, if this is not possible, surgical iridectomy. The fellow eye should be treated prophylactically in the near future, since it is at high risk for developing acute angle closure as well.

Ocular Chemical Burn

Chemical burns of the eye are among the few true ocular emergencies in which every minute matters. In cases of chemical burns, begin eye irrigation immediately, even before completing the patient history or measuring vision.

Acid burns cause denaturation of tissue proteins, which then act as a barrier to prevent further diffusion of acid. For this reason, acid burns are generally less devastating than alkali burns, but they can still be very severe. Alkali burns cause saponification of tissue and therefore tend to penetrate deeper than acid burns and be more destructive to ocular tissues. They can cause limbal ischemia, severe corneal and conjunctival scarring, and intraocular complications such as uveitis and secondary glaucoma (Figure 14-11).

Clinical findings in mild burns of either type include conjunctival hyperemia, chemosis, corneal epithelial erosions, and mild haziness. More severe cases show limbal ischemia and corneal opacification.

Treatment

The most important step in the treatment of acute chemical burns of any type is immediate and copious irrigation. Clinical Protocol 14-3 presents instructions for eye irrigation.

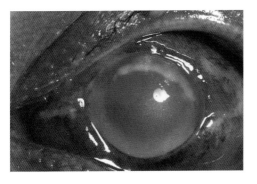

Figure 14-11 Alkali burn.

After irrigation, examine the eye carefully, checking for epithelial defects, corneal haze, and limbal ischemia, and measure IOP. For mild to moderate burns, administer topical cycloplegics and antibiotic ointment. With severe burns, additional medications may be administered to decrease inflammation, promote collagen synthesis, inhibit the enzyme collagenase, and enhance epithelialization (eg, topical corticosteroids, oral tetracyclines, oral ascorbate, topical citrate 10%, and acetylcysteine 10% eyedrops). If IOP is elevated, an oral carbonic anhydrase inhibitor may be given.

Central Retinal Artery Occlusion

Patients with central retinal artery occlusion present with sudden onset of unilateral, painless, severe loss of vision. It results from obstruction of blood flow due to an embolus or thrombus formation. It is associated with a number of conditions, including carotid or cardiac disease, arteriolosclerosis, giant cell (temporal) arteritis, collagen vascular disease, hypercoagulation disorders, and talc emboli with intravenous drug abuse.

   Affected patients show an afferent pupillary defect. Fundus examination reveals retinal arterial narrowing and blood column segmentation. The retina is white or gray except for a cherry-red spot at the fovea, which is perfused by the choroid (Figure 14-12). In the 25% of patients with a cilioretinal artery, the visual acuity will be 20/20 with sparing of this small area. Hollenhorst plaques or other types of emboli are sometimes visible on examination (Figure 14-13). Over time, patients will develop inner retinal atrophy and optic atrophy. The prognosis of central retinal artery occlusion is generally poor.

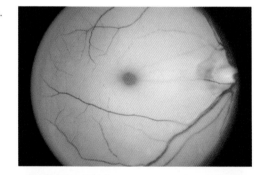

Figure 14-12   Central retinal artery occlusion. Note retinal pallor and cherry-red spot at fovea.

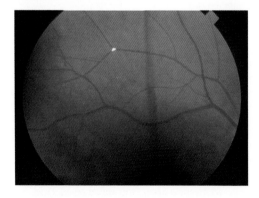

Figure 14-13   Hollenhorst plaque. Note the typical location of the yellow cholesterol embolus at the bifurcation of the arteriole. (© 2014 American Academy of Ophthalmology.)

Treatment

There are no proven therapies that have been shown to improve the outcomes of a central retinal artery occlusion, but certain maneuvers may be considered if the patient presents within 24 hours of the onset of symptoms. The goals of these maneuvers are to restore retinal blood flow and to move a potential retinal embolus distally.

1. Lower IOP to improve retinal perfusion in one or more of the following ways:
   a. Massage the globe either digitally or with a fundus contact lens. In addition to lowering the intraocular pressure, this might also dislodge an embolic plaque.
   b. Administer acetazolamide (500 mg intravenously) and/or instill topical timolol 0.5%.
   c. Consider performing anterior chamber paracentesis (Clinical Protocol 14-4).
2. Give the patient an oxygen mask to try to increase oxygen perfusion in the choroid. In the past, patients were given 95% oxygen and 5% carbon dioxide to breathe in order to produce arterial dilation, but this is no longer recommended due to complications.
3. Intravenous tissue plasminogen activator (tPA) is controversial but may be given in some centers if the patient presents within 6 hours of symptom onset. Serious systemic complications are associated with tPA administration.

A central retinal artery occlusion should be treated like an acute stroke. Neurology consultation should be obtained and workup should be performed for a possible embolic stroke. In patients older than 55 years, erythrocyte sedimentation rate should be measured at the time of presentation to rule out giant cell arteritis if an embolus is not visible. If the patient's sedimentation rate and symptoms suggests temporal arteritis, immediate high-dose intravenous corticosteroids should be administered.

Arteritic Anterior Ischemic Optic Neuropathy

Arteritic anterior ischemic optic neuropathy (AAION) presents as painless, unilateral visual loss that develops over hours to days. It occurs in patients older than 50 years (70 years is the average), and is more common in women. Vision loss is often accompanied by other symptoms, such as headache (most sensitive), jaw claudication (most specific), scalp tenderness, proximal muscle aches, weight loss, or fever.

Clinical exam for AAION reveals severe monocular vision loss; over 60% of patients have visual acuity of less than 20/200 in the affected eye. An afferent pupillary defect will be present with unilateral disease, and an altitudinal visual field defect may also be observed. Funduscopic examination typically demonstrates a pale, swollen optic nerve head with flame-shaped hemorrhages along the disk margin (Figure 14-14).

If AAION is suspected, emergency laboratory evaluation with an erythrocyte sedimentation rate (ESR), C-reactive protein (CRP), and platelet count should be ordered. The ESR should be considered positive if it is greater than the value obtained from the following formulas:

Men: ESR > (Patient age)/2

Women: ESR > (Patient age +10)/2

Figure 14-14 Anterior ischemic optic neuropathy. Note pale swelling of the optic disc with associated flame-shaped hemorrhages. (© 2014 American Academy of Ophthalmology.)

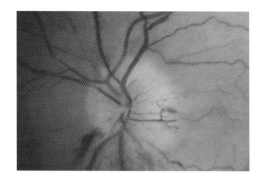

ESR is a nonspecific marker, however, as it can be elevated in any acute inflammatory process (ie, infection, vasculitis, malignancy). CRP can provide additional support for a diagnosis of AAION, with a specificity of 97% in patients with both a positive ESR and CRP. Thrombocytosis is often found in patients with AAION. Steroid treatment should be initiated immediately. A definitive diagnosis is made through temporal artery biopsy, which should be performed within a week of presentation in all patients suspected of having AAION.

Treatment

Any patient who is suspected of having AAION and has a positive ESR or CRP should be started on high-dose corticosteroids immediately, with the goal of preventing ischemic visual loss in the contralateral eye. A typical therapeutic regimen begins with 3–5 days of IV methylprednisolone (1 g/day), followed by oral prednisone (80–100 mg/day). If the temporal artery biopsy is positive, the patient is continued on prednisone, which is slowly tapered over the course of 3–12 months. If left untreated, up to 95% of patients experience visual loss in the fellow eye within days to weeks. Therefore, corticosteroid therapy should not be delayed until temporal artery biopsy. Corticosteroids are usually discontinued in patients without evidence of arteritis in adequate temporal artery biopsy specimens, unless the clinical presentation or the response to treatment is highly characteristic of the disease.

Retinal Tears and Rhegmatogenous Retinal Detachments

As people age, the central vitreous undergoes syneresis, and a posterior vitreous detachment (PVD) slowly develops. The vitreous gel usually remains attached at the vitreous base, a circumferential zone that straddles the ora serrata and extends about 2 mm anterior and 4 mm posterior to the ora. As the liquefied portion of the PVD moves within the globe, traction is created at the posterior vitreous base and other points of firm attachment to the retina (eg, blood vessels, margins of lattice degeneration) and can sometimes produce a retinal tear or break. A majority of retinal breaks occur in the superotemporal quadrant. Symptoms of a PVD and retinal tears include the entopic phenomena of photopsias (from mechanical traction of the retina) and new floaters. Figure 14-15 shows a horseshoe retinal tear with associated retinal detachment.

Once a tear has formed in the retina, liquefied vitreous is able to pass through to the potential subretinal space between the neurosensory retina and RPE, which causes a rhegmatogenous retinal detachment (RRD). As the retina is detaching, a patient will

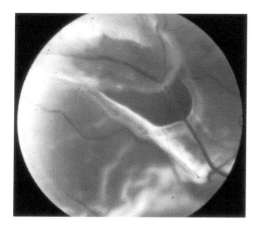

Figure 14-15 Horseshoe retinal tear with associated retinal detachment. (© 2014 American Academy of Ophthalmology.)

have the sensation of a veil, curtain, or shadow being pulled across their visual field. Other risk factors for RRD include lattice degeneration, high myopia, previous intraocular surgery, and trauma.

After taking a careful history, testing the visual acuity, and performing a thorough pupil, adnexal, alignment, motility, confrontation visual field, and anterior segment examination, the examiner should dilate the patient's eyes. Performing accurate tonometry is important as well, given that the IOP is often relatively decreased in eyes with RRDs when compared to the fellow eye. After the eyes are dilated, use a slit lamp to examine the anterior vitreous. The presence of blood or pigment (also known as "tobacco dust" or Schaffer sign) suggests a possible retinal break. One should then proceed with a thorough posterior segment examination via indirect ophthalmoscopy with a 20 D or 28 D lens with scleral depression to visualize to the ora serrata. A Goldmann 3-mirror lens can also allow for visualization of the ora serrata.

Examination for a retinal tear or retinal detachment in the presence of cloudy ocular media such as a vitreous hemorrhage can be aided with the use of ultrasonography.

Treatment

If after thorough examination no break or tear is found, the patient should be given specific instructions to return immediately if they experience a change in symptoms, such as new photopsias or an increase in floaters, or if a veil, curtain, or shadow develops. Repeated dilated fundus examination should be performed in 3–4 weeks.

If a symptomatic retinal tear is found, it should be treated, especially if there is residual traction on the retina. The goal of treatment is to create a chorioretinal scar around each break to prevent liquefied vitreous from entering the subretinal space and creating an RRD. Tears can be treated either with laser demarcation or with cryotherapy. If subretinal fluid is present, the treatment area should extend beyond the fluid to an area of attached retina. After treatment, the patient should be advised to return immediately if they experience new photopsias, an increase in floaters, or a veil, curtain, or shadow develops. Otherwise, repeat dilated fundus examination should be performed at 1 week, and then again at 1 month. The patient should also be advised that they are at risk of developing a tear in the fellow eye as well and to return immediately if symptoms develop. The fellow eye should also be thoroughly examined with scleral depression for the presence of asymptomatic tears.

If an RRD has already occurred, it requires prompt treatment in order to prevent vision loss. A detailed discussion of retinal detachment repair is beyond the scope of this book; however, one should detail the physical examination findings as best as possible and obtain a consultation from a vitreoretinal specialist as soon as possible. Depending on the location of the break(s), lens status, presence of lattice degeneration, and degree of myopia, the repair strategies may include a combination of any of the following: laser, cryotherapy, pneumatic retinopexy, scleral buckling, and pars plana vitrectomy.

Vitreous Hemorrhage

The onset of floaters and flashing lights or photopsias with associated vision loss may indicate the presence of vitreous hemorrhage. Vitreous hemorrhage is commonly associated with retinal neovascularization from proliferative diabetic retinopathy or a prior vein occlusion. Neovascularization of the iris or angle may accompany either of these conditions. The patient's other eye should be examined for evidence of proliferative diabetic retinopathy. Hemorrhage may also complicate a PVD in patients over the age of 50 whose ocular health is otherwise normal.

A thorough retinal examination to rule out retinal tears and detachment (as above) is indicated. If there is no view of the posterior segment, B-scan ultrasonography to rule out a retinal tear or detachment is indicated. In the presence of retinal neovascularization, panretinal laser photocoagulation should be performed as soon as the view is adequate. The patient may be a candidate for pars plana vitrectomy if the hemorrhage fails to clear or if the patient is monocular.

Pitfalls and Pointers

- Give priority to the treatment of life-threatening conditions over the treatment of ophthalmic trauma.
- Make appropriate follow-up arrangements after evaluating the patient in the emergency department.
- Make the medical records sufficiently detailed for later medicolegal and insurance purposes (see Chapter 3).
- Do not allow a patient who might require surgery to eat or drink.
- Perform CT scans in the setting of suspected IOFBs, orbital fractures, or occult open globe injuries.
- MRIs are contraindicated in patients with metallic (magnetic) foreign bodies.
- If significant head trauma exists, avoid dilating the patient's pupils for ophthalmoscopy until neurologic evaluation is completed. When you do dilate, be sure to notify other health care personnel and document the dilation in the chart.
- Do not apply pressure (eg, ocular palpation, scleral depression) to a globe that might be open or an eye that has a hyphema.
- Do not use a papoose board to restrain a child with an open or potentially ruptured globe. Give priority to the treatment of life-threatening conditions over the treatment of ocular trauma.

- Do not prescribe or give a patient a bottle of anesthetic eyedrops. Keep all ophthalmic medications out of reach.

- Do not administer acetazolamide to individuals with sickle-cell disease or trait, or patients with a sulfonamide allergy.

- Most important, do no harm. Know your limits and don't hesitate to call for help when you need it.

Suggested Resources

Bacterial Keratitis [Preferred Practice Pattern]. American Academy of Ophthalmology; 2019. Accessed September 20, 2020. https://www.aaojournal.org/article/S0161-6420(18)32644-7/fulltext

Conjunctivitis [Preferred Practice Pattern]. American Academy of Ophthalmology; 2018. Accessed September 27, 2020. https://www.aao.org/preferred-practice-pattern/conjunctivitis-ppp-2018

Flynn HW, Scott IU. Legacy of the Endophthalmitis Vitrectomy Study. *Arch Ophthalmol.* 2008;126(4):559–561.

Gerstenblith AT, Rabinowitz MP, eds. *The Wills Eye Manual: Office and Emergency Room Diagnosis and Treatment of Eye Disease.* 6th ed. Lippincott, Williams & Wilkins; 2012.

Posterior Vitreous Detachment, Retinal Breaks, and Lattice Degeneration [Preferred Practice Pattern]. American Academy of Ophthalmology; 2019. Accessed September 27, 2020. https://www.aao.org/preferred-practice-pattern/posterior-vitreous-detachment-retinal-breaks-latti

Primary Angle Closure [Preferred Practice Pattern]. American Academy of Ophthalmology; 2015. Accessed September 27, 2020. https://www.aao.org/preferred-practice-pattern/primary-angle-closure-ppp-2015

CLINICAL PROTOCOL 14-1

Applying Patches and Shields

1. Set out sterile eye pads and adhesive surgical tape. Tear the tape into lengths of 5–6 inches.
2. Instruct the patient to close both eyes.
3. Clean the forehead and zygoma with an alcohol pad to remove the skin oils. This helps the tape stick to the skin.
4. Any of 3 techniques may be used, depending on the amount of pressure desired and what is most comfortable for the patient:
   a. 1 pad unfolded (minimal pressure)
   b. 2 pads unfolded (a bit more pressure)
   c. 2 pads, underlying one folded (moderate pressure)

Figure 1 Positioning and taping the unfolded pad.

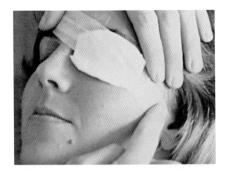

Figure 2 Taping the aluminum shield over the pad.

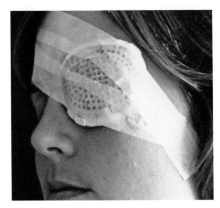

5. Tape the unfolded pad firmly to the forehead and zygoma (Figure 1). To prevent blinking, further bleeding, or swelling, the patch must exert some mild pressure on the lids. The patient should not be able to open the eyelid beneath the patch. The tape should not extend to the mandible or near the corner of the mouth because jaw movement could loosen the patch.

6. If the patient has any an open-globe injury, hyphema, or eyelid laceration, apply and tape a Fox shield, instead of a patch, over the globe, to protect these tissues from further damage until healing occurs or definitive repair is performed. Rest the shield on the bony superior orbital ridge and zygoma (Figure 2).

CLINICAL PROTOCOL 14-2

Removing Foreign Bodies from the Cornea

1. Apply eyedrops of topical anesthetic solution to the affected eye.

2. While holding the patient's upper and lower eyelids apart with your thumb and index finger, remove a loose, nonembedded foreign body as appropriate in either of the following 2 ways:

   a. Wipe the corneal surface gently with a cotton swab moistened with saline solution or any bland ophthalmic eyedrop.

   b. Perform saline lavage, inspecting the cornea periodically, until the foreign body is no longer apparent. (See Clinical Protocol 14-3).

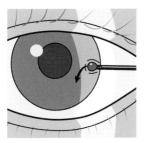

Figure 1   Extracting the foreign body.

3. Remove a firmly embedded foreign body by careful extraction with a small-gauge needle on a tuberculin syringe under slit-lamp magnification. Use a flicking motion with the needle and avoid pushing the foreign body deeper into the cornea or inserting the needle any deeper into the cornea than is absolutely necessary (Figure 1).

4. If a rust ring remains, you may try to curette it with the needle or remove it with a corneal burr. It is not necessary to remove the entire rust ring. It is better to leave a small rust ring in the visual axis than to risk creating a dense stromal scar after the removal.

5. Treat the abrasion that results from the foreign body as for a typical corneal abrasion.

CLINICAL PROTOCOL 14-3

Irrigating the Ocular Surface

1. With the patient supine, instill eyedrops of topical anesthetic solution into the cul-de-sac.

2. Gently keep the eyelids open, either manually or with a Desmarres retractor or an eyelid speculum.

   a. Topical anesthetics allow effective irrigation with minimal discomfort to the patient.

   b. Inspect quickly the ocular surface and conjunctival cul-de-sac for particulate chemical substances. Remove small particles by rolling a moistened cotton-tipped applicator across the conjunctiva; remove large particles with forceps.

3. Begin irrigating the eye copiously with normal saline solution or other similarly isotonic solution.

   a. You may use a Morgan lens or normal saline connected to plastic tubing (such as intravenous tubing) to irrigate the eye.

   b. Ask the patient to shift gaze periodically so that the entire cul-de-sac is flushed.

4. After irrigating for at least 20 minutes and using a minimum of 1 liter of fluid, reexamine the eye, especially the fornices, for particulate matter. You might need to evert the upper eyelid to irrigate or manually remove

particulate matter that is lodged there. If particulate matter is found, irrigate further after removing the particles.

5. Continue irrigation until the pH of the conjunctival sac is neutral (7.0–7.4). The test strips should be periodically checked with controls.

CLINICAL PROTOCOL 14-4

Performing Anterior Chamber Paracentesis

1. Instill topical anesthetic solution (eg, proparacaine) and an eyedrop of betadine 5% to the eye.

2. Place an eyelid speculum.

3. Place the patient either sitting at the slit lamp or supine under the operating microscope.

4. With a 30-gauge short needle on a tuberculin syringe, enter the anterior chamber at the temporal limbus, with the bevel of the needle pointing up and with the needle parallel to the iris plane. Keep the tip of the needle over the midperiphery of the iris, and avoid the lens throughout the procedure.

5. An assistant can withdraw fluid slowly from the anterior chamber into the syringe until you observe that it shallows slightly (0.1–0.2 cc of aqueous fluid).

6. Withdraw the needle.

15 Common Ocular Medications

This chapter includes related videos, which can be accessed by scanning the QR codes provided in the text or going to aao.org/PracticalOphthalmologyvideo.

This chapter presents an abbreviated overview of the most common categories of medications the beginning resident is likely to encounter.

- anesthetic agents
- dyes
- anti-infective agents
- anti-inflammatory agents
- mydriatic/cycloplegic agents
- glaucoma medications
- decongestant, vasoconstrictive, and anti-allergy agents
- lubricating agents and tear substitutes
- corneal dehydration medications
- agents delivered by intravitreal injection

Ocular medications are used for both ophthalmic diagnosis and treatment. They can be delivered to the eye by 4 routes:

- as topical eyedrops or ointments
- as thin drug-containing wafers deposited in the conjunctival sac for timed release of medication
- as injectable drugs administered directly subconjunctivally, intravitreally, intracamerally, into the sub-Tenon capsule, or into the peribulbar or retrobulbar spaces
- as systemic medications, especially for treating serious intraocular, optic nerve, or orbital inflammations and infections

Video 15-1 demonstrates the instillation of eyedrops.

VIDEO 15-1 Instilling Eyedrops
Courtesy of Richard C. Allen, MD, PhD.
Access all *Practical Ophthalmology* videos at
aao.org/PracticalOphthalmologyvideo.

Anesthetic Agents

Topical anesthesia is used in the performance of routine procedures such as measuring intraocular pressure and removing corneal foreign bodies. Instill 1 or 2 eyedrops in the eye for temporary anesthesia (15–20 minutes) to facilitate ocular examination. Common agents include tetracaine HCl 0.5% (Altacaine, Tetcaine, TetraVisc), proparacaine HCl 0.5% (Alcaine, Ocu-Caine, Ophthetic), and benoxinate 0.4% with fluorescein (Altafluor, Fluorox, Fluress). These agents are toxic to the corneal epithelium when used habitually and can even cause corneal melting and/or perforation with prolonged use. These agents should never be dispensed to the patient to take home.

Dyes

Certain dyes are useful for ophthalmic diagnosis. Fluorescein is a yellow-orange dye that emits a green color when exposed to a blue light. It is used topically for applanation tonometry and to diagnose corneal abrasions, punctate epithelial erosions, and other epithelial defects. The dye stains the corneal or conjunctival stroma in areas where the epithelium is absent, and it is also used intravenously for fluorescein angiography. Rose bengal is a red dye that stains devitalized epithelium and mucus. It is picked up by abnormal epithelial cells (but not areas of absent epithelial cells) in diseases such as keratoconjunctivitis sicca. Lissamine green is another dye that stains dead and devitalized epithelial cells; however, it is far less irritating than rose bengal. Rose bengal and lissamine green are usually available in prepackaged strips that can be wetted with a topical anesthetic and applied to the ocular surface.

Anti-Infective Agents

Medications for ocular infections comprise mainly antifungal, antibacterial, and antiviral agents. Antiprotozoal and antiparasitic agents are available but uncommonly used. The names and attributes of common antifungal, antibacterial, and antiviral medications are summarized in Tables 15-1, 15-2, and 15-3, respectively. Topical antibacterial agents should be used judiciously to avoid sensitization and emergence of resistant organisms. Agents that combine an antibiotic and an anti-inflammatory agent, such as tobramycin plus dexamethasone (TobraDex) and sulfacetamide plus prednisolone acetate (Blephamide), are available but should be used with caution due to the significant side effects of corticosteroids outlined below.

Anti-Inflammatory Agents

These drugs are used either topically or systemically to reduce ocular inflammation.

Corticosteroids

Topical corticosteroids are used for anterior segment inflammation, including refractory cases of allergic conjunctivitis, iridocyclitis, episcleritis, scleritis, and both noninfectious and infectious keratitis (once the infection has been adequately treated). Many different

Table 15-1   Common Antifungal Agents

Name	Preparation	Comments
Amphotericin B	0.15%–0.3% solution Intravitreal (5 µg/0.1 mL)	Solution may be made in hospital pharmacy (reconstitute amphotericin B deoxycholate in sterile water). May be extremely uncomfortable to the patient when administered topically. Administered as intravitreal injection for fungal endophthalmitis, although narrow therapeutic window due to retinal toxicity. Systemic administration achieves minimal intraocular penetration
Fluconazole (Diflucan)	Oral	Effective against *Candida*.
Ketoconazole (Nizoral)	Oral	Effective against *Candida, Cryptococcus,* and *Histoplasma.*
Miconazole (Monistat)	1% intravenous solution	Intravenous solution may be used topically.
Natamycin (Natacyn)	5% suspension	Used topically for yeast and filamentary forms (corneal ulcers).
Voriconazole	Oral; 0.05% solution	Solution may be made in hospital pharmacy for topical use. Effective against *Aspergillus, Candida,* and *Fusarium.*

corticosteroid preparations are available for topical ocular use; some of the most common are listed below:

- prednisolone:
  - prednisolone acetate suspension 0.125% (Econopred, Pred Mild)
  - prednisolone acetate suspension 1% (Econopred Plus, Omnipred, Pred Forte)
  - prednisolone sodium phosphate solution 0.125% (AK-Pred, Inflamase Mild, Pred Mild)
  - prednisolone sodium phosphate solution 1% (AK-Pred, Inflamase Forte, Orapred)
- dexamethasone
  - dexamethasone sodium phosphate solution 0.1% (AK-Dex, Decadron Phosphate)
  - dexamethasone sodium phosphate ointment 0.05% (AK-Dex, Baldex, Decadron Phosphate, Maxidex)
  - dexamethasone suspension 0.1% (Maxidex)
- progesteronelike agents
  - medrysone 1.0% (HMS)
  - fluorometholone suspension 0.1% (FML Liquifilm)

Table 15-2   Common Topical Ophthalmic Antibacterial Agents

Antibiotic	Commercial Name	Preparation	Spectrum of Coverage
Aminoglycosides:			*Enterobacteriaceae, P aeruginosa, S aureus.*
Gentamicin	Garamycin, Genoptic	Ointment or solution	Fortified eyedrops may be formulated from intravenous preparations for topical use. Widely used in serious ocular infections (eg, corneal ulcers in which G— organisms are implicated). Covers many G+ staphylococci but not streptococci.
Tobramycin	Tobrex	Solution or ointment	Fortified eyedrops may be formulated from intravenous preparations for topical use. More effective against streptococci and *Pseudomonas* than gentamicin.
Bacitracin	AK-Tracin	Ointment	G+ cocci (*Staphylococcus, Streptococcus*).
Bacitracin/ polymyxin B	Polysporin	Ointment	See action of each drug separately.
Chloramphenicol	Chloromycetin, Ocu-Chlor, Chloroptic	Solution or ointment	Broad-spectrum: G—bacilli (*H influenzae, N meningitidis*), *S pneumoniae, Salmonella,* and anaerobes (β *fragilis*). Rare cases of aplastic anemia have been reported.
Erythromycin	Ak-Mycin, Ilotycin	Ointment	G+ organisms, chlamydiae, mycoplasmas, some atypical mycobacteria, *H ducreyi, C jejuni, N gonorrhoeae, Actinomyces.* Particularly good in staphylococcal conjunctivitis. Bacteriostatic.
Fluoroquinolones:			
Ciprofloxacin	Ciloxan	Solution or ointment	Broad-spectrum; anaerobes usually resistant; may not be effective against some G+ cocci (streptococci).
Gatifloxacin	Zymar, Zymaxid	Solution	Same as ciprofloxacin, but improved coverage of G+ and atypical mycobacteria.
Levofloxacin	Quixin	Solution	Similar to ofloxacin.
Moxifloxacin	Vigamox	Solution	Same as ciprofloxacin, but improved coverage of G+ and atypical mycobacteria.
Ofloxacin	Ocuflox	Solution	Same as ciprofloxacin, but also covers *Chlamydia* and *Bacteroides.*
Besifloxacin	Besivance	Solution	Only fluoroquinolone not available systemically; may have fewer issues with resistance than other eyedrops in this class
Neomycin/ bacitracin/ polymyxin B	Neosporin	Ointment	Neomycin can cause contact allergies in up to 10% of users. Neomycin has broad-spectrum activity in G+ and G— organisms.
Neomycin/ gramicidin/ polymyxin B	Neosporin	Solution	Polymyxin: G— enteric bacteria, *P aeruginosa.* Inactive against G+ organisms. See above regarding neomycin.
Sulfacetamide	Bleph-10, Sulf-10, Sulamyd, Vasosulf	Solution or ointment	Sulfonamides: G+ and G— organisms but not *P aeruginosa* or enterococci. Bacteriostatic.
Tetracycline	Achromycin	Solution or ointment	G+ organisms, Enterobacteriaceae, vibrios, rickettsia. Inactive for *P aeruginosa, Bacteroides,* and group B streptococci.
Trimethoprim/ polymyxin B	Polytrim	Solution	Trimethoprim: G+ and G— organisms but not *P aeruginosa* or enterococci

Table 15-3   Common Antiviral Medications

Name of Drug	Other Names	Chemical Composition	How Administered	Mode of Action	Main Clinical Uses
Acyclovir	Zovirax	Purine analog	Ointment, oral, parenteral	Blocks viral DNA polymerase, thus selectively attacks viral replication in infected cell. Oral form (400–800 mg 5 times daily) reduces severity of skin and eye involvement. Particularly helpful in herpetic uveitis.	Herpes simplex (HSV), varicella-zoster (VZV), Epstein Barr virus (EBV), cytomegalovirus (CMV)
Famciclovir	Famvir	Purine analog	Oral	Same as ganciclovir	HSV, VZV
Foscarnet	Foscavir	Pyrophosphate analog	Parenteral (IV) Intravitreal (2.4 mg/0.1 mL)	Interferes with viral DNA polymerase and reverse transcriptase	CMV, HSV, EBV, Acute Retinal Necrosis
Ganciclovir	Cytovene	Purine analog	Oral, parenteral (IV), Intravitreal (2 mg/0.1 mL)	Interferes with viral DNA synthesis	CMV retinitis
Idoxuridine	IDU, Stoxil, Herplex	Thymidine analog	0.1% ophthalmic eyedrops q1h, 0.5% ointment q4h	Inhibits thymidine incorporation into DNA	HSV keratitis
Trifluridine	Viroptic	Thymidine analog	1% solution, usually given q2h to a maximum total of 9 eyedrops daily	Inhibits viral DNA synthesis	HSV keratitis; some activity against VZV
Vidarabine	Vira-A	Purine analog	3% ophthalmic ointment, applied q3h or 5 times daily for 6–10 days	Inhibits viral DNA synthesis	HSV keratitis
Zidovudine	Retrovir	Thymidine analog	Oral, parenteral	Interferes with RNA-directed DNA polymerase	HIV

- – fluorometholone suspension 0.25% (FML Forte Liquifilm)
- – fluorometholone acetate 0.1% (Flarex)
- – fluorometholone ointment 0.1% (FML S.O.P)
- loteprednol
  - – loteprednol etabonate 0.2% (Alrex)
  - – loteprednol etabonate 0.5% (Lotemax)
- difluprednate
  - – difluprednate 0.05% (Durezol)

Some corticosteroids may also be given by subconjunctival, sub-Tenon capsule, intravitreal, peribulbar or retrobulbar, and systemic routes. Dosage and route of administration depend on the location and severity of the inflammation. Eyedrops or ointment may be instilled every 1, 2, or 4 hours (among other regimens), with tapering according to response. Even brief exposure to topical corticosteroids can worsen herpes simplex epithelial keratitis and fungal keratitis, and can sometimes provoke severe ulceration or even perforation. In some people, corticosteroid use causes ocular hypertension or glaucoma, also called a steroid response. The likelihood of steroid response depends on the potency of the steroid and the duration of its use. Long-term use of corticosteroids can cause posterior subcapsular cataracts. Other adverse effects include delayed wound healing, corneal melting (keratolysis), prolongation of the natural duration of the disease, mydriasis, and ptosis.

Immunomodulating Drugs

Cyclosporine (Restasis) is an immunomodulating drug with anti-inflammatory effects. It is available as a 0.05% ophthalmic emulsion for use twice daily for keratoconjunctivitis sicca. Cyclosporine is immunosuppressive when given systemically.

Lifitegrast (Xiidra) is another anti-inflammatory drug used to treat keratoconjunctivitis sicca. It is available in a 5% formulation.

Nonsteroidal Anti-Inflammatory Drugs

Nonsteroidal anti-inflammatory drugs (NSAIDs) reduce inflammation primarily by inhibition of the cyclo-oxygenase enzyme, which is involved in prostaglandin synthesis. Topical ophthalmic preparations with widening indications have become available recently. Certain agents such as flurbiprofen (Ocufen) are used topically to reduce pupillary constriction during intraocular surgery. Ketorolac tromethamine (Acular, Acular LS) has been approved for treatment of ocular allergies. Diclofenac sodium (Voltaren), nepafenac (Ilevro, Nevanac), and bromfenac (Bromday, Prolensa) are used for postoperative inflammation. Corneal melting has been described as a complication of topical NSAID use.

Mydriatics and Cycloplegics

Mydriasis (dilation of the pupil) is achieved either by paralyzing the iris sphincter (with parasympatholytic [cycloplegic] agents) or by stimulating the iris dilator (with sympathomimetic [mydriatic] agents). Maximal mydriasis is achieved with a combination of both types of agents. In addition to causing mydriasis, parasympatholytic agents paralyze the ciliary muscle, which controls accommodation. Cycloplegia is useful when refracting children, whose active accommodation precludes accurate measurement of refractive errors. Cycloplegic (but not mydriatic) agents are also useful for relieving the pain of ciliary muscle spasm, which accompanies epithelial defects of the cornea, corneal inflammation, and intra-ocular inflammation. Dilating the pupils also helps prevent posterior synechiae in patients with anterior segment inflammation. Agents that dilate the pupil should be used with caution in patients with narrow anterior chamber angles, as they can precipitate angle-closure glaucoma. Table 15-4 lists commonly used agents and their characteristics.

Table 15-4   Common Mydriatics and Cycloplegics

Agent	How Available	Maximum Effect (Minutes)	Duration of Action	Comments
Atropine 0.25%, 0.5%, 1%	Ointment or solution	30	1–2 weeks	Systemic absorption can result in flushing, fever, tachycardia, restlessness, and excited behavior/acute psychosis possible.
Cyclopentolate (Cyclogyl) 0.5%, 1%, 2%	Solution	30	12–24 hours	Adequate for most cycloplegic refractions. Neurotoxicity (incoherence, visual hallucination, ataxia, slurred speech, and seizures) can occur, particularly in children.
Homatropine 1%, 2%, 5%	Solution	40	2–3 days	Side effects are rare.
Phenylephrine (Neo-Synephrine) 2.5%, 10%	Solution	20	3 hours	Produces mydriasis, but no cycloplegia; avoid 10% solution. May cause angina, increased blood pressure, myocardial infarction, stroke (mainly with 10%).
Scopolamine 0.25%	Solution	30	4–7 days	CNS side effects; dizziness, disorientation.
Tropicamide (Mydriacyl) 0.5%, 1%	Solution	25	4–6 hours	Inadequate for cycloplegic refraction of children.

Glaucoma Medications

Glaucoma medications lower intraocular pressure to prevent optic nerve damage. Seven different classes of drugs are used to treat open-angle glaucoma. In addition, hyperosmotic agents are used to lower the intraocular pressure in acute glaucoma. These 8 classes of glaucoma medications are discussed below and reviewed in Table 15-5. Agents that combine glaucoma medications from different classes are available, including timolol plus dorzolamide (Cosopt), timolol plus brimonidine (Combigan), brinzolamide plus brimonidine (Simbrinza), and netarsudil plus latanoprost (Rocklatan). Benzalkonium chloride is a common preservative in most glaucoma medications. However, some

Table 15-5   Common Glaucoma Medications

Name of Agent	Concentration and Dosage	Comments
Adrenergic agonists:		
Apraclonidine (Iopidine)	0.5% and 1% solution	Commonly used for prophylaxis of postlaser IOP spikes. High rate of tachyphylaxis and allergy limits its use in long-term glaucoma therapy.
Brimonidine (Alphagan P)	0.1%, 0.15%, or 0.2% solution, given bid–tid	Useful in long-term glaucoma therapy. Can cause apnea in infants.
Beta-adrenergic antagonists:		
Timolol (Timoptic, Betimol)	0.25% and 0.5% solution, given bid	A nonselective beta-blocker should be prescribed with care in patients with asthma, heart failure, and heart block. Has some corneal toxicity; also available as a once-daily-dose (Timoptic XE).
Levobunolol (Betagan)	0.25% and 0.5% solution given bid	Comparable effects to timolol.
Carteolol (Ocupress)	1% solution given bid	Comparable effects to timolol.
Metipranolol (OptiPranolol)	0.3% solution given bid	Comparable effects to timolol.
Betaxolol (Betoptic S)	0.25% suspension or 0.5% solution given bid	A selective beta-blocker, should reduce the risk of pulmonary side effects, particularly in patients with reactive or restrictive airway disease.
Carbonic anhydrase inhibitors (CAI):		
Acetazolamide (Diamox)	125 mg and 250 mg tablets, sustained-release 500 mg capsule (sequel); tablets given bid–qid, capsules given once or twice daily	May also be given intravenously in 500 mg ampules.
Methazolamide (Neptazane)	25–50 mg given bid–tid	
Dorzolamide (Trusopt)	A topical ophthalmic CAI (2% solution), given bid–tid	10% incidence of allergy.
Brinzolamide (Azopt)	A topical ophthalmic CAI (1% solution) given bid–tid	
Cholinergic agonists:		
Pilocarpine	0.5%–6% solution, 4% gel, also as sustained-release wafer (Ocusert)	1%–4% strengths are in widest use; instilled qid.
Hyperosmotic agents:		
Mannitol	20% intravenous solution given 1.5–2 g/kg	Maximum ocular hypotensive effect occurs at 1 hour intravenously and lasts 5–6 hours.

Table 15-5   Common Glaucoma Medications (continued)

Name of Agent	Concentration and Dosage	Comments
Glycerin (Glyrol, Osmoglyn)	50% solution usually given orally with water, orange juice, or flavored normal saline solution over ice, 1–1.5 g/kg	Maximum ocular hypotensive effect occurs in 1 hour and lasts 4–5 hours. Can occasionally produce nausea, vomiting, and headache.
Urea (Ureaphil)	Powder or 30% intravenous solution given 0.5–2 g/kg intravenously	
Prostaglandin analogues (PGAs):		
Bimatoprost (Lumigan)	0.01% solution given qPM; also available in 0.03% concentration (more likely to cause hyperemia)	May cause ocular redness, increased pigmentation of the iris and eyelids, and eyelash growth.
Latanoprost (Xalatan)	0.005% solution given qPM	Similar efficacy and side effects as bimatoprost.
Latanoprost (Xelpros)	0.005% ophthalmic solution	Preservative-free
Travoprost (Travatan)	0.004% solution given qPM	Similar efficacy and side effects as bimatoprost.
Tafluprost (Zioptan)	0.0015% solution given qPM	Only preservative-free PGA available; similar efficacy and side effects as other PGAs
Prostaglandin analog + nitric oxide metabolite:		
Latanoprostene bunod (Vyzulta)	0.024% solution given qPM	Common side effects include increased pigmentation of the iris and periorbital tissue, conjunctival hyperemia.
Rho Kinase Inhibitors:		
Netarsudil dimesylate (Rhopressa)	0.02% solution given qPM	Common side effects include conjunctival hyperemia, blurred vision.

glaucoma medications contain different preservatives thought to be less toxic to the ocular surface. For example, Alphagan P contains Purite, a stabilized oxychloro complex (sodium chlorite). Travatan Z is preserved with SofZia, which contains borate, zinc, and sorbitol. Other medications that are preservative-free include Timoptic in Ocudose, Cosopt PF, Zioptan (tafluprost), and Xelpros (Latanoprost). These options are particularly useful in glaucoma patients who are prone to benzalkonium chloride toxicity.

More Commonly Used Agents

Prostaglandin analogues
Prostaglandin analogues are a newer class of glaucoma medication and commonly used as first-line therapy. They lower intraocular pressure by increasing aqueous outflow

through the uveoscleral pathway. Examples include latanoprost (Xalatan, Xelpros), bimatoprost (Lumigan), bimatoprost ophthalmic implant (Durysta), travoprost (Travatan Z), tafluprost (Zioptan), and latanoprostene bunod (Vyzulta—combination drug; see below). Ocular side effects include conjunctival hyperemia, iritis, increased pigmentation of the iris and eyelid skin, eyelash growth, cystoid macular edema (CME), and atrophy of periorbital fat. This class of medication is generally considered safer systemically. These drugs should be used with caution in cases of active ocular inflammation, as they may promote inflammation and/or contribute to CME.

β-adrenergic antagonists

β-adrenergic antagonists, also known as *beta-blockers*, lower intraocular pressure by reducing aqueous production in the ciliary epithelium. Timolol (Betimol, Istalol, Timoptic, Timoptic XE), levobunolol (AK Beta, Betagan, Vistagan), carteolol (Ocupress), and metipranolol (Optipranolol) are nonselective beta-blockers; betaxolol (Betoptic, Betoptic S) selectively blocks β_1 receptors. Systemic side effects include bradycardia, decreased cardiac output, exercise intolerance, bronchiolar spasm, hypotension, syncope, decreased libido, lethargy, and depression. These adverse effects can be additive to those associated with systemic beta-blockers that the patient might be taking for high blood pressure. Selective β_1 blockers are less closely associated with bronchospasm and therefore safer to use in patients with chronic obstructive pulmonary disease.

Topical carbonic anhydrase inhibitors

Carbonic anhydrase inhibitors reduce aqueous production by inhibiting the enzyme carbonic anhydrase. They are sulfonamide derivatives and should be avoided in patients with sulfonamide allergies. Examples of topical carbonic anhydrase inhibitors include dorzolamide (Trusopt) and brinzolamide (Azopt). Because they are thought to have at least mildly adverse effects on the function of corneal endothelial cells, caution should be taken with their use in patients who have compromised endothelial function, such as in Fuchs endothelial dystrophy.

α_2-adrenergic agonists

α_2-adrenergic agents lower intraocular pressure by reducing the production of aqueous humor and possibly by increasing uveoscleral outflow. Examples include apraclonidine (Iopidine) and brimonidine (Alphagan P). Side effects include fatigue, dry mouth, and allergic conjunctivitis. One should avoid using this class of medications in infants and young children due to the risk of respiratory depression and apnea.

Newer agents

Rho kinase inhibitors decrease intraocular pressure by increasing outflow: they increase permeability of cells in the trabecular meshwork and Schlemm canal, thus decreasing resistance to aqueous outflow. Netarsudil dimesylate is a rho kinase inhibitor available as a single agent (Rhopressa) or in combination with latanoprost (Rocklatan). Adverse effects may include conjunctival hemorrhages and hyperemia.

Latanoprostene bunod (Vyzulta) combines the effects of a prostaglandin analog with the action of nitric oxide. Nitric oxide, released by the metabolism of latanoprostene bunod in the eye, acts to promote relaxation of trabecular meshwork cells, thus increasing outflow. Adverse effects are similar to those of other prostaglandin analogs.

Cholinergic agonists

These agents, also known as *miotics* or *parasympathomimetics,* act by increasing outflow of aqueous humor through the trabecular meshwork. Examples include pilocarpine, carbachol, and echothiophate iodide. Ocular adverse effects include pupillary constriction and ciliary spasm (which results in brow ache and a myopic shift in refraction). Young people particularly are sensitive to ciliary spasm.

Sympathomimetics

Sympathomimetics lower intraocular pressure by increasing conventional trabecular and uveoscleral outflow. Examples include epinephrine (Epifrin, Glaucon) and dipivefrin (Propine, Thilodrin). Ocular adverse effects include rebound hyperemia that leads to a red eye, CME in aphakic patients, and pupillary dilation that can trigger an acute attack of angle-closure glaucoma in patients with narrow angles. Systemic adverse effects are uncommon but include tachycardia, hypertension, tremor, anxiety, and premature ventricular contractions. These drugs are rarely used now, and are mostly of historical significance.

Systemic carbonic anhydrase inhibitors

Oral carbonic anhydrase inhibitors are given systemically to patients with glaucoma who do not respond sufficiently to topical medication Examples include acetazolamide (Diamox) and methazolamide (Neptazane). Acetazolamide can also be given intravenously, usually pre- or postoperatively. Adverse effects include nausea, tingling of the fingers and toes, anorexia, peculiar taste sensations (metallic/bitter taste, especially with carbonated beverages), hypokalemia, renal lithiasis, acidosis, lethargy, loss of libido, depression, and (very uncommonly) aplastic anemia.

Hyperosmotic agents

Urea, glycerin, and mannitol reduce intraocular pressure by making the plasma hypertonic to aqueous and vitreous humor, with the result that fluid is drawn from the eye into the intravascular space. These agents are used orally or intravenously to lower the intraocular pressure in cases of acute glaucoma, and they are used pre- and postoperatively in selected patients. Caution must be exercised in patients with diabetes mellitus, congestive heart failure, or kidney damage.

Decongestant, Vasoconstrictive, and Anti-Allergy Agents

Several nonprescription ophthalmic preparations (vasoconstrictors) are available to reduce ocular redness, itching, and irritation. Most contain naphazoline, tetrahydrozoline, or phenylephrine. Some of these also have an added antihistamine, such as pheniramine maleate or antazoline phosphate.

Antihistamine-decongestant combinations include naphazoline HCl 0.025% plus pheniramine maleate 0.3% (Visine A, Naphcon-A, Opcon-A) and naphazoline HCl 0.05% plus antazoline phosphate 0.5% (Vasocon-A). Antihistamines (without decongestant) include levocabastine (Livostin), emedastine (Emadine), and bepotastine besilate (Bepreve).

Mast cell stabilizers are used for allergic disorders such as vernal conjunctivitis. These include cromolyn sodium (Cromal), ketotifen fumarate (Zaditor, Alaway), lodoxamide tromethamine (Alomide), nedocromil (Alocril) and pemirolast potassium (Alamast). Combination antihistamines and mast cell stabilizers include azelastine (Optivar), epinastine (Elestat, Relestat), and olopatadine (Patanol, Pataday, Pazeo).

Lubricating Medications and Tear Substitutes

Many formulations of artificial tears and ointments are useful in patients with dry eyes. These are available over the counter in most cases. Basic ingredients include hypotonic or isotonic buffered solution, surfactants, and viscosity agents such as methylcellulose and carboxymethylcellulose, which prolong corneal contact time. In general, ointments and viscous solutions adhere better to the cornea and require less frequent administration, but they have the disadvantage of temporarily degrading vision. Oily medications (such as ointments) can also destabilize the tear film. Artificial tears often have preservatives (eg, benzalkonium chloride), which can cause epithelial toxicity if overused. This is especially problematic in patients with dry eyes and chronic users of artificial tears, but preservative-free preparations have been developed. Examples of artificial tears include Bion Tears, Celluvisc, GenTeal PF, Refresh Endura, Refresh Plus, Systane, and Tears Naturale Free.

Corneal Dehydration Medications

Hypertonic medications may be instilled on the eye to clear corneal edema osmotically. Patients may be placed on hypertonic sodium chloride 2% or 5% (Muro 128, Hyper-Sal, Adsorbonac).

Agents Delivered by Intravitreal Injection

The delivery of medications directly into the vitreous cavity by injection (intravitreal injection) has revolutionized many aspects of clinical ophthalmology. Intravitreal injections can be performed in the office with a 27-, 30-, or 32-gauge needle with an anesthetic to minimize patient discomfort and an antiseptic to minimize the risk of infection. Injections are performed through the pars plana in order to avoid the vascular ciliary body anteriorly and the neurosensory retina posteriorly. Care is taken to direct the needle posteriorly toward the midvitreous cavity to avoid trauma to the crystalline lens. Although these procedures are relatively safe, intravitreal injections carry risks, including endophthalmitis, sterile inflammation, retinal detachment, lens trauma, hemorrhage, increased intraocular pressure, wound leak, and hypotony.

Anti-Vascular Endothelial Growth Factor (anti-VEGF) Agents

Intravitreal anti-VEGF pharmacotherapy has become the standard of care treatment for multiple sight-threatening retinal diseases. VEGF is a family of diffusible cytokines that stimulate angiogenesis and promote vascular permeability. VEGF A, in particular, plays an important role in the pathogenesis of wet age-related macular degeneration (AMD), also known as exudative or neovascular AMD, as well as diabetic retinopathy, retinal venous occlusion, and other retinal vascular diseases.

Ranibizumab
Ranibizumab (Lucentis) was approved by the US Food and Drug Administration (FDA) in 2006 for the treatment of wet AMD. Ranibizumab is a monoclonal antibody fragment that binds to and inhibits all subtypes of VEGF A. Ranibizumab was the first wet AMD treatment to show a mean improvement in visual acuity; this initiated a paradigm shift toward intravitreal anti-VEGF pharmacotherapy as the first-line treatment for multiple retinal diseases. It is now approved by the FDA for the treatment of retinal venous occlusion (2010), diabetic macular edema (2012), myopic choroidal neovascularization (2017), and diabetic retinopathy with or without diabetic macular edema (DME) (2017).

Bevacizumab
Bevacizumab (Avastin) was approved by the FDA for intravenous use in metastatic colon cancer in 2004. It is a humanized monoclonal antibody derived from the same murine antibody as ranizibumab, and it neutralizes all VEGF A isoforms. Bevacizumab is administered as an off-label (non-FDA–approved) intravitreal treatment for a broad range of retinal vascular diseases. The multicenter, prospective Comparison of Age-related Macular Degeneration Treatment Trials (CATT), which was sponsored by the National Institutes of Health (NIH), has shown that bevacizumab and ranibizumab produce similar clinical outcomes in patients with wet AMD.

Aflibercept
Aflibercept (Eylea), which was approved by the FDA in 2011 for wet AMD, is a fusion protein composed of key extracellular domains from VEGF receptors 1 and 2 fused to the immunoglobulin fragment of human immunoglobulin G-1. Aflibercept (called "VEGF Trap-Eye" in earlier studies) has a high binding affinity for VEGF A and also inhibits the activity of VEGF B and placental growth factor (PlGF). It is now approved by the FDA for the treatment of retinal venous occlusion (2012), diabetic macular edema (2014), and diabetic retinopathy (2019).

Brolucizumab
Brolucizumab (Beovu) was approved by the FDA in 2019 for wet AMD. It is a single-chain antibody fragment that binds to and inhibits all isoforms of VEGF A. Initial clinical trial results demonstrated its efficacy as an intravitreal injection given every 12 weeks. However, retinal vasculitis and retinal vascular occlusion have been reported with use.

Anti-Inflammatory Agents
Corticosteroids are used extensively in ophthalmology, and several sustained-release platforms are now available for intravitreal delivery of these medications. Intraocular corticosteroid pharmacotherapy is a highly effective treatment for multiple sight-threatening ocular conditions; however, they carry significant risks that physicians and patients must weigh. A majority of patients treated with intraocular sustained-release corticosteroids will develop a cataract within 2 years, and a significant number of those

patients will develop elevated intraocular pressure that requires medical and/or surgical treatment for glaucoma.

Intravitreal triamcinolone acetonide (Kenalog) and dexamethasone are used in an off-label fashion to decrease ocular inflammation and macular edema. The preservative-free synthetic corticosteroid Triesence (triamcinolone acetonide) was approved by the FDA in 2007 for visualization during vitrectomy and for the treatment of certain ocular inflammatory conditions. Retisert (fluocinolone acetonide 0.59 mg) is an FDA-approved surgical implant that slowly releases a high-potency corticosteroid to the posterior segment of the eye at a steady rate over more than 2 years. Iluvien (0.19 mg) and Yutiq (0.18 mg) are also fluocinolone implants that are injected through the pars plana for treatment of DME and uveitis, respectively. Ozurdex is a sustained-release dexamethasone intravitreal implant (0.7 mg) that is approved by the FDA for the treatment of DME, macular edema from retinal vein occlusion, and noninfectious uveitis that affects the posterior segment of the eye.

Anti-Infective Agents

The administration of antibiotics into the vitreous cavity to treat endophthalmitis was first reported in the 1940s. It was not until the 1970s and 1980s, however, that this practice became widespread. Anti-infective agents are now routinely given intravitreally in the setting of endophthalmitis and infectious retinitis.

The most commonly administered intravitreal antibiotics are vancomycin (1.0 mg in 0.1 mL), ceftazidime (2.2 mg in 0.1 mL), and amikacin (0.2 or 0.4 mg in 0.1 mL). Voriconazole (100–200 µg in 0.05–0.1 mL) and amphotericin B (5 µg in 0.1 mL) are both used in the treatment of fungal endophthalmitis that involves the vitreous (see Table 15-1).

Antiviral agents may be administered intravitreally as an alternative or adjunct to the systemic treatment of acute retinal necrosis (ARN), progressive outer retinal necrosis (PORN), and cytomegalovirus (CMV) retinitis. The most commonly employed agents are ganciclovir (0.2–2.0 mg) and foscarnet (2.4 mg) (see Table 15-3). A sustained-release surgical ganciclovir implant (Vitrasert) is also used in specific circumstances for the treatment of CMV retinitis.

Suggested Resources

Glaucoma. Basic and Clinical Science Course, Section 10. American Academy of Ophthalmology; published annually.

Comparison of Age-related Macular Degeneration Treatments Trials (CATT) Research Group, Maguire MG, Martin DF, Ying G, et al. Five-year outcomes with anti-vascular growth factor treatment of neovascular age-related macular degeneration: the Comparison of Age-Related Macular Degeneration Treatments Trials. *Ophthalmology.* 2016;123:1751–1761.

Heier JS, Brown DM, Chong V, Korobelnik J-F, Kaiser PK, Nguyen QD, et al. Intravitreal aflibercept (VEGF Trap-Eye) in wet age-related macular degeneration. *Ophthalmology.* 2012;119:2537–2548.

Intravitreal Injections - 2015 [Clinical Statement]. American Academy of Ophthalmology; 2015. Accessed September 27, 2020. https://www.aao.org/clinical-statement/intravitreal-injections-statement

CLINICAL PROTOCOL 15-1

Performing an Intravitreal Injection

1. Observe a procedural pause to confirm laterality, medication, allergies, and lens status. Consider subconjunctival or retrobulbar anesthesia for patients with inflamed eyes.

2. Collect all necessary materials, including a needle (30 g or 32 g, ½" or ⅝"), a 1 cc syringe, povidone iodine 5% eyedrops for the ocular surface, povidone iodine for the skin (eg, 10% swabs), topical anesthetic (eg, proparacaine, tetracaine), an eyelid speculum, caliper, sterile cotton-tipped applicators, and medication (prepackaged or drawn up sterile with a filter needle). Consider gloves and a mask, although they are not required.

3. If subconjunctival anesthesia will be used, administer it now. Place the patient in the supine position and instill topical anesthetic into the eye. Have the patient close their eyes for 30 seconds.

4. Instill one eyedrop of povidone iodine solution into the eye. Prepare the eyelashes and eyelids with povidone Iodine solution.

5. Place an eyelid speculum.

6. Identify the inferotemporal injection site with a sterile caliper (4 mm posterior to the limbus if the eye is phakic, 3.5 mm posterior to the limbus if the eye is pseudophakic or aphakic).

7. Place povidone iodine eyedrops over the planned injection site, and then wait at least 30 seconds.

8. Ask the patient and care team to refrain from speaking once the needle is uncapped.

9. Direct the needle toward the center of the eye and slowly inject the medication. The hand that is holding the syringe should be stabilized by also touching the brow or cheek.

10. Withdraw the needle, carefully remove the speculum, and irrigate the eye.

11. Confirm ocular perfusion by testing for hand-motion vision.

Video 1 demonstrates intravitreal injection.

VIDEO 1 Intravitreal Injection Technique
Courtesy of Jed H. Assam, MD, and Jaafar El-Annan, MD.

Index

Page numbers followed by "*f*" denote figures; "*t*," tables; "*c*," clinical protocols

A

Abbreviations
   ophthalmic evaluation, 14
   strabismus evaluation, 87*t*
   visual acuity examination, 29, 30*t*
Abduction, 86
Abrasion, corneal, 281–282
Absolute scotoma, 119
Accommodation
   cycloplegia effects on, 64
   definition of, 53
   near point of, 32, 43*c,* 71
   relaxing of, 66
Accommodative convergence, 96
Accommodative convergence/accommodation
   ratio, 96
Accommodative esotropia, 68
Accreditation Council for Graduate Medical
   Education, 3
Acetazolamide, 312*t,* 315
Achromycin. *See* Tetracycline
Acid burns, 295
Activities of daily living, 14
Acular. *See* Ketorolac tromethamine
Acute angle-closure glaucoma, 114, 293–295, 294*f*
Acute conjunctivitis, 288
Acute retinal necrosis, 318
Acyclovir, 291, 309*t*
Adduction, 86
Adie syndrome, 110*t*
Adie tonic pupil, 112, 113–114
Aflibercept, 317
Against-the-rule astigmatism, 53
Age-related macular degeneration (AMD, 263
Aging, 261*t*
Air-puff tonometer, 224
AK-Dex. *See* Dexamethasone
AK-Mycin. *See* Erythromycin
AK-Pred. *See* Prednisolone
AK-Tate. *See* Prednisolone
AK-Tracin. *See* Bacitracin
Alignment testing
   considerations with, 95–96
   corneal light reflection test, 91–92, 92*f,* 101*c*

cover tests, 92–94
description of, 90–96
red reflex test, 91, 91*f*
Alkali burns, 295, 295*f*
Allen picture chart, 28*f*
Allergic conjunctivitis, 189
Allergies
   eyedrop-induced, 217*f*
   history-taking, 23–24
α_2-adrenergic agonists, 312*t,* 314
Alphagan P. *See* Brimonidine
Altitudinal defect, 128
Amaurotic pupil, 111
Amblyopia
   bilateral, 39
   causes of, 39
   crowding phenomenon associated with, 39
   definition of, 38, 85
Amblyopia Treatment Study visual acuity testing
   protocol, 29, 34
AMD. *See* Age-related macular degeneration
American Academy of Ophthalmology (AAO)
   Code of Ethics, 5–6
   Low Vision Rehabilitation Committee, 37
   Ophthalmic Knowledge Assessment Program
     (OKAP) examination, 6
   resources of, 7–8
American Board of Ophthalmology
   (ABO), 1, 6
Ametropia, 53
Amikacin, 318
Aminoglycosides, 308*t*
Amphotericin B, 307*t*
Amsler grid, 119, 121–122, 122*f,* 133*c*
Anesthetic agents, 306
Angioedema, 180
Angiography, 257–258
Angle-closure glaucoma, 114, 201, 293–295, 294*f*
Angle recess, 214
Angular blepharitis, 183
Aniridia, 111
Anisocoria
   definition of, 21, 105
   essential, 109, 110*t*